1987
YEAR BOOK OF
SPORTS
MEDICINE®

The 1987 Year Book Series

Anesthesia: Drs. Miller, Kirby, Ostheimer, Roizen, and Stoelting

Cancer: Drs. Hickey, Saunders, Clark, and Cumley

Cardiology: Drs. Schlant, Collins, Engle, Frye, Gifford, and O'Rourke

Critical Care Medicine: Drs. Rogers, Allo, Dean, Gioia, McPherson, Michael, Miller, and Traystman

Dentistry: Drs. Cohen, Hendler, Johnson, Jordan, Moyers, Robinson, and Silverman

Dermatology: Drs. Sober and Fitzpatrick

Diagnostic Radiology: Drs. Bragg, Keats, Kieffer, Kirkpatrick, Koehler, Miller, and Sorenson

Digestive Diseases: Drs. Greenberger and Moody

Drug Therapy: Drs. Hollister and Lasagna

Emergency Medicine: Dr. Wagner

Endocrinology: Drs. Bagdade, Ryan, Molitch, Braverman, Robertson, Halter, Kornel, Horton, Korenman, Morley, Rogol, Burger, and Metz

Family Practice: Drs. Rakel, Couchman, Driscoll, Avant, and Prichard

Hand Surgery: Drs. Dobyns, Chase, and Amadio

Hematology: Drs. Spivak, Bell, Ness, Quesenberry, and Wiernik

Infectious Diseases: Drs. Wolff, Tally, Keusch, Klempner, and Snydman

Medicine: Drs. Rogers, Des Prez, Cline, Braunwald, Greenberger, Wilson, Epstein, and Malawista

Neurology and Neurosurgery: Drs. DeJong, Currier, and Crowell

Nuclear Medicine: Drs. Hoffer, Gore, Gottschalk, Sostman, and Zaret

Obstetrics and Gynecology: Drs. Mishell, Kirschbaum, and Morrow

Ophthalmology: Drs. Ernest and Deutsch

Orthopedics: Dr. Coventry

Otolaryngology–Head and Neck Surgery: Drs. Paparella and Bailey

Pathology and Clinical Pathology: Drs. Brinkhous, Dalldorf, Grisham, Langdell, and McLendon

Pediatrics: Drs. Oski and Stockman

Perinatal/Neonatal Medicine: Drs. Klaus and Fanaroff

Plastic and Reconstructive Surgery: Drs. McCoy, Brauer, Haynes, Hoehn, Miller, and Whitaker

Podiatric Medicine and Surgery: Dr. Jay

Psychiatry and Applied Mental Health: Drs. Freedman, Lourie, Meltzer, Nemiah, Talbott, and Weiner

Pulmonary Disease: Drs. Green, Ball, Menkes, Michael, Peters, Terry, Tockman, and Wise

Rehabilitation: Drs. Kaplan and Szumski

Sports Medicine: Drs. Krakauer, Shephard, and Torg, Col. Anderson, and Mr. George

Surgery: Drs. Schwartz, Jonasson, Peacock, Shires, Spencer, and Thompson

Urology: Drs. Gillenwater and Howards

Vascular Surgery: Drs. Bergan and Yao

1987
The Year Book of
SPORTS MEDICINE®

Editor-in-Chief

Lewis J. Krakauer, M.D., F.A.C.P.
Adjunct Professor of Health, Oregon State University; Assistant Clinical Professor of Medicine, University of Oregon Medical School

Editors

Col. James L. Anderson, PE.D.
Professor, Director of Physical Education, United States Military Academy

Frank George, A.T.C., P.T.
Head Athletic Trainer, Brown University

Roy J. Shephard, M.D., Ph.D.
Director, School of Physical and Health Education, and Professor of Applied Physiology, Department of Preventive Medicine and Biostatistics, University of Toronto

Joseph S. Torg, M.D.
Professor of Orthopedic Surgery, and Director, Sports Medicine Center, University of Pennsylvania School of Medicine

Year Book Medical Publishers, Inc.
Chicago • London • Boca Raton

Editorial Director, Year Book Publishing: Nancy Gorham
Sponsoring Editor: Judy L. Plazyk
Literature Surveillance Supervisor: Laura J. Shedore
Assistant Director, Manuscript Services: Frances M. Perveiler
Associate Managing Editor, Year Book Editing Services: Linda H. Conheady
Production Manager: H.E. Nielsen
Proofroom Supervisor: Shirley E. Taylor

Table of Contents

The material covered in this volume represents literature reviewed through February 1987.

Journals Represented 9

Publisher's Preface 11

1. Exercise Physiology and Medicine 13

Cardiovascular Physiology 13

Respiratory Physiology 55

Metabolism 62

Physiology of Specific Sports 119

Physiology of Drugs 144

Miscellaneous Topics 158

2. Biomechanics 183

3. Sports Injuries 207

Epidemiology 207

Head, Neck, and Spine Injuries 217

Upper Extremity Injuries 225

Lower Extremity Injuries 262

Knee Injuries 272

Knee Arthroscopy 306

Foot and Ankle Injuries 317

Miscellaneous Topics 331

4. Pediatric Sports Medicine 341

5. Women in Sports 351

6. Athletic Training 383

Introduction 383

Journals Represented

Acta Medica Scandinavica
Acta Orthopaedica Scandinavica
Acta Physiologica Scandinavica
American Heart Journal
American Journal of Cardiology
American Journal of Clinical Nutrition
American Journal of Diseases of Children
American Journal of Gastroenterology
American Journal of Medicine
American Journal of Physiology
American Journal of Public Health
American Journal of Roentgenology
American Journal of Sports Medicine
Annales Chirurgiae et Gynaecologiae
Annales d'Oto-Laryngologie et de Chirurgie Cervico-Faciale
Annals of Emergency Medicine
Annals of Sports Medicine
Archives of Environmental Health
Archives of Internal Medicine
Archives of Orthopedic and Traumatic Surgery
Archives of Physical Medicine and Rehabilitation
Arthroscopy
Athletic Training
Australian Journal of Science and Medicine in Sport
British Heart Journal
British Journal of Dermatology
British Journal of Sports Medicine
British Medical Journal
Canadian Journal of Applied Sports Sciences
Canadian Journal of Public Health
Chest
Clinical Nuclear Medicine
Clinical Orthopaedics and Related Research
Clinical Pharmacology and Therapeutics
Clinical Science
Contemporary Orthopedics
Critical Care Medicine
Digestive Diseases and Sciences
Endocrinology
European Journal of Applied Physiology and Occupational Physiology
European Journal of Clinical Investigation
European Journal of Clinical Pharmacology
European Journal of Respiratory Diseases
Exercise and Sports Sciences Reviews
Fertility and Sterility
Foot and Ankle
Geriatrics
International Journal of Oral and Maxillofacial Surgery
International Journal of Sports Cardiology
International Journal of Sports Medicine
International Orthopaedics

Journal of the American College of Cardiology
Journal of the American Dental Association
Journal of the American Medical Association
Journal of Applied Physiology: Respiratory, Environmental and Exercise
  Physiology
Journal of Bone and Joint Surgery (American vol.)
Journal of Bone and Joint Surgery (British vol.)
Journal of Cardiopulmonary Rehabilitation
Journal of Chronic Diseases
Journal of Clinical Endocrinology and Metabolism
Journal of Clinical Investigation
Journal of Clinical Pathology
Journal of Neurosurgery
Journal of Orthopaedic Research
Journal of Orthopaedic and Sports Physical Therapy
Journal of Pediatrics
Journal of Sports Medicine and Physical Fitness
Journal of Sports Sciences
Journal of Trauma
Journal of Urology
Klinische Wochenschrift
Lancet
Life Sciences
Medecine Du Sport
Medicine and Science in Sports and Exercise
New England Journal of Medicine
Orthopaedic Review
Orthopedics
Paraplegia
Perceptual and Motor Skills
Physical Therapy
Physician and Sportsmedicine
Physiotherapy Canada
Postgraduate Medicine
Practitioner
Primary Cardiology
Psychosomatic Medicine
Quarterly Journal of Experimental Physiology
Quarterly Journal of Medicine
Radiology
Research Quarterly for Exercise and Sport
Revue de Chirurgie Orthopedique et Reparatrice de l'Appareil Moteur
S.A.M.J./S.A.M.T.–South African Medical Journal
Scandinavian Journal of Rehabilitation Medicine
Skeletal Radiology
Sports Medicine
Sportsmedicine Digest
Virchows Archiv B: Cell Pathology
Western Journal of Medicine

Publisher's Preface

After nearly a decade of excellent contribution to the YEAR BOOK OF SPORTS MEDICINE, Lewis J. Krakauer, M.D., will be retiring as Editor-in-Chief with the completion of this edition.

His contribution, an invaluable and lasting one, has been greatly appreciated by Year Book Medical Publishers. We extend our deepest appreciation for the service he has provided and for his unending support and enthusiasm for the YEAR BOOK. We wish him the very best in the future.

Dr. Krakauer's Year Book Editorial colleagues will be editing his sections for the 1988 Year Book Edition.

1 Exercise Physiology and Medicine

Cardiovascular Physiology

Physical Activity, Other Life-Style Patterns, Cardiovascular Disease and Longevity
Ralph S. Paffenbarger, Jr., Robert T. Hyde, Chung-Cheng Hsieh, and Alvin L. Wing (Stanford Univ. and Harvard Univ.)
Acta Med. Scand. Suppl. 711:85–91, 1986   1–1

There is a marked inverse relationship between physical activity and the incidence of fatal and nonfatal coronary heart disease (CHD). Health-oriented participation in recreational activity has become increasingly popular, and health professionals have become more interested in prescribing health regimens for young and old. Yet there is much uncertainty regarding actual practices, the extent of physical activities and their effects upon cardiovascular disease and general health.

We reviewed the findings of 16,936 Harvard University alumni who entered college between 1916 and 1950. Their life experiences with regard to cardiovascular health and estimated survival were followed. Data were obtained from college physical examinations and records of athleticism. Data on postcollege physical activity, disease, and life-style were obtained by questionnaires sent in 1962 or 1966 and again in 1972 regarding the development of CHD. Deaths between 1962 and 1978 were recorded from official death certificates.

The cardiovascular benefits of continuing exercise were evident in the results. Men with an energy expenditure of 8.4 ± MJ (2,000 + kcal) per week were 39% less at risk of CHD than classmates with a lower index. The incidence rates and relative risks of death from CHD were 31% greater in men with sedentary life-styles, 84% greater in smokers, 118% greater in men with hypertension, 18% greater in overweight men, and 33% greater in men whose parents had a history of CHD. Risk estimates suggested that there might have been 16% fewer deaths if every man had exercised 8.4 + MJ per week; 25% fewer with cigarette abstinence; 9% with abolition of hypertension; 6% without obesity; and 11% minus parental CHD factor. If all five risk factors were removed, the death risk might have been 65% less, a loss of only 224 alumni instead of 640.

An age-adjusted average advantage was calculated for the active men. With all factors considered, the average advantage gained during the 16-year interim survival period for the active men over the less active group was 1¼ years.

▶ This updated summary of more than 16,000 Harvard University alumni of the classes of 1916 through 1950 has been cited in various forms previously and was the lead article in the 1985 YEAR BOOK. The broad comments still stand. Hypertension may be the strongest single predictor for coronary disease in the individual, but inadequate exercise remains a very strong predictor in the communal perspective. Ongoing epidemiologic studies will have to distinguish between strength and power exercise as opposed to endurance and aerobic activity. This distinction is not made in the Paffenbarger series in a clear sense. Prior British studies, namely those of Morris, have suggested that there is an intensity level of activity that is critical beyond activity per se.—L.J. Krakauer, M.D.

Sudden Death and Vigorous Exercise: A Study of 60 Deaths Associated With Squash
Robin J. Northcote, Clare Flannigan, and David Ballantyne (Victoria Infirm., Glasgow, Scotland)
Br. Heart J. 55:198–203, February 1986   1–2

Squash is a popular pastime among middle-aged businessmen and older persons. Data were reviewed on 60 sudden deaths in 1976 to 1984 that were associated with playing squash. The 59 men and 1 woman had a mean age of 46 years. Autopsy findings were available in 51 cases.

All deaths occurred within 1 to 24 hours of the onset of symptoms. All but one occurred within 1 hour of playing squash. Forty-six subjects collapsed on the court, ten of them in the first 10 minutes of play. Cardiopulmonary resuscitation was attempted in 46 instances, but only 1 subject was defibrillated.

All subjects had played squash for 1 year or longer, most of them about twice a week. In 42 cases there was severe stenosis of at least one main coronary vessel. Eighteen subjects had evidence of healed infarction, but this had been diagnosed in only two cases. The left anterior descending artery was the single vessel most often affected. Forty-five subjects had reported prodromal symptoms within a week of dying, but only nine were known to have consulted a physician. Hypertension was documented in 14 cases, and 14 other subjects had medical disorders that were relevant to the cardiovascular system.

Many subjects were considered by relatives to have been very fit, and none was considered unfit. Many subjects clearly had ignored prodromal symptoms and known medical disorders and continued to play squash. Many were professional or executive persons and were competitive and hard driving.

Most sudden deaths associated with vigorous sports are due to coronary artery disease. The risk in squash is small, but an appreciable number of such deaths have occurred, and consideration of how the sport may be made safer is necessary. Both the public and the medical profession must become more aware of the risks of exhaustive exercise in unsuitable subjects.

Causes of Sudden Death in Competitive Athletes

Barry J. Maron, Stephen E. Epstein, and William C. Roberts (Natl. Heart, Lung, and Blood Inst., Bethesda, Md.)
J. Am. Coll. Cardiol. 7:204–214, January 1986   1–3

Causes of sudden unexpected death due to cardiovascular disease in competitive athletes in the United States are largely related to the athlete's age at time of death. While sudden death in athletes less than 35 years old is usually due to congenital heart disease, sudden death in athletes more than 35 years of age is mainly caused by coronary artery disease. The authors review the underlying etiology of sudden cardiac death in athletes for each age category.

The highest incidence rate of sudden cardiovascular death in athletes in the under-35 age group is found among male junior high school or high school students. A lower rate is found on the collegiate level of athletics, and an even lower rate on the professional level of competition. Death usually occurs during or just after exertion on the athletic field. Evidence of structural congenital cardiovascular disease as the cause of death was found at autopsy in almost all of the cases under review, with hypertrophic cardiomyopathy occurring in almost half of the cases. The mechanism of sudden death in these cases is not clear, but it is presumed that congenital structural and functional abnormalities present in patients with hypertrophic cardiomyopathy predispose certain individuals to malignant ventricular arrhythmia.

Other young athletes exhibited an unexplained increase in left ventricular mass at autopsy, classified as idiopathic concentric left ventricular hypertrophy, which differs from hypertrophic cardiomyopathy in several important respects. Other causes of sudden death include the presence of potentially lethal, congenital malformations of the coronary artery system, and rupture of the aorta due to cystic medial necrosis. Coronary heart disease as a cause of death is found infrequently in young athletes, but it is the leading cause of death in older athletes. Myocarditis, mitral valve prolapse, aortic valve stenosis and sarcoidosis appear to be very uncommon causes of sudden death in young athletes.

Most athletes who die suddenly have not experienced previous cardiac symptoms, and cardiovascular disease is usually not suspected. In only about 25% of all sudden deaths is any underlying cardiovascular disease detected or suspected before competitive athletic participation, while a correct clinical diagnosis is rarely made at all.

▶ In most young competitive athletes, sudden death will be due to congenital cardiovascular disease, of which the most common cause is hypertrophic cardiomyopathy. Less common may be congenital coronary artery anomalies, ruptured aorta, and idiopathic left ventricular hypertrophy. In contrast, in the older athletes, of which the Northcote paper is more representative (see preceding abstract), sudden death is usually due to coronary artery disease and rarely results from congenital heart disease. It is distressing in a preventative sense that in the young only a very small percentage have any cardiac symptoms and the disease is usually unsuspected during life.—L.J. Krakauer, M.D.

Sudden Cardiac Death in Air Force Recruits: A 20-Year Review
Matthew Phillips, Max Robinowitz, James R. Higgins, Kevin J. Boran, Thomas Reed, and Renu Virmani (Wilford Hall Med. Ctr., Lackland Air Force Base, Texas, and Armed Forces Inst. of Pathology, Washington, D.C.)
JAMA 256:2696–2699, Nov. 21, 1986   1–4

Sudden cardiac death is rare in young healthy adults. The authors report the incidence and specific causes of sudden cardiac death among 1,606,167 healthy, medically screened U.S. Air Force recruits (90% male), aged 17 to 28 years. These subjects participated in a 42-day basic training period between 1965 and 1985 that included a minimum of 1 hour per day of exercise.

There were 21 cardiac deaths, of which 19 were sudden and 2 nonsudden. Of the 19 sudden cardiac victims, 16 had underlying structural heart disease, and 3 had no anatomical cause of death. Myocarditis was the most common cause of sudden death; others were the result of anomalous origin of a coronary artery, hypertrophic cardiomyopathy, mitral valve prolapse, Shone's syndrome, and focal subendocardial fibrosis and calcification with normal coronary arteries. Exercise was associated with sudden cardiac death in 17 cases, for an incidence of 0.17 deaths per 50,000 exercise-hours. There were 32 nonsudden, noncardiac deaths; only 2 cases involved structural heart disease.

Sudden cardiac death in young healthy adults is usually associated with exertion. Nevertheless, the risk of exercise-related sudden death is no greater than deaths occurring by chance alone.

▶ Thompson et al. (*JAMA* 242:1265–1267, Sept. 21, 1979) reported on the autopsy findings of 18 deaths that occurred while jogging or running. The subjects were over 42 years of age, and of these 13 had autopsy findings of coronary artery disease. In the present study sudden cardiac death in 21 young healthy persons, of which 16 had underlying structural heart disease, is noteworthy. The authors do not deal with screening indicators that may identify the individual predisposed to sudden cardiac death with exertion. It should be noted that persons who experience unexplained syncopy or dizziness with exertion should be subjected to complete cardiac evaluation.—J.S. Torg, M.D.

Sudden Death and Myocarditis During Activities and Sports Performance
J.B. Bouhour and C. Borgat (Ctr. Hosp. Univ., Nantes, France)
J. Sports Cardiol. 2:81–85, July–Dec. 1985   1–5

Besides coronary disease and obstructions of the left ventricular ejection pathway, acute and subacute myocarditis are classic causes of sudden death in young athletes during or after competition. However, since the term "myocarditis" is often used to describe cases of sudden death that have not been confirmed on a criterion of anatomicopathologic certainty, namely, the presence of an inflammatory infiltrate associated with signs of myocardial degeneration in the absence of coronary artery lesions, the authors believed that the number of reported cases of sudden death in athletes due to acute or subacute myocarditis might be too high. They reviewed the literature for reported cases of acute or subacute myocarditis resulting in sudden death due to physical effort or exercise to find out how well-documented these cases really were and to assess the true incidence of sudden death in athletes caused by acute or subacute myocarditis.

It was found that myocarditis as a cause of sudden death in athletes has been overreported. In fact, well-documented myocarditis as a cause of sudden death in athletes is extremely rare. However, on the basis of experimental studies, the authors advise against sports training or competition during rhinopharyngitis or any flulike state or febrile diarrhea, since any of these illnesses could contribute to the development of myocarditis.

▶ The diagnosis of acute myocarditis is often made in retrospect—a person dies while exercising, and it is then discovered or remembered that they had complained of flulike symptoms the day previously; I have encountered two such incidents, one in a close friend, and another in a postcoronary patient who died in the fifth mile of a fun run. However, as Bonhour and Borgat point out, there is a danger of overdiagnosis of acute myocarditis in the absence of pathologic confirmation. While some early studies attributed as many as 5.5% of sudden deaths to an acute myocarditis, well-documented autopsy studies such as that of P. Wentworth et al. (*Can. Med. Assoc. J.* 120:676–680, 1979) have quoted much lower figures of 2.0% to 2.5%. Incidents during exercise may be even less frequent (perhaps 1% of all exercise deaths); however, even this low figure remains a significant argument against exercising in the presence of an acute viral infection.—R.J. Shephard, M.D., Ph.D.

Effect of Exercise on Acute Myocardial Infarction in Rats
Judith S. Hochman and Bernardine Healy (Johns Hopkins Hosp.)
J. Am. Coll. Cardiol. 7:126–132, January 1986   1–6

Early ambulation, rehabilitation exercise programs, and early exercise testing are currently encouraged before discharge of patients after acute myocardial infarction. However, infarct expansion, the time-related thinning and dilatation of acute transmural infarct leads to aneurysm formation and cardiac rupture in humans. The effect of moderate exercise on acute infarct expansion early after myocardial infarction was evaluated in 129 rats who underwent left coronary artery ligation to achieve infarction. Ninety rats exercised on a treadmill for 1.5 hours daily for 1 week beginning on the day of coronary ligation; the remaining 39 rats did not exercise.

There was no difference in the prevalence or degree of infarct expansion between groups; infarct wall thickness, left ventricular diameter, and expansion grade were similar in both groups. Infarct size or aneurysmal shape changes did not differ between groups. No hearts ruptured, and the two groups had a similar incidence of intramural hemorrhage, a histologic finding associated with cardiac rupture. However, there was a nonsignificant trend toward higher mortality in the exercised group, with five animals dying between days 1 and 7, including three who died during exercise on the treadmill, compared to none in the unexercised group.

Moderate exercise early after myocardial infarction is safe, with no significant detrimental effect on infarct size or left ventricular topography in the rat model.

▶ One of the original reasons for bed rest following myocardial infarction was a fear that premature exercise might cause aneurysmal dilatation or even rupture of the infarcted area of ventricular wall.

Most authors currently believe that such fears are unwarranted, and current hospital practice thus calls for early ambulation (Bloch, A., et al.: *Am. J. Cardiol.* 34:152, 1974), with assessment of prognosis from treadmill testing within a few weeks of infarction (DeBusk, R.F., and Haskell, W.R.: *Circulation* 61:738, 1980).

The present study was conducted on rats. The use of small mammals enables complete and well-controlled randomization, but on the other hand the coronary obstruction is artificial, and it is difficult to equate times between an animal with a 2- to 3-year life span and a human with 70 to 80 years of life expectancy. The animal experiments suggest no pathologic disadvantage if moderate exercise is begun on the same day as coronary artery ligation. However, two notes of caution should be sounded. First, early exercise did lead to a statistically insignificant increase in mortality (5 versus 0 incidents). Second, since the ligation of the coronary vessels was experimental, the rest of the heart was in better condition than would be anticipated in the average postcoronary patient. Certainly, it seems important to monitor the heart rhythm of human subjects in the first few days after infarction, as the activity of the postinfarct patient is increased.—R.J. Shephard, M.D., Ph.D.

Ventricular Tachycardia Induced by Exercise
Alan Woelfel (Univ. of North Carolina)
Primary Cardiol. 12:35–42, July 1986   1–7

The widespread use of treadmill testing has identified more patients with exercise-induced ventricular tachycardia (VT). The pathogenesis, clinical features, and treatment of this disorder are discussed.

Exercise-induced VT can occur in young patients without evident organic heart disease, in older patients with recurrent coronary artery disease, and in those with a variety of cardiac disorders such as hypertensive heart disease, cardiomyopathies, and valvular heart disease. Symptoms vary from palpitations to syncope or even cardiac arrest, and most often are related to exertion. A few patients may have no symptoms, and diagnosis is established when VT is observed during a treadmill test performed for other indications. The rate and duration of exercise-induced VT varies widely. The induced VT may show a right or left bundle-branch block configuration, and it may occur early in exercise, at or near peak, or after exercise. The mechanism of exercise-induced VT remains unknown, but delayed afterpotentials, reentry, and catecholamine-sensitive automaticity have been postulated as responsible for exercise-induced VT.

After diagnosis, the exercise test should be repeated to document arrhythmia reproducibility and to identify patients with a consistent relationship between a critical sinus rate and onset of VT. In marked contrast to their ineffectiveness in patients with VT unrelated to exercise, β-adrenergic blocking agents are highly effective in about 90% of patients with exercise-induced VT. It should be administered orally for at least five half-lives to achieve steady-state levels. Therapy is effective if no VT occurs, and the duration of exercise equals or exceeds that of the pretreatment level. Effectiveness of β-blockade therapy in patients who exhibit a critical sinus rate-VT relation is assessed by its ability to prevent increase of the rate during maximal exercise to the point at which VT is triggered. The calcium-channel blocking agents, i.e., verapamil, are useful should alternative drug therapy be indicated. Yearly exercise tests are recommended to assess continuing efficacy of treatment.

Ventricular Tachycardia in the Young Athlete: A Systematic Approach to Selection of Drug Therapy
Philip J. Podrid (Harvard Univ.)
Physician Sportsmed. 14:69–73, February 1986   1–8

Sudden cardiac death has been reported in young athletes who were found to have had underlying heart disease at autopsy, including hypertrophic cardiomyopathy or congenital structural heart disease. Such pa-

DRUGS, DOSAGE, AND BLOOD LEVEL IN PATIENTS WITH
VENTRICULAR TACHYCARDIA

Drug	Dose (mg) Acute	Maintenance	Blood Level ($\mu g \cdot ml^{-1}$)
Quinidine	600	300–400 4 times/day	2–5
Disopyramide	300	100–200 3–4 times/day	2–4
Procainamide	1,500	500–1,500 4 times/day or every 4 hr	6–10
Tocainide	800	400–800 3 times/day	6–10
Mexiletine	400	200–400 3 times/day	0.7–1.6
Long-lasting preparations available:			
Quinidine gluconate		324 3 times/day	
Disopyramide		100–300 2 times/day	
Procainamide		500–1,500 3–4 times/day	

(Courtesy of Podrid, P.J.: Physician Sportsmed. 14:69–73, February 1986. Reprinted by permission. A McGraw-Hill publication.)

tients often experience serious ventricular arrhythmias during exercise. However, little has been written about the management of such patients. A young man treated successfully for exertion-related ventricular tachyarrhythmia is described.

Man, 24, a professional tennis player, had several episodes of tachycardia followed by syncope while playing championship tennis matches and had been treated with quinidine before hospitalization. Electrophysiologic studies were performed after quinidine therapy was stopped, but programmed premature stimulation failed to induce ventricular tachycardia. Cardiac catheterization showed normal left ventricular function with normal hemodynamics. An echocardiogram showed no evidence of coronary artery disease, asymmetric hypertrophy, or mitral valve prolapse, and a treadmill test showed only occasional ventricular premature beats. The patient was released taking propranolol and quinidine.

Because he continued to experience recurrent episodes of tachycardia and syncope, the patient was referred to the author's institution, where arrhythmogenic right ventricular dysplasia was diagnosed. A time-saving, four-phase approach to acute drug testing with single antiarrhythmia drugs and electrophysiologic testing was used quickly to find an optimum regimen (table). The patient was discharged on a program of tocainide and metoprolol and has done well over the past 3 years, without recurrence of ventricular tachycardia.

▶ Ventricular tachycardia as isolated episodes or repetitive episodes may be completely unsuspected and picked up on routine stress testing. On the other hand, some individuals will have symptoms of palpitations, rarely syncope relating to exertion. This seems to be less common. The therapy remains in dispute and many, such as Woelfel, are of the belief that β-blockade is effective in 90% of exercise-induced VT (see preceding abstract). Others use a multidrug approach in the given patient; the article by Podrict (Abstract 1–8) is an example. Some leave isolated episodes untreated. Bricker and colleagues have reported in the *American Heart Journal* (July 1986) the uncommon finding of ventricular tachycardia with exercise in children. In their series, this occurred in 22 of 2,761 cases and was sustained in only five cases. Therapy may change significantly in the next year or two as calcium channel blockade interrelates with the present dominant β-blockade and the other empirical agents used to date.—L.J. Krakauer, M.D.

Exercise Training Following Cardiovascular Surgery
Carl Foster
Exerc. Sport Sci. Rev. 14:303–323, 1986   1–9

Exercise-based rehabilitation in patients with coronary heart disease (CHD) and patients recovering from coronary artery bypass grafting (CABG) has gained wide acceptance during the past decade. Success with exercise programs for post-CABG patients has led to the inclusion of patients recovering from other cardiovascular operations, including valve repair and repair of congenital abnormalities in children, and in postautologous transplant patients.

Patients who have undergone cardiovascular operations are somewhat less difficult to rehabilitate than postmyocardial infarction (MI) or angina patients, since the former may generally be in somewhat more stable condition than post-MI patients. In postsurgical patients, rehabilitation should be focused on minimization of bed rest, treatment of the sequelae of sternotomy, and close surveillance for new or changing medical problems. It is likely that physiologic adaptations to exercise training in patients who are recovering from cardiovascular operations follow those observed in post-MI patients, although it is unlikely that postsurgical patients will show improved myocardial perfusion as a result of exercise training, given the magnitude of improvement known to occur with CABG. Only patients with exertional myocardial ischemia are likely to show improved myocardial perfusion from exercise training.

The potential of exercise for preventing a return of symptoms in patients who have undergone CABG, either through graft closure or because of progress of the disease in the native circulation, is about equal to that observed in post-MI patients. Follow-up studies on secondary prevention after other types of cardiovascular operation are not yet available.

▶ Although the title suggests a discussion covering the broad sweep of cardiovascular surgery, the main focus of this review is upon cardiac bypass patients, where much of the available research has been concentrated. One might take issue with one conclusion—that an improvement of coronary perfusion is unlikely to be observed after cardiovascular surgery. In fact, much of the improvement of coronary perfusion in all cardiac patients is due to a slowing of the exercise heart rate, with a lengthening of the diastolic phase; there seems no reason why this could not develop as the patient recovers from the hospital phase of cardiac surgery, with further benefit from any training which may have been undertaken.

There are interesting discussions relating to the relative importance of catecholamines and the Frank/Starling mechanism to the increase of cardiac output when the denervated heart is exercised. In some patients who have undergone rejection, performance may also be limited by pulmonary vascular changes, and there seem differences of response between a simple cardiac replacement and the use of the donor heart to assist the existing myocardium. Much of the deterioration of performance appears related to loss of muscle function during prolonged bed rest, and there is evidence that an appropriate training regimen improves peripheral blood flow and thus performance through a strengthening of the limb muscles.

Fascinating issues remain to be explored with respect to the training responses of patients following the various types of cardiac transplantation; here is scope for another review!—R.J. Shephard, M.D., Ph.D.

Cardiac Size and $\dot{V}O_{2Max}$ Do Not Decrease After Short-Term Exercise Cessation

Eileen M. Cullinane, Stanley P. Sady, Louise Vadeboncoeur, Michael Burke, and Paul D. Thompson (Miriam Hosp., Providence, R.I.)

Med. Sci. Sports Exerc. 18:420–424, 1986   1–10

Cross-sectional echocardiographic studies which compared endurance athletes and sedentary controls have revealed larger right and left ventricular diameters and calculated left ventricular masses in the athletes. However, such studies cannot determine whether increased cardiac dimensions are an effect of or a selection factor for physical activity. Although the influence of physical activity on cardiac dimensions can be examined in studies of reduced physical activity, few studies have examined the effects of detraining on the cardiovascular dimensions of endurance athletes. The goal of the present study was to describe the effects of exercise cessation on the cardiac dimensions and maximum oxygen uptake of athletes who ceased training.

The authors measured maximum oxygen uptake, estimated changes in plasma volume, and the cardiac dimensions of 15 male competitive distance runners (28.2 ± 5.6 years of age) before and after 10 days of exercise cessation. The subjects were habitually active but adjusted their training to run 16 km daily for 2 weeks before the study; they were maintained on defined diets for the week before and during the detraining period. Average body weight decreased within 2 days of exercise cessation and

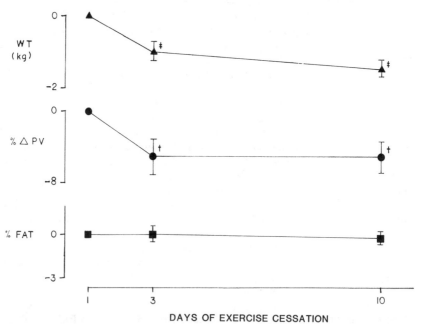

ABSOLUTE CHANGES FROM BASELINE

DAYS OF EXERCISE CESSATION

Fig 1–1.—Absolute changes (mean ± SE) in body weight (kg), percent change in plasma volume (% PV), and percent body fat during 10 days of exercise cessation. Significant changes from day 1 are indicated by † ($P < .01$) and ‡ ($P < .001$). (Courtesy of Cullinane, E.M., et al.: Med. Sci. Sports Exerc. 18:420–424, 1986. Copyright 1986, the American College of Sports Medicine. Reprinted by permission.)

was accompanied by a 5.0 ± 5.9% decrease in plasma volume. During the study, there were no further changes in plasma volume, and estimated percent body fat did not change (Fig 1–1). Furthermore, resting heart rate, blood pressure, and cardiac dimensions were also unchanged with physical inactivity. Finally, maximum oxygen uptake was not altered although peak exercise heart rate was found to be an average of 9 ± 5 beats per minute (5%) higher subsequent to detraining.

It is concluded that short periods of exercise cessation decrease estimated plasma volume and increase the maximum exercise heart rate of endurance athletes but do not alter their cardiac dimensions or maximum oxygen uptake.

▶ B. Saltin and G. Grimby (*Circulation* 38:1104–1115, 1968) looked at the long-term effects of detraining on the radiographic heart volume a number of years ago; they concluded that the effects of training persisted for quite a number of years, although eventually the size of the heart shadow reverted to that found in the sedentary population. However, radiographs cannot distinguish clearly between an enlargement of the heart due to ventricular muscle and that due to an increase in the dimensions of the ventricular cavity. One more recent echocardiographic paper (Ehsani et al.: *Am. J. Cardiol.* 42:52, 1978) concluded that there were decreases of wall thickness with as little as four days of detraining. This was surprising information in view of the relatively long time required to induce ventricular hypertrophy, and the present report, which finds no change after ten days of detraining, sounds much more plausible.—R.J. Shephard, M.D., Ph.D.

Enlarged Left Atrial Dimension in Former Endurance Athletes: An Echocardiographic Study
C. Höglund (Södersjukhuset, Stockholm, and Univ. of Lund, Mälmo, Sweden)
Int. J. Sports Med. 7:133–136, June 1986   1–11

It is well known that highly active endurance athletes have larger hearts on x-ray examination than do sedentary persons. Echocardiographic studies have shown that cardiac enlargement in this group of athletes involves both the ventricles and the left atrium. Although x-ray films made several years after all competition was stopped have shown that former endurance athletes may also have enlarged hearts, this group has not yet been studied by echocardiography. The author examined the echocardiographic dimensions of the left atrium and ventricle and left ventricular wall thickness in former endurance athletes and in age-matched sedentary controls.

Thirteen formerly well-trained endurance athletes, aged 54 to 74 years (mean, 66), who had competed until age 35, were matched with 21 randomly selected, sedentary controls, with a mean age of 69 years, who had never participated in athletic competitions. None of the participants had a history of heart disease or hypertension.

The former athletes had a significantly larger left atrial dimension than did controls. No statistically significant difference was found between former athletes and controls in left ventricular end-diastolic dimension, both as absolute values and in relation to body surface area, in the thickness of the interventricular septum, or in the thickness of the left ventricular posterior wall.

Former endurance athletes have an enlarged left atrium, but a normal-sized left ventricle.

▶ There are two major difficulties in dealing with radiographic estimates of cardiac volume—one is uncertain whether the shadow is due to cardiac muscle or to blood content, and even if muscle, it remains unclear whether the increment is ventricular or atrial in origin. The present echocardiographic study finds a very similar overall cardiac volume to that reported in the radiographic studies of B. Saltin and G. Grimby (*Circulation* 38:1104–1115, 1968), but it suggests that the persistent cardiac enlargement of the former athletes has an atrial rather than a ventricular origin. While the cross-sectional comparison with sedentary controls is reasonably convincing, the experiment deserves repeating with longitudinal data collection on a population of former athletes during the first few years after they have abandoned rigorous training.

The reason why the atrium should remain enlarged remains unexplained. Höglund speculates that fibrosis of the left atrium may have developed in response to atrial dilatation during the active phase of the athletes' lifespans; he notes further that the atrial enlargement can give rise to supraventricular arrhythmias and AV blocks, which can cause clinical problems in former athletes (Holmgren, A., and Strandell, T.: *Acta Med. Scand.* 163:149–160, 1959).— R.J. Shephard, M.D., Ph.D.

Cardiopulmonary Stress Testing: A Review of Noninvasive Approaches
Juliette Wait (Eastern Virginia Med. School)
Chest 90:504–510, October 1986   1–12

Dyspneic patients often have coexisting pulmonary and cardiac diseases. However, since patients are routinely tested at rest, it is often difficult to pinpoint the exact cause of the exercise limitation because of vague clinical clues and inconclusive laboratory results. The introduction of computerized laboratory equipment has permitted measurement of pulmonary gas exchange during exercise, and radionuclide computer-assisted cardiac imaging techniques and echocardiography allow noninvasive cardiac function testing. The author reviews the practical aspects of noninvasive incremental exercise testing to characterize precisely cardiac and pulmonary disease in patients with exercise limitation and to assess accurately response to treatment.

Pulmonary gas exchange data, including the rate of oxygen consumption ($\dot{V}O_2$), minute ventilation ($\dot{V}E$), and rate of carbon dioxide production ($\dot{V}CO_2$) are correlated to assess the physiologic response to exercise. By comparing the measured pulmonary gas exchange data with predicted normal values, characteristic patterns of disease can be identified (Fig 1–

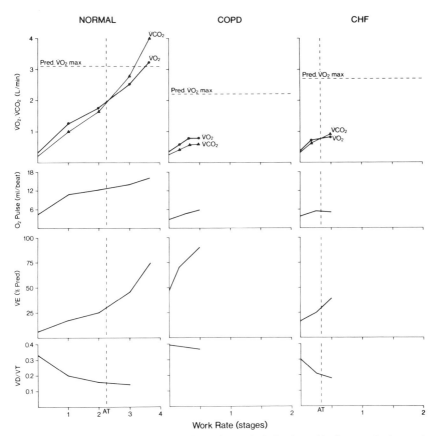

Fig 1–2.—Changes in pulmonary gas exchange data and calculated variables for normal subject and patients with chronic obstructive pulmonary disease *(COPD)* and congestive heart failure *(CHF)* studied in author's laboratory. Changes in $\dot{V}O_2$, $\dot{V}CO_2$, $\dot{V}E$, oxygen pulse, and dead space to tidal volume ratio (VD/VT) are plotted against increasing work rate on treadmill. Normal subject was exercised according to 3-minute incremental protocol on treadmill. The two patients were studied by use of modified incremental protocol on treadmill. Stages 1 and 2 are comparable workloads for both protocols. (Courtesy of Wait, J.: Chest 90:504–510, October 1986.)

2). Pulmonary gas exchange data are also useful in determination of the anaerobic threshold, which is important in evaluating cardiovascular responses to incremental exercise.

Results of cardiopulmonary exercise testing should be interpreted on the basis of available clinical information, but they should not be used to make a primary diagnosis.

▶ A good review of noninvasive techniques used with exercise when the issue is to clarify whether causation is cardiac or pulmonary. This cannot always be done easily, and sometimes both systems are involved. In such testing, the most prominent abnormality demonstrated is likely to be the primary source of exercise limitation at the time of testing.—L.J. Krakauer, M.D.

Vigorous Physical Activity and Cardiovascular Risk Factors in Young Adults

James F. Sallis, William L. Haskell, Peter D. Wood, Stephen P. Fortmann, and Karen M. Vranizan (Univ. of California, San Diego)
J. Chronic Dis. 39:115–120, 1986   1–13

It has been shown that regular participation in vigorous activity (i.e., at least 7.5 kcal per minute) is protective against fatal and non-fatal cardiovascular disease (CVD). Although the mechanism of this protective effect is not known, it has been hypothesized that physical activity may benificially affect other established factors in CVD, such as serum levels of lipoproteins, obesity, blood pressure, or cigarette smoking. However, epidemiologic data have not conclusively supported the relationship between physical activity and these risk factors.

In an attempt to clarify the inconsistent findings of previous studies, the authors carried out both cross-sectional and longitudinal analyses of the relationship between vigorous exercise and risk factors for CVD in a representative sample of male and female subjects aged 20 to 35 years. A self-report measure of habitual vigorous physical activity was validated by pulse rate.

It was found there were relationships, in both cross-sectional and longitudinal analyses, between self-reported vigorous physical activity and ratio of high-density lipoproteins to low-density lipoproteins, particularly for women. In addition, in cross-sectional analyses relationships were found among physical activity and diastolic blood pressure, and levels of total cholesterol, high-density lipoprotein cholesterol, triglycerides, and alveolar carbon monoxide.

These findings tend to confirm the results of investigations of other samples which showed physical activity is related to levels of high-density lipoprotein cholesterol but is unrelated to most other health behaviors.

Prognostic Value of Exercise Electrocardiogram in Men at High Risk of Future Coronary Heart Disease: Multiple Risk Factor Intervention Trial Experience

Pentti M. Rautaharju, Ronald J. Prineas, William J. Eifler, Curt D. Furberg, James D. Neaton, Richard S. Crow, Jeremiah Stamler, and Jeffrey A. Cutler (for the Multiple Risk Factor Intervention Trial Research Group) (Dalhousie Univ., Halifax, N.S., Univ. of Minnesota, Natl. Heart, Lung, and Blood Inst., Bethesda, Md., and Northwestern Univ., Evanston, Ill.)
J. Am. Coll. Cardiol. 8:1–10, July 1986   1–14

The prognostic usefulness of the exercise electrocardiogram (ECG) was evaluated from data from the Multiple Risk Factor Intervention Trial, a primary prevention trial designed to test the effect of a multifactor intervention program on mortality from coronary heart disease. A total of 12,866 men aged 35 to 57 years were assigned to an intervention program or to standard community care.

An insignificant 7% reduction in coronary mortality was found in the intervention group, but men with an abnormal ECG response to exercise had nearly a four-fold increase in 7-year coronary mortality when they were assigned to usual care, compared with those who had normal ST-segment responses to exercise.

More than 80% of men reached the age-specific target heart rate on exercise testing. Men with abnormal responses to exercise had higher overall mortality and more angina, but the trend for nonfatal infarctions was not significant. The relative risk increased with the extent of depression of the ST segment. Abnormalities on resting ECGs were of no demonstrable prognostic value, and the risk associated with abnormalities at exercise testing was not altered by considering the presence or absence of abnormalities on resting ECGs.

Abnormalities in early ventricular repolarization at peak exercise have prognostic significance for middle-aged men at risk of coronary heart disease. Excess risk is present in men who have normal findings on resting ECGs, and the risk increases with the degree of depression of the ST segment.

▶ This thorough study demonstrates the prognostic value of early ventricular repolarization abnormality occurring at peak exercise in middle-aged men at high risk of future coronary heart disease. An abnormal ST depression integral in a submaximal heart rate-limited exercise test at high risk of future heart episodes is an independent predictor of coronary heart disease death. The authors stress that this excess risk is present among those with minor ECG abnormalities at rest as well as among those with normal ECG at rest and that the risk may be progressive with the amount or level of ST depression.—L.J. Krakauer, M.D.

The Changing Role of the Exercise Electrocardiogram as a Diagnostic and Prognostic Test For Chronic Ischemic Heart Disease
Bernard R. Chaitman (St. Louis Univ.)
J. Am. Coll. Cardiol. 8:1195–1210, November 1986   1–15

Many different ECG lead systems and parameters have been used to diagnose chronic ischemic heart disease and for prognostic purposes. Tracings now can be acquired during and after exercise. The diagnostic accuracy of the exercise ECG has been improved by the use of Bayesian theory, multivariate models, and new non–ST-segment criteria. Posttest coronary risk estimates are best made in terms of conditional probability, rather than simple statements of "positive" or "negative." Newer criteria include the maximal ST/heart rate slope and quantitative treadmill exercise score. Computer software programs are available which incorporate clinical and exercise test variables into a model to obtain posttest estimates of coronary risk and estimates of the likelihood of subsequent coronary events.

Exercise test results must be interpreted in light of the clinical findings.

An abnormal test result does not indicate obstructive coronary disease in most asymptomatic, apparently healthy subjects. Cardiac event rates are relatively low when patients with known coronary disease achieve a high exercise workload. Exercise testing of patients with typical angina provides a baseline, helps assess antianginal treatment, and aids in making decisions concerning coronary angiography and revascularization. Marked exercise ECG abnormalities in persons with typical angina call for early coronary angiography and revascularization if clinically indicated.

▶ ST segmental depression was once thought diagnostic of myocardial ischemia and an increased risk of myocardial infarction, but in recent years there has been increasing recognition that diagnosis and prognostication are complicated by a large number of false negative and false positive test results. If electrocardiography is applied indiscriminately, then as many as two of every three positive results is likely to be "incorrect" relative to an angiographic criterion; indeed, the poor clinician would be better advised to base prognosis on the simple toss of a coin!

There has thus been interest in the possibility of improving diagnostic and prognostic accuracy by the incorporation of other electrocardiographic criteria. An increase in R-wave amplitude after exercise has not proved very helpful, but the R-wave can be used to standardize the extent of ST depression; regression of Q-wave amplitude and an inversion of the U wave during exercise are also associated fairly consistently with myocardial perfusion defects. Finally, the clinical precision of the ST change is improved if it is related to heart rate. A multiple regression analysis based on all of these various electrocardiographic indicators is considerably more useful than a simple ST measurement. However, the real remedy for false-positive diagnoses is to avoid making unnecessary "fishing trips" on asymptomatic persons; in this connection, there is a great deal to commend the Canadian position of not requiring an exercise ECG on everyone who has the idea of undertaking a moderate increase of personal physical activity.—R.J. Shephard, M.D., Ph.D.

Exercise Thallium-201 Scintigraphy in Men With Nondiagnostic Exercise Electrocardiograms: Prognostic Implications

Abdulmassih S. Iskandrian, Abdul-Hamid Hakki, and Sally Kane-Marsch (Hahnemann Univ.)
Arch. Intern. Med. 146:2189–2193, November 1986   1–16

Previous studies have shown that exercise ^{201}Tl imaging is useful in the differentiation of false positive from true positive exercise ECGs. The authors examined the usefulness of exercise ^{201}Tl imaging in the identification of patients at high risk of cardiac events.

The patients were 196 men, aged 45 to 65 years, including 90 (46%) with a history of hypertension, 85 (43%) with a history of myocardial infarction (MI), 46 (23%) with previous Q wave MI, 19 (10%) being treated with digitalis, and 93 (47%) being treated with β-blockers at the time of exercise testing. Typical angina pectoris was present in 82 patients

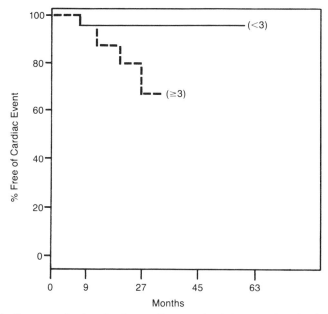

Fig 1–3.—Percentage of patients free from cardiac events in relation to number of perfusion defects (in parentheses). Difference between groups is highly significant (Mantel-Cox, $P = .009$). (Courtesy of Iskandrian, A.S., et al.: Arch. Intern. Med. 146:2189–2193, November 1986. Copyright 1986, American Medical Association.)

(42%) and atypical angina in 42; the rest had nonanginal chest pain, dyspnea, or palpitations. Exercise ^{201}Tl imaging results were normal in 72 patients (37%) and abnormal in the rest.

At follow-up, which ranged from 1 to 66 months (mean, 15), 5 patients had died of cardiac causes and 7 had sustained nonfatal acute MIs. Only the number of perfusion defects significantly predicted cardiac events. Neither clinical presentation, nor history of MI, presence of Q-wave MI, exercise duration, exercise heart rate, or double product could predict cardiac events. These factors added no information to that already provided by the number of perfusion defects found with exercise ^{201}Tl imaging. The prognosis for patients with three or more perfusion defects was significantly worse than that for patients with fewer defects on exercise ^{201}Tl imaging (Fig 1–3).

Exercise ^{201}Tl imaging is useful for risk stratification in men who have nondiagnostic exercise ECGs.

▶ This study goes a step further in differentiating false- from true-positive exercise ECG and states that patients at high risk for cardiac events can then be stratified with some accuracy. This must be viewed as a further noninvasive test which, if positive, may well lead to cardiac catheterization and surgical decisions. At this time, it should be a backup test to the nondiagnostic exercise ECG in men, and possibly for women in the future.—L.J. Krakauer, M.D.

Effects of Aerobic Training on Exercise Tolerance and Echocardiographic Dimensions in Untrained Postmenopausal Women

Douglass A. Morrison, Thomas W. Boyden, Richard W. Pamenter, Beau J. Freund, William A. Stini, Richard Harrington, and Jack H. Wilmore (Univ. of Arizona and VA Med. Ctr., Tucson)
Am. Heart J. 112:561–567, September 1986   1–17

Physical activity among persons of all ages has increased considerably. Although exercise training has been evaluated extensively in younger populations, little is known about the consequences of exercise training in older persons, especially older women. A prospective, controlled training study was conducted to evaluate whether an exercise program of sufficient intensity can safely increase maximal oxygen consumption (Vo_{2max}) in healthy postmenopausal women, and whether such a training program can lead to significant changes in cardiac function.

Thirty-four untrained postmenopausal women were randomly assigned to an aerobic exercise training program or to a control group. The exercise group performed supervised exercises at least three times a week in 40-minute sessions over an 8-month period.

Twenty-five women completed the study, including 8 in the control group and 17 in the training group. Maximal oxygen consumption and maximal treadmill time (MTT) increased significantly in the exercise group, in which other variables are maximal ventilation (VE_{max}), maximal respiratory exchange ratio (RER_{max}), and maximal heart rate (HR_{max}). Although there was no significant change in MTT in the controls, the group had a slight increase in Vo_{2max}. Controls showed no significant changes in left ventricular dimensions of wall thickness on echocardiography, but the exercise group showed significant increases.

Previously untrained postmenopausal women can safely participate in exercise programs that are sufficiently vigorous to increase Vo_{2max} and MTT.

▶ The echocardiogram was used as the guide in this series of untrained postmenopausal, healthy women. Training had a clear effect on the echocardiograms in these women, and in the trained group there was an enhanced resting left ventricular ejection fraction and an increased resting left ventricular end-diastolic dimension. This suggests that the training benefits were due to true cardiac factors and not just peripheral factors.—L.J. Krakauer, M.D.

Is Peak Quadriceps Blood Flow in Humans Even Higher During Exercise With Hypoxemia?

Loring B. Rowell, Bengt Saltin, Bente Kiens, and Niels Juel Christensen (Univ. of Copenhagen, Herlev Hosp., Herlev, Denmark, and Univ. of Washington)
Am. J. Physiol. 251:H1038–H1044, November 1986   1–18

Muscle blood flow can increase without apparent limit as a muscle group works up to capacity. If the total mass of active muscle is large, as in whole-body maximal exercise, the rise in vascular conductance can exceed the ability of cardiac output to increase, and vasoconstriction is necessary to maintain blood pressure. Quadriceps blood flow was measured by thermal dilution in six normal males 22–29 years of age during rest and dynamic exercise of one leg in normoxic and hypoxemic conditions. Hypoxemia of 10% to 11% oxygen was utilized. Exercise was performed at loads of 20 W and 30 to 40 W, and at the highest load sustained for about 5 minutes in normoxic and hypoxic conditions, averaging 52 W and 49 W, respectively. Femoral venous flow was measured by the constant-infusion thermal-dilution method.

Both quadriceps blood flow and vascular conductance were higher under hypoxemic conditions. Arterial pressure and levels of lactate and catecholamines increased at work levels above 20 W. Both muscle blood flow and muscle vascular conductance were maximal at the highest work intensity (Fig 1–4). Muscle oxygen delivery was unchanged by hypoxemia,

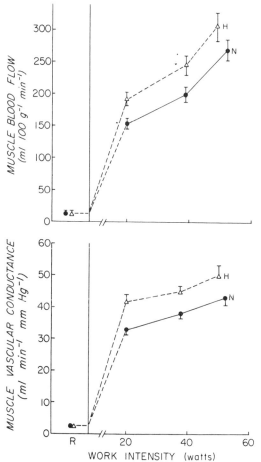

Fig 1–4.—**Upper panel,** average (with SE) muscle blood flow per 100 gm of estimated quadriceps muscle mass at rest and 3 work intensities. **Lower panel,** average (with SE) muscle vascular conductances. (Courtesy of Rowell, L.B., et al.: Am. J. Physiol. 251:H1038–H1044, November 1986.)

although oxygen extraction decreased. Femoral venous oxygen content remained much higher than with whole-body exercise at all work loads.

Muscle blood flow can rise to higher peak levels in hypoxemia, without apparent limit, when the mass of active muscle is too small to overwhelm the pumping capacity of the heart. With strenuous whole-body exercise there is a "threat" of hypotension because of the disparity between maximal cardiac output and muscle vascular conductance, and intense vasoconstriction is needed to limit the fall in blood pressure. Working muscle may be the major source of high circulating norepinephrine during exercise with hypoxemia.

▶ Physiologists have for many years debated whether the factor ultimately limiting performance is the pumping ability of the heart or the capacity of the periphery to accept the oxygen which is thus delivered. P. Andersen and B. Saltin recently presented evidence (*J. Physiol.* [*Lond.*] 366:233–249, 1985) suggesting that there was no apparent ceiling on the ability of the muscles to accept an increase of blood flow, provided a ceiling of cardiac output was not exceeded. Their studies were, however, based on the relatively large extensor muscles of the thigh, and it seems likely that with a smaller group of muscles such as those used in elbow flexion the contractions could become sufficiently intense to prevent perfusion. In association with H. Vandewalle, E. Bouhlel, and H. Monod, I recently demonstrated that central hypoxia (breathing 12% oxygen) reduced the peak oxygen usage in one or two leg ergometry, but not in single arm flexion or single arm plus shoulder movements.

The present article extends this debate, suggesting that part of the problem in perfusing a large muscle mass is not the force exerted by the vigorously contracting fibers, but rather a catecholamine-induced vasoconstriction, which can be partially reversed by hypoxia. Certainly, the immediate response to exercise is a general vasoconstriction which is reversed by a local accumulation of metabolites in the active muscles; it is thus reasonable to postulate that this local reversal is incomplete and can be further modulated by hypoxia.—R.J. Shephard, M.D., Ph.D.

Incidence of Heart Rate Overshoot
Keiji Yamaji, and Roy J. Shephard (Toyama Univ., Japan, and Univ. of Toronto)
J. Sports Med. 26:157–161, June 1986   1–19

In supramaximal exercise, where a steady-state heart rate is not achieved, the rate continues to increase for several seconds after exercise. Occurrence of the "overshoot" phenomenon was studied in 20 young men in a physical education program who performed maximal and heavy submaximal work on a cycle ergometer. The mean age was 20 years, and the average body mass was 63 kg. All subjects did sports or recreational activities two to four times per week, and they were accustomed to the experimental routine.

Fourteen of the 20 subjects exhibited overshoot in maximal exercise tests. The incidence was highest for beat 4 after exercise. At heart rates below 140 beats per minute in submaximal tests, overshoot occurred only once in 52 studies. At higher instantaneous heart rates the prevalence of overshoot increased and, at the highest level, the incidence of 65% approached that associated with maximal exercise.

An overshoot of heart rate is demonstrable after both maximal and submaximal aerobic work in healthy young men. The effect most likely represents relative underperfusion of the active muscles during exercise, rather than a lag in cardiovascular response, venous pooling, or respiratory change. The heart rate during vigorous exercise may be approximated from immediate postexercise values, but these should be averaged over about 10 seconds to obtain the most accurate results.

▶ Accumulated anaerobic metabolites must be cleared from the working muscles immediately after exercise, and this seems at least one reason why there is a brief "overshoot" of heart rate during the recovery period. It is important to note this phenomenon if the immediate recovery pulse is used to test cardiac function or regulate training; taking account of both the overshoot and the subsequent rapid decline of heart rate, the best approximation to the end-exercise value is obtained if data are averaged over the first 10 seconds following exercise.—R.J. Shephard, M.D., Ph.D.

Exercise Training and Hypertension

James M. Hagberg and Douglas R. Seals (Washington Univ., St. Louis, and Univ. of Arizona, Tucson)
Acta Med. Scand, Suppl. 711:131–136, 1986   1–20

Hypertension is a major problem in the world today and may exist in up to 25% of some populations. Cardiovascular complications associated with elevated blood pressure are important factors in cardiovascular mortality and morbidity. There are numerous drugs on the market today that are very effective in reducing blood pressure; however, they present some negative aspects such as side effects, high cost, and poor compliance. As a result, nonpharmacologic approaches to treatment of hypertension include reductions in weight, sodium intake, and stress. Cessation of smoking and initiation of an exercise program have been proposed as initial therapy of essential hypertension.

The results of 16 studies comparing the effects of exercise on diastolic and systolic blood pressure were reviewed. Eleven of the 16 studies reported a significant reduction in systolic blood pressure at rest with exercise training. The average systolic blood pressure in the 16 studies before training was 153 mm Hg and the reduction due to exercise averaged 11 mm Hg. The average reduction in diastolic blood pressure induced by exercise was 8 mm Hg from an initial value of 94 mm Hg. Although these data are suggestive of the beneficial effect of exercise upon arterial hypertension, many of the studies suffer from design deficiencies, such as lack of inclusion of a nonexercising hypertensive control group, that may adversely influence the outcome.

While studies have shown that intensive exercise improves myocardial function in coronary artery patients, the same may not be true for the antihypertensive effect of exercise. Reduction in blood pressure appears to be unrelated to increased maximal O_2 consumption and lower intensity exercise training may be as, or more, effective in reducing blood pressure in hypertensive patients. It is evident that further investigation on the effect of exercise in hypertension is needed. Whether or not cardiac output and/ or total peripheral resistance are decreased during exercise and by what mechanisms remain to be determined.

▶ This is an important baseline paper to evaluate the role of exercise training in the nonpharmacologic setting. Exercise exerts some favorable effect in the 17 studies which were assessed in the order of both systolic and diastolic blood pressure (approximately 10 mm Hg each, following training). The authors acknowledge the possible presence of design deficiencies in the studies evaluated, and there is the suggestion that mild to moderate intensity training may be as useful as higher intensity training in lowering blood pressure. Lacking are significant data to indicate whether cardiac output or total peripheral resistance or both are reduced in the process of the total blood pressure reduction. Few would argue that exercise is a useful adjunct to pharmacology for hypertension. The responsible mechanisms are still not clear.—L.J. Krakauer, M.D.

Physical Activity and Blood Pressure in Normotensive Young Women
E. Saar, R. Chayoth, and N. Meyerstein (Kaye Coll. of Educ. and Ben Gurion Univ. of the Negev, Beer Sheva, Israel)
Eur. J. Appl. Physiol. 55:64–67, April 1986 1–21

Habitual physical activity has been associated with lower blood pressure (BP) in normotensive subjects. To evaluate the influence of aerobic physical activity on BP in young women, BP and heart rate (HR) were measured in 22 physically active and 25 physically non-active normotensive women in supine, sitting, and standing positions. Mean ages of patients were 20 ± 1.7 and 20.9 ± 1.7 years, respectively.

Physically active young women had significantly lower heart rates and mean BP in all body positions and lower diastolic BP in the supine and sitting positions than the non-active women. A significant negative correlation was evident between maximal oxygen consumption and blood pressure. There was no correlation between age or body weight and blood pressure.

Aerobic physical training can be a nonpharmacologic therapy in young women with moderate and borderline hypertension. The decrease in BP may be due to the lower sympathetic tone induced by aerobic training.

▶ This would serve as an example of one of the papers considered in the extensive summary cited above. This adds women to the data base since the numbers have been disproportionately weighted toward men in prior years. The comments and conclusions mentioned above would stand.—L.J. Krakauer, M.D.

Sex- and Age-Related Blood Pressure Response to Dynamic Work With Small Muscle Masses
U. Kobryn, B. Hoffmann, and E. Ransch (Zentralinstitut für Arbeitsmedizin der DDR, Berlin)
Eur. J. Appl. Physiol. 55:79–82, April 1986   1–22

For a given load, the smaller the active muscle mass involved, the higher the heart rate will be. With isometric hand exercises, there are sex- and age-related differences in blood pressure response. This group investigates blood pressure alterations during fatiguing dynamic hand exercises, and studies the effects of sex and age.

Four groups consisting of men or women of ages 20 to 29 years or 30 to 39 years each contained ten subjects. Each did one-handed dynamic work on a dynamometer at 40%, 60%, and 80% of maximum voluntary contraction (MVC). Tests were repeated after 1-hour rests. Indirect arterial blood pressure was measured during exercise and rest. Heart rate was determined from continuous ECG signals.

After a few minutes of fatiguing dynamic one-hand exercise, large increases in systolic and diastolic blood pressure were noted in both sexes (table). Men always had higher systolic blood pressure than women. Diastolic blood pressure was higher in the older groups than in the younger groups. Heart rate showed moderate increases with increased loading, and was higher in men.

Both sex and age appear to play a role in blood pressure response to dynamic work performed by small muscle masses. Sex-related effects may be due to different levels of catecholamine release in men and women. The increased diastolic pressure associated with increased age may be the result of arteriosclerotic changes which lead to increased peripheral resistance.

▶ The rise of blood pressure during isometric exercise has frequently been cited as an argument against prescribing this type of activity for older adults. The present article concerns heavy rhythmic exercise, at large fractions of maximum voluntary force. At first inspection the fact that the diastolic pressure rise during such exercise is greater in the older men seems to substantiate the hazard of any type of muscle building in the elderly, thythmic or isometric (although a larger age discrepancy in pressure increments would have helped to prove the point). On the other hand, if the sole content of an exercise prescription is a moderate endurance activity such as jogging, there is a danger that the arm muscles will actually become weaker, and then an emergency which calls for isometric arm work will be very liable to provoke a major rise of blood pressure, leading to a heart attack. The key to exercise prescription is the fact that the rise of blood pressure during vigorous muscle contraction is almost linearly related to the duration of effort. Thus, if the exercise is

MEAN VALUES AND STANDARD DEVIATIONS OF SYSTOLIC AND DIASTOLIC BLOOD PRESSURE AND HEART RATE MEASURED WITH LOADS BETWEEN 40% AND 80% MVC

Test groups	I Women, 20—29 years	II Men, 20—29 years	III Women, 30—39 years	IV Men, 30—39 years
Blood pressure (kPa)				
systolic	20.40 ± 1.87	23.86 ± 2.27	20.80 ± 2.67	24.00 ± 1.99
diastolic	13.30 ± 0.93	13.60 ± 1.47	14.00 ± 1.60	15.20 ± 1.47
Heart rate (beats · min^{-1})	106 ± 8.7	113 ± 11.9	102 ± 12.6	113 ± 13.0

(Courtesy of Kobryn, U., et al.: Eur. J. Appl. Physiol. 55:79–82, April 1986.)

rhythmic, or a vigorous isometric effort is only held for a few seconds per repetition, muscle training can be assured without placing an excessive load upon an aging myocardium.

The authors may be correct in suggesting that women react differently than men during muscular exercise. However, it is important to note that experiments were conducted at fixed percentages of the individual's experimentally determined maximum isometric force; thus, if the men made a better 100% effort, they would also be working harder at an estimated 40%, 60% and 80% of maximum. It is very difficult to be sure that levels of motivation were identical in the two groups.—R.J. Shephard, M.D., Ph.D

Abnormal Blood Pressure Response During Exercise

Radha J. Sarma and Miguel E. Sanmarco (Univ. of California, Los Angeles, and Univ. of Southern California)
Primary Cardiol. 12:23–34, September 1986   1–23

Exertional hypotension is an abnormal drop in blood pressure (BP) or a failure of BP to rise with exercise. A review of the literature (table) showed that exertional hypotension is suggestive of coronary artery disease (CAD) and ischemic left ventricular dysfunction. It is also a highly specific indicator of severe triple-vessel disease and left main coronary artery stenosis. The incidence of exertional hypotension was studied in 378 consecutive patients who were evaluated for CAD by a treadmill exercise test and coronary arteriography. The 321 men and 57 women were aged 30 to 72 years. All patients underwent exercise testing; blood pressure was recorded after each minute of the Bruce multistage exercise protocol.

Of the 378 patients, 90 (24%) had exertional hypotension. Of these 90, 40 had a repeated exercise test at an average of 12 months, including 23 who had been managed medically and 17 who had undergone bypass

---

ABNORMAL BLOOD PRESSURE RESPONSE DURING EXERCISE TESTING IN REPORTED SERIES

Author	Total Patients	Patients with Abnormal BP	Comments
Bruce et al	26	10	Direct recording of arterial pressure was made during exeriose
Thomson et al	—	17	15 patients had angiograms showing coronary artery disease (CAD)
Irving et al	10,700	6	6 patients had nonfatal ventricular fibrillation
McHenry	600+	5%	5% of all patients with multivessel CAD had a drop in BP
Morris et al	460	22	None of the 560 normal men and 107 women tested had an abnormal BP response
Levites et al	1,105	30	25 patients had angiograms; 13 had CAD
Li et al[12]	360	37	Retrospective study of 360 patients who had coronary artery bypass surgery
Sanmarco et al	378	90	240 patients had myocardial infarction; 63 of 90 patients with abnormal BP had triple-vessel or left main stenosis
Weiner et al	436	47	46 patients had CAD; 26 had triple-vessel or left main disease

(Courtesy of Sarma, R.J., and Sanmarco, M.E.: Primary Cardiol. 12:23–34, September 1986.)

grafting. There were no significant differences in exercise performance or resting hemodynamics between the medical and the surgical groups at first, but follow-up tests show that surgical patients improved their exercise duration and maximal heart rate, whereas the medically managed patients were essentially unchanged.

Continued medical management of patients with severe CAD does not improve exercise duration or exertional hypotension.

► While this was a preselected group with suspected coronary artery disease, the fact that more than 25% of these persons had exertional hypotension strongly emphasizes the point that when present this is a highly specific indicator of severe coronary artery disease. Revascularization of diseased coronary arteries can correct this abnormal blood pressure response in most. As an isolated observation during routine treadmill testing, it must not be ignored and mandates further intensive testing and probably therapy of a major order.—L.J. Krakauer, M.D.

Exercise During Therapeutic Beta-Blockade: A Two-Year Study in Hypertensive Patients
M. Frisk-Holmberg and G. Ström (Uppsala Univ., Stockholm)
Pharmacol. Ther. 40:395–399, October 1986   1–24

The issue of whether β-blockers impair physical performance is much debated. Previous studies have produced varying results, depending on the type of subjects investigated, the dose or route of administration used, and the size of the work load used in each study. Because of extensive clinical use of some β-blockers by young, active hypertensive patients, the issue is an important one that needs further clarification. The authors studied patients with mild to moderate essential hypertension under submaximal exercise testing after treatment with a placebo and after treatment with the β-blocker betaxolol.

The study was done in 12 otherwise healthy, sedentary, hypertensive patients, 11 men and 1 woman, ranging in age between 38 and 58 years, who were treated with betaxolol in doses of 20 to 40 mg per day after an initial 1- to 2-week run-in period with a placebo. The patients performed a submaximal exercise test at the end of the placebo period, after 3 months of drug treatment, and again after at least 24 months of drug treatment. No one participated in any exercise programs.

A reduction in resting heart rate by 24% to 15% and a reduction in systolic and diastolic blood pressures was observed after 3 months of treatment with betaxolol. This reduction was maintained 24 hours after the last dose had been taken at the 2-year follow-up visit. Blood pressure was reduced during exercise only in patients who had mild hypertension. However, the working capacity as measured by the exercise test did not decrease in any of the patients.

Treatment with β-blockers does not impair short-term physical performance in sedentary patients with mild to moderate hypertension.

▶ It has been argued that β-blocking drugs may impair physical performance. In this study of 12 patients extending for 2 years, this did not occur using a single drug, betaxolol, in therapeutic dosage.—L.J. Krakauer, M.D.

Blood Pressure and Catecholamines Following Exercise During Selective Beta-Blockade in Hypertension
R. Vandongen, B. Margetts, L.J. Beilin, N. deKlerk, and P. Rogers (Univ. of Western Australia and Royal Perth Hosp., Perth, Australia)
Eur. J. Clin. Pharmacol. 30:283–287, May 1986   1–25

Varied effects of β-blocking drugs on plasma epinephrine and norepinephrine have been reported. Some of the β-blockers currently available are cardioselective, while others are nonselective. If peripheral β-receptors are blocked, exercise-induced sympathetic stimulation may cause a pressor effect by stimulation of unopposed α-receptors. Despite this theoretical prediction, several studies have failed to show an advantage of cardioselective agents over nonselective drugs in this respect. Therefore, in the present study, the effects of equipotent doses of metoprolol and propranolol were compared during cardiovascular responses to exercise in 13 patients with essential hypertension. Plasma norepinephrine and epinephrine concentrations were measured as well. Propranolol, 80 or 160 mg, or metoprolol, 100 or 200 mg, was given twice daily for two weeks each while a third group of patients received placebo on the same dose schedule. Patients were then crossed over to the other treatments. Exercise was by bicycle ergometer.

Immediately following exercise, systolic blood pressure and heart rate increased to the same extent in both drug groups. Diastolic pressure in the metoprolol group did not change, as it did in the propranolol group. Thus, the change in systolic and diastolic blood pressure immediately and 20 minutes after exercise was consistently smaller during metoprolol treatment. The differences were particularly notable at 20 minutes after exercise. Both plasma norepinephrine and epinephrine increased after exercise and returned to baseline levels at 20 minutes. Although the levels of these compounds were higher during propranolol and metoprolol treatment, compared with placebo, there were no differences between the two drugs for these parameters.

This study shows that both plasma norepinephrine and epinephrine release are enhanced after exercise by β-blockers. Further, the effect does not seem to be related to cardioselectivity, since similar increases were seen for both propranolol and metoprolol. The mechanism for this increase may be related to a fall in cardiac output, altering blood flow to the liver and lungs, and decreasing norepinephrine and epinephrine elimination. The value of a selective β-blocker is seen by the blunted response to these catecholamine levels in the patients during metoprolol treatment as opposed to propranolol treatment. Other studies have shown conflicting results, but this may be due to methodologic differences.

The balance between dilator and constrictor activities is likely to be important in situations where sympathoadrenal activity is stimulated, such as during exercise. With cardioselective agents, β-2-adrenoceptors in the periphery are stimulated and oppose the vasoconstrictor effects of norepinephrine. This may be an important consideration when treating the active hypertensive patient.

▶ β-Blockade, selective and nonselective, has received extensive comment in the past (note the 1986 YEAR BOOK OF SPORTS MEDICINE pp. 28–38.) The argument for cardioselectivity probably relates to the action of epinephrine on peripheral vascular β-2-adrenoceptors opposing the vasoconstrictor effects of norepinephrine. Cardioselectivity is only relative, and at high dosages it is lost. Vidt of the Cleveland Clinic Foundation makes the point that β-blocker–induced interruption of glycogenolysis mandates that these drugs be used with caution in patients with diabetes mellitus (insulin dependent or receiving oral hypoglycemic drugs).—L.J. Krakauer, M.D.

β-Blockade Used in Precision Sports: Effect on Pistol Shooting Performance

Peter Kruse, Jørgen Ladefoged, Ulla Nielsen, Poul-Erik Paulev, and Jean Pierre Sørensen (Univ. of Copenhagen and Rigshospitalet, Copenhagen)
J. Appl. Physiol. 61(2):417–420, August 1986   1–26

Many artists and athletes use β-adrenergic receptor blockers (BB) in an attempt to improve performance. Nevertheless, such use is probably not based on facts about the effects of the drugs, and it appears to be largely the product of ignorance, credulity, and psychological pressure from the surroundings. Although the effect of BB on the central nervous system is controversial, BB are known to have anxiolytic effects and to be able to reduce different types of tremor. Moreover, BB reduces O_2 consumption and increases the arteriovenous O_2 content during exercise, as does training. A null hypothesis, that BB would not change the performance of pistol marksmen, was tested.

The study population consisted of 33 amateur marksmen who used a standard pistol at a distance of 25 m. There were 2 women and 31 men and the median age was 40 years (range, 20 to 60 years). In a double-blind cross-over study the effect of the adrenergic $β_1$-receptor blocker, metoprolol, was compared to placebo. Metoprolol improved pistol shooting performance when compared with placebo. Shooting improved by 13.4% of possible improvement as an average. The most skilled athletes showed the clearest metoprolol improvement. There was no correlation between the shooting improvement and changes in measured cardiovascular variables (i.e., changes of heart rate and systolic blood pressure) nor any correlation with the estimated maximum O_2 uptake.

The shooting improvement is an effect of metoprolol on hand tremor. Metoprolol was able to eliminate the emotional increase of heart rate and systolic blood pressure; it is likely, then, that these are $β_1$-receptor phenomena.

▶ Anyone who has watched competitive pistol shooting cannot but be impressed at the rise of tension as the final line of targets is presented, and whereas the first line can be hit dead center with casual abandon, the final target may be missed completely. There is thus tremendous pressure to find some agent that will conquer anxiety-induced tremor in the final moments of a competitive performance. Metoprolol can readily penetrate the blood/brain barrier. It is probable that it acts mainly by reducing central arousal, and thus activity in the gamma loop to the arm muscles. However, pistol shooters also try to slow their heart rate during competition, with a view to firing "between beats," and some effect of the β-blocker on heart rate could conceivably contribute to the increased accuracy of shooting.

Others reportedly using β-blocking drugs for similar reasons include archers, ski-jumpers, musicians, and ballet dancers (Beckett, A.H.: *Br. J. Hosp. Med.* 29:221–223, 1983; Burks, T.F.: *Fed. Proc.* 40:2680–2681; Percy, E.C.: *West. J. Med.* 133:478–484, 1980). It is thus important that doping controls counter the use of such potent medications for nontherapeutic purposes. Since contestants in archery and pistol shooting may include older coronary-prone and hypertensive competitors who have legitimate need of β-blockers, the rules of any contest in these sports will need very careful consideration.—R.J. Shephard, M.D., Ph.D.

Effects of β-Blockade on Exercise Capacity of Trained and Untrained Men: A Hemodynamic Comparison
Michael J. Joyner, Beau J. Freund, Sarah M. Jilka, Gregory A. Hetrick, Elkin Martinez, Gordon A. Ewy, and Jack H. Wilmore (Univ. of Arizona, Tucson)
J. Appl. Physiol. 60:1429–1434, April 1986   1–27

It is well established that exercise heart rate (HR) is reduced during β-adrenergic blockade (BAB). In untrained subjects, BAB-mediated reductions in HR have been shown to have little effect on maximal O_2 uptake ($\dot{V}O_{2max}$). It is thought that increases in stroke volume (SV) and arterial mixed venous O_2 difference compensate for the potentially negative effects of HR reduction on $\dot{V}O_{2max}$. These compensatory changes associated with BAB in untrained subjects are qualitatively similar to the increases in SV and arterial-mixed venous O_2 difference that result from prolonged intense endurance exercise training. It is possible that the large exercise SV values observed in endurance-trained subjects partially result from changes in cardiac loading conditions, i.e., increased preload and reduced after load. In addition, the increased SV observed during exercise after BAB in untrained subjects may also be due to changes in cardiac loading. The consequences of BAB on the cardiovascular systems of highly trained subjects were studied.

The authors investigated hemodynamic responses during BAB by collecting submaximal and maximal treadmill exercise data in 11 trained and 11 untrained male subjects. The study subjects completed two maximal control tests followed by a randomized, double-blind series of maximal tests after 1-week treatments with placebo, propranolol (160 mg per day,

Hemodynamic and Metabolic Responses to Exercise
at 60% $\dot{V}O_{2max}$

	PLAC	PROP	ATEN
$\dot{V}O_2$, ml·kg^{-1}·min^{-1}			
T	37.4±2.8	37.2±2.5	36.7±2.4
UT	25.8±3.2	25.5±2.5	25.3±2.5
$\dot{V}E$, l/min			
T	66.6±8.8	65.0±9.8	65.3±9.8
UT	44.1±8.0	44.2±8.6	43.3±7.7
$\dot{Q}$, l/min			
T	17.3±2.8	16.9±2.8	16.5±2.5*
UT	12.2±1.7	11.7±1.4*	11.5±1.3*
HR, beats/min			
T	134.8±8.8	107.0±6.7*	107.9±7.0*
UT	141.1±12.9	106.1±10.2*	105.0±8.3*
SV, ml/beat			
T	129.8±26.9	158.6±31.1*	156.2±32.4*
UT	86.8±12.1	110.0±11.3*	109.8±11.2*
SBP, mmHg			
T	186.8±17.8	153.6±15.9*	153.2±6.6*
UT	165.2±11.5	143.3±11.6*	135.6±9.2*†
DBP, mmHg			
T	70.0±15.6	72.2±10.3	67.4±7.2†
UT	69.6±7.2	67.4±5.9	66.5±5.4
MAP, mmHg			
T	108.9±8.1	99.3±7.2*	96.0±5.3*†
UT	100.5±7.6	92.7±6.8*	89.5±6.2*†
TPR, PRU			
T	6.42±0.99	6.02±0.99*	5.94±1.02*
UT	8.44±1.03	8.03±0.84*	7.92±0.56*

*Significantly different from PLAC (*P* < .05).
†ATEN significantly different from PROP (*P* < .05).
‡Values are means ± SD. For HR, change from PLAC elicited by ATEN significantly different between T and UT (*P* < .05). $\dot{V}O_{2max}$ = maximum O_2 uptake, PLAC = placebo, PROP = propanolol, ATEN = atenolol, $\dot{V}O_2$ = O_2 uptake, T = trained, UT = untrained, $\dot{V}E$ = minute ventilation, $\dot{Q}$ = cardiac output, HR = heart rate, SV = stroke volume, SBP = systolic blood pressure, DBP = diastolic blood pressure, MAP = mean arterial pressure, and TPR = total peripheral resistance.
(Courtesy of Joyner, M.J., et al.: J. Appl. Physiol. 60:1429–1434, April 1986.)

β_1 and β_2 blockade), and atenolol (100 mg per day, β_1 blockade). At submaximal exercise, none of the subjects experienced a reduction in O_2 uptake with either drug; however, submaximal heart rate fell in both trained and untrained subjects in response to both drugs. Cardiac output fell slightly in all subjects in response to both drugs, and stroke volume rose significantly in all subjects in response to both drugs (table). The maximum heart rate fell markedly in both trained and untrained subjects. In addition, maximum O_2 uptake fell in all subjects in response to both drugs, but the drop was greater in trained subjects when compared to untrained subjects during propranolol treatment.

Trained as well as untrained subjects experience large increases in exercise stroke volume during BAB, and these increases suggest that factors other than central hemodynamics may cause the somewhat larger reductions in maximum O_2 uptake in trained subjects during exercise with BAB.

▶ The present study confirms earlier reports that whereas β-blockade has little impact on the maximum oxygen intake of untrained subjects, it does induce an appreciable reduction of maximal performance in those who are already well trained (Hughson, R.L., et al.: *J. Cardiac Rehabil.* 4:27–30, 1984; MacFarlane, B.J., et al.: *Can. J. Physiol. Pharmacol.* 61:1010–1016, 1983; Tesch, P.A., and Kaiser, P.: *Acta Physiol. Scand.* 112:351–352, 1981).

It is interesting that effects (particularly depression of maximal heart rate) are greater with the non-specific blocker propranolol than with the specific β_1 antagonist atenolol. Possible explantations of this include an action against cardiac β_2 receptors normally stimulated by systemic catecholamines, problems in mobilization of metabolic fuels, and loss of normal bronchodilatation, the last response leading to a cessation of the maximum exercise test from breathlessness before a true limitation of cardiac performance is realized.—R.J. Shephard, M.D., Ph.D.

The Effect of Verapamil on Cardiovascular and Metabolic Responses to Exercise

H. Petri, B.G. Arends, and M.A. van Baak (Univ. of Limburg and Inst. for Sports Med. Limburg, Maastricht, The Netherlands)
Eur. J. Appl. Physiol. 55:499–502, September 1986   1–28

The calcium entry blocker verapamil has been shown to have antianginal and antiarrhythmic activity, and recently it has been used to treat hypertension. Beta-receptor blocking agents are also used for antihypertensive therapy, and these agents have been reported to have substantial hemodynamic and metabolic effects during exercise. Beta-blockers have been shown to reduce maximal and submaximal exercise tolerance in normotensive and in hypertensive subjects. Because many patients who are treated with beta blockers are young and physically active, it is of interest to ascertain whether other antihypertensive agents have a less negative effect

VARIABLES DURING MAXIMAL EXERCISE (MEAN ± SEM)				
	Placebo	Verapamil (mg·d^{-1})		
	0	3 × 40	3 × 80	3 × 120
Perceived Exertion (Borg scale)	19.3 ±0.3	19.4 ±0.3	19.6 ±0.2	19.0 ±0.2
Systolic BP (mm Hg)	177.6 ±7.5	176.8 ±8.2	190.6 ±7.2	182.0 ±8.6
Diastolic BP (mm Hg)	71.6 ±2.4	73.6 ±3.8	71.4 ±2.0	67.4 ±3.0
HR (beats·min^{-1})	183.3 ±3.5	178.9 ±4.9	174.8 ±3.1	170.7 ±3.8*
$\dot{V}_{O_2}$ (l·min^{-1})	3.43 ±0.13	3.42 ±0.13	3.45 ±0.14	3.41 ±0.14
$\dot{V}_{CO_2}$ (l·min^{-1})	3.77 ±0.16	3.81 ±0.18	3.78 ±0.16	3.77 ±0.17
$\dot{V}_E$ (l·min^{-1})	118.0 ±6.2	122.6 ±8.0	116.4 ±7.1	119.2 ±6.7
Lactate (mmol·l^{-1})	10.7 ±0.9	11.4 ±1.0	11.4 ±1.0	11.0 ±0.7
Glucose (mmol·l^{-1})	4.8 ±0.3	5.1 ±0.3	4.7 ±0.3	4.9 ±0.4
Glycerol (mmol·l^{-1})	0.145±0.025	0.141±0.029	0.160±0.037	0.121±0.020
FFA (mmol·l^{-1})	0.133±0.016	0.165±0.021	0.172±0.026	0.124±0.018

*$P < .001$.
(Courtesy of Petri, H., et al.: Eur. J. Appl. Physiol. 55:499–502, September 1986.)

on exercise tolerance. The goal of the present study was to determine the effects of verapamil on cardiovascular and metabolic responses to exercise in normotensive subjects.

The study population consisted of 12 subjects (aged 22 to 32 years) who were normotensive and had no history of cardiovascular disease. Each subject was treated with placebo and verapamil in three different dosages: 3×40, 3×80, and 3×120 mg per day in random order. The drugs were given for 2 days and on the third day, 2 hours after the final dose, a progressive exercise test until exhaustion was performed on a bicycle ergometer. There were no significant differences in maximal exercise capacity between the different groups of medication. Furthermore V_{O_2}, V_{CO_2}, and ve were shown to be unaffected by verapamil administration. However, heart rate during exercise was decreased in a dose-dependent manner: with the highest dose of verapamil, the maximal heart rate was reduced by 13 ± 1 beats per minute. There was no detectable effect of verapamil on parameters of carbohydrate and fat metabolism (table). Finally, perceived exertion, estimated by the Borg scale, did not differ between placebo and the three medication groups.

Despite a distinct reduction of heart rate, maximal exercise capacity remains unaffected after verapamil use.

▶ Calcium blockers have been getting a bad press lately, and some authors have suggested that because of their effects on myocardial contractility, physicians using such agents have increased the mortality of "postcoronary" patients by an unnecessary 20%!

Much probably depends on the age of the patient, and this report suggests that in those aged 22 to 32 years, the doses of calcium blocker commonly adopted in the treatment of hypertension have no adverse effects upon maximal working performance. Moreover, the adverse effects on tissue metabolism which might have been anticipated with β-blockers were not seen. The one disquieting feature was that blood pressure was not reduced, either during rest or exercise. The authors argue that verapamil will reduce blood pressure, but only in hypertensive patients (Leonetti, G., et al.: *J. Cardiovasc. Pharmacol.* 4:(suppl. 3) 319–324, 1982). However, this means that it is necessary to repeat the experiment described here and show that the working capacity and the peripheral metabolism of hypertensive patients is not adversely affected by use of verapamil in a dose that provides effective control of hypertension.—R.J. Shephard, M.D., Ph.D.

Enzymatic Adaptation to Physical Training Under β-Blockade in the Rat: Evidence of a β₂-Adrenergic Mechanism in Skeletal Muscle
Li L. Ji, Doris L.F. Lennon, Robert G. Kochan, Francis J. Nagle, and Henry A. Lardy (Univ. of Wisconsin at Madison)
J. Clin. Invest. 78:771–778, September 1986   1–29

Many well-established physiologic changes occur during prolonged exercise, including a high level of sympathoadrenergic activity. Because a high level of activation of the sympathoadrenergic system alone has been shown to induce the activities of oxidative enzymes, some physiologists have proposed that functional adrenoceptors are necessary for a metabolic adaptation of physical training. However, this hypothesis has been controversial. This discrepancy is of significant clinical importance because most cardiac patients who take β-blocking agents are also physically active. Although it is thought that during exercise training, cardiovascular functions are suppressed by the β-blocking drugs, whether or not the whole-body adaptational changes observed after training occur at the level of peripheral tissues has not been clearly resolved. The goal of the present study was to determine whether a functional β-adrenergic system is required in the training-induced enzyme adaptation in skeletal muscle, and to investigate the influence of chronic physical exercise and β-adrenergic blockade on the activities of hepatic gluconeogenic enzymes and other related enzymes.

The study was carried out using 30 male Sprague-Dawley rats aged 2 months, body weight 250 to 275 gm. Both nonselective (propranolol, which has β_1 and β_2 blocking effects) and β_1-selective (atenolol) adrenergic antagonists were tested for their effects on enzymatic adaptation to exercise training as follows: trained + placebo (TC); trained + propranolol (TP); trained + atenolol (TA); and corresponding sedentary groups, SC and SP. The trained rats ran 1 hour per day at 26.8 m per minute, 15% grade, 5

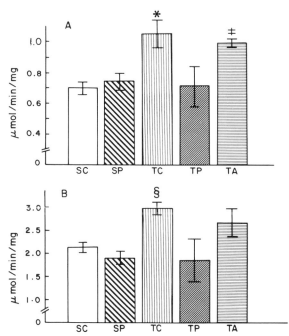

Fig 1–5.—**A,** skeletal muscle citrate synthase and **B,** cytochrome *c* oxidase specific activities (μmole/min/mg mitochondrial protein) in the SC, SP, TC, TP, and TA rats. *Bars* show standard error. *$P < .01$ (TC vs. SC); ‡$P < .05$ (TA vs. SC); §$P < .05$ (TC vs. SC). (Courtesy of Ji, L.L., et al.: J. Clin. Invest. 78:771–778, September 1986. Reproduced from the Journal of Clinical Investigation, Copyright permission of The American Society for Clinical Investigation.)

days per week, for 10 weeks. Both of the β-antagonists were administered at doses that decreased exercise heart rates by 25%. It was found that training increased skeletal muscle citrate synthase, cytochrome c oxidase (Fig 1–5), carnitine palmitoyltransferase, β-hydroxyacyl coenzyme A dehydrogenase, mitochondrial malate dehydrogenase, and alanine aminotransferase significantly in the TC groups, but not in the TP group. These enzyme activities, excluding cytochrome c oxidase and carnitine palmitoyltransferase, were also markedly increased in the TA group. Hepatic phosphoenolpyruvate carboxykinase activity did not change with training or with β blockade. Furthermore, fructose 1,6-bisphosphatase activity was observed to be lower in TC than in SC, but unchanged in TP or TA. Hepatic mitochondrial malate dehydrogenase and alanine aminotransferase activities were enhanced with training only in TC.

β$_2$-Adrenergic mechanisms play an essential role in the training-induced enzymatic adaptation in skeletal muscle. The data suggest that hepatic enzymes which function solely in gluconeogenesis do not adapt to chronic physical training by increasing total activities, as is the case with skeletal muscle mitochondrial enzymes. However, chronic training did increase the activities of hepatic enzymes indirectly involved in gluconeogenesis, and β-blockade inhibited the training adaptation of these enzymes, suggesting that the liver does play a central role in the interorgan cooperation under metabolic stress.

▶ At one time there was much controversy as to whether a patient treated by β-blocking drugs could increase maximum oxygen intake through participation in an endurance training program. It is now generally agreed that this is the case, despite the fact that the training bouts induce a relatively low heart rate in such individuals.

However, in terms of adaptation to long-term exercise, an increase in the activity of aerobic enzymes and a resultant ability to oxidize an increased proportion of fat is also an important aspect of adaptation. It is interesting that the activity of the aerobic enzymes can be increased by any powerful sympathoadrenergic stimulus, incuding exposure to intense heat or cold (Harri, M.N.E.: Acta Physiol. Scand. 95:391–399, 1975). Moreover, the response to all of these forms of stimulation, including endurance training, is inhibited by the use of nonspecific β-blocking drugs. On the other hand, the response is relatively unimpaired when using a selective β$_1$ blocker such as atenolol. While the mechanism is still debated, it is probable that lipid flux depends on the activity in an adrenergic cyclic-AMP dependent pathway, and if the lipid flux is not boosted during exercise, there may be less incentive for the body to increase the activity of its aerobic enzymes. These data seem an important argument for the use of specific rather than non-specific β-blocking preparations.—R.J. Shephard, M.D., Ph.D.

Effect of Chronic β-Adrenergic Blockade on Exercise-Induced Leukocytosis
L. Röcker and I.-W. Franz (Univ. of Berlin)
Klin. Wochenschr. 64:270–273, March 17, 1986   1–30

Physical exercise can enhance the total number of leukocytes in the peripheral blood. Because exercise-induced leukocytosis can be almost completely prevented by the acute intravenous injection of propranolol, leukocytosis has been thought to be mediated by a β-adrenergic receptor mechanism. Research was conducted to determine whether chronic β-receptor blockade can prevent exercise-induced leukocytosis; whether there are differences between blockade of specific β_1-receptors and both β_1/β_2-receptors; and whether short-term exercise leads to lymphocytosis and long-term exercise leads to granulocytosis.

The study population consisted of 11 males (mean age, 37 years) who had stage 1–2 essential hypertension according to the criteria of the World Health Organization. Blood samples for determinating leukocytes were drawn before and during the 6th and the 30th minutes of submaximal exercise, and 5 and 15 minutes after work. Lymphocytosis and granulocytosis were dependent upon the intensity and duration of exercise.

Leukocytosis during short-term and long-term exercise was the result of both a lymphocytosis and a granulocytosis. Under resting conditions, the chronic β-receptor blockade caused a significant decrease of neutrophil granulocytes. Nevertheless, both patients and controls exhibited the same percent increase in leukocytes compared with the untreated control study. Therefore, the adrenergic system does not play the primary role in exercise-induced leukocytosis.

▶ It has been known since the early 1930s that vigorous exercise will induce a leukocytosis (Edwards, H.T., and Wood, W.B.:*Arbeitsphysiologie* 6:73–83, 1933; Andersen, K.: *J. Appl. Physiol.* 7:671–674, 1955), although it has been less clear whether this should be attributed to hormonal mechanisms, or whether it should be regarded merely as a byproduct of hemoconcentration, increased blood flow, and a decrease in plasma pH. Certainly, injections of epinephrine can induce a leukocytosis, and the exercise response can be blocked by acute administration of propranolol (Ahlborg, B., and Ahlborg, G.: *Acta Med. Scand.* 187:241–246, 1970).

While the present investigation did not show suppression of the exercise repsonse with chronic β-blockade, it is worth stressing that after administration of propranolol, the subjects were starting from a substantially lower baseline white cell count. There does appear to be a chronic harmful effect of propranolol upon granulopoiesis, and regular white cell counts are advisable where chronic treatment with propranolol is envisaged.—R.J. Shephard, M.D., Ph.D.

Thermogenesis in Human Skeletal Muscle as Measured by Direct Microcalorimetry and Muscle Contractile Performance During β-Adrenoceptor Blockade
Birger Fagher, Hans Liedholm, Marip Monti, and Ulrich Moritz (Univ. Hosp., Lund, Sweden)
Clin. Sci. 70:435–443, May 1986   1–31

Several studies have suggested that β-receptors mediate a thermogenic effect. For example, it has been shown that temperature regulation in resting subjects exposed to cold conditions could be suppressed by the nonselective β blocker oxprenolol. Others have shown that the thermogenic response to insulin and glucose infusion decreased after intravenously administered propranolol, whereas the basal metabolic rate after an overnight fast was not altered. Finally, in the postprandial state, propranolol has been observed to reduce thermogenesis, measured as the inhibitory effect on the increase in metabolic rate that normally occurs after food intake. The goal of the present study was to evaluate thermogenesis of human skeletal muscle with a microcalorimeter to determine whether medication with various β-adrenergic blockers could have an inhibiting influence.

The study population consisted of ten healthy males who were given propranolol (nonselective), atenolol (β_1-selective) and pindolol (nonselective with partial β_2-agonist activity) randomly for 8 days each in a crossover double-blind test. After 7 days on each agent, muscle function was evaluated by an isokinetic dynamometer. Thermogenesis in biopsy samples taken from vastus lateralis after low-grade exercise was investigated after 8 days on each drug by direct calorimetry with a perfusion microcalorimeter. Prior to drug administration, a median heat production rate of 0.67 mW per gram of muscle was measured. This value was markedly reduced by 25% during propranolol administration, but exhibited no significant change during atenolol or pindolol administration. The peak torque decline during isokinetic endurance test changed markedly in knee flexor but not in extensor muscles, from 15–27% after propranolol and from 15–23% after pindolol. Conversely, the maximum dynamic strength was not changed.

Blockade of sympathetic β_2-receptors decreases thermogenesis in human skeletal muscle and impairs isokinetic endurance.

▶ This article reports some more negative effects of nonspecific β-blocking drugs such as propranolol. The enhanced responsiveness of the body to norepinephrine plays an important part in the normal adaptation to cold, and if this form of heat production is checked by nonselective β-blockade, the individual concerned will be at an increased risk of hypothermia.

Adverse effects on muscle performance are also gaining increasing recognition. The selective deterioration of isokinetic endurance in the knee flexors but not the knee extensors can probably be explained on the basis that there are more type II (glycolytic) fibers in the flexor muscles about the knee joint (Garrett, W.E., et al.: *Am. J. Sports Med.* 12:98–103, 1984). It is probable that β_2 receptors play an important role in the breakdown of glycogen and thus the provision of fuel for the type II fibers (Juhlin-Dannfeldt, A.: *Acta Med. Scand. Suppl.* 672, 49–54, 1983).—R.J. Shephard, M.D., Ph.D.

Alpha-2-Adrenoreceptor Density on Intact Platelets and Adrenaline-Induced Platelet Aggregation in Endurance- and Nonendurance-Trained Subjects

M. Lehmann, K. Hasler, E. Bergdolt, and J. Keul (Univ. of Freiburg, Germany)
Int. J. Sports Med. 7:172–176, June 1986   1–32

It is generally accepted that there is an endurance training-related control of sympathetic drive, and that β-adrenoreceptor density on intact blood cells or myocardial cells of healthy subjects and cardiac patients is negatively regulated to circulating free catecholamines. These results suggest an increased endurance training-related sensitivity to β-adrenergic agonists and a decreased sensitivity in cardiac patients dependent upon left-ventricular function. However, it is not known whether α-adrenoceptors exhibit a similar endurance training-associated increase in sensitivity. The goal of the present study was to investigate the behavior of α-2-adrenoceptors on intact platelets and the adrenaline-induced platelet aggregation in vitro in endurance and nonendurance-trained subjects.

The study population consisted of 17 sportsmen (mean age, 25 ± 6 years), 8 of whom were endurance-trained athletes. Receptor density was assayed by measuring ^{3}H-Yohimbine binding to intact platelets, and adrenaline-induced aggregation of platelets in vitro was also determined. It was found that maximal binding and dissociation constant (K_D) for adrenaline were significantly decreased in platelets isolated from the endurance-trained athletes (148 fmol/10^9 platelets; $K_D = 0.92$ nmol) than in the 9 nonendurance-trained individuals (284 fmol; $K_D = 1.79$ nmol)

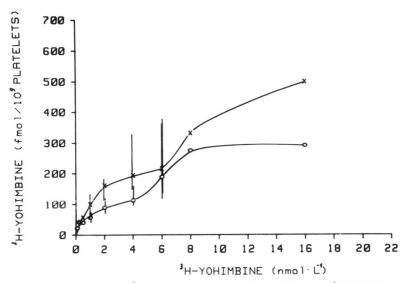

Fig 1–6.—Specific binding of ^{3}H-Yohimbine to intact platelets as a function of ^{3}H-Yohimbine concentration in eight endurance-trained subjects and in nine nonendurance-trained individuals (x). Data point to high affinity binding sites related to low radioligand concentrations up to 4 nmole/L or up to 6 nmole/L, respectively, and additionally to not yet well-defined low affinity binding sites at high ligand concentrations of more than 8 nmole/L. Specific binding was significantly lower in endurance-trained than in nonendurance-trained subjects at low radioligand concentrations of 1, 2, and 4 nmole/L ($P < .05$). Each point represents median value (and 50% range of confidence) of eight duplicate determinations or nine determinations, respectively. (Courtesy of Lehmann, M., et al.: Int. J. Sports. Med. 7:172–176, June 1986.)

(Fig 1–6). These values translated into 89 receptors per cell in the endurance-trained subjects and 171 receptors per cell in the nonendurance-trained subjects. There was no significant change of receptor density or affinity subsequent to exhaustive exercise in the group of eight endurance-trained individuals. It was found that the maximal binding values and oxygen uptake capacity correlated negatively, but that the maximal binding values and induced platelet aggregation in vitro correlated positively.

There may be a reduced sensitivity of platelets in endurance-trained subjects. At present, it is not known whether these results represent only one in vitro phenomenon or point to a biologic and clinical significance of a changed endurance training-related platelet sensitivity.

▶ The α-receptors are in general associated with excitatory responses to both norepinephrine and epinephrine, including both a general vasoconstriction and a stimulation of mechanisms of platelet aggregation; in the latter connection, there is plainly an interaction with the clotting and lytic actions of the prostaglandins.

The authors demonstrate by the somewhat fallible method of a cross-sectional comparison that the α-receptor density on the platelets is lower in those who are athletes, and the liability that norepinephrine will induce clotting is lessened. This observation could have some relevance to the benefits of exercise in the coronary-prone patient.

Some investigators have drawn a parallel between the binding sites measured on the platelets and responses elsewhere in the body. Thus, O.-E. Brodde et al. (*Therapiewoche* 34:6372, 1984) pointed to a positive correlation between platelet-binding sites and the mean arterial pressure of hypertensives. This could explain why exercise is helpful to the patient with hypertension. However, Lehmann et al. quite properly caution that the evidence regarding the generalization of platelet binding site data is as yet relatively weak.—R.J. Shephard, M.D., Ph.D.

Plasma Catecholamines at Rest and Exercise in Subjects With High- and Low-Trait Anxiety
Francois Peronnet, Pierre Blier, Guy Brisson, Pierre Diamond, Marielle Ledoux, and Michel Volle (Univ. of Montreal and Univ. of Quebec)
Psychosom. Med. 48:52–58, January–February 1986   1–33

Earlier studies showed that changes in plasma catecholamine concentrations after short-duration dynamic exercise are directly related to the size of the workload. Although this is thought to reflect increased activity of the sympathoadrenal system in response to the homeostatic challenge of exercise, part of that increased activity might also be the result of exercise- or test-related psychologic stress. If so, plasma catecholamine concentrations would vary in subjects with different psychologic characteristics. The authors tested this hypothesis in 6 subjects with high trait anxiety (TA) and 6 with low TA, selected from among 149 male college students on the basis of psychologic tests. Plasma norepinephrine (NE) and epinephrine (E) concentrations were measured during supine rest and during light and moderate exercise of 5 minutes' duration on a cycle ergometer.

Plasma E concentrations at rest and during light and moderate exercise did not differ significantly between subjects with low and high TA. However, though plasma NE concentrations did not differ significantly at rest and during light exercise between both groups, high-TA subjects had significantly higher plasma NE values than low-TA subjects in response to moderate exercise.

Plasma E and NE concentrations at rest and in response to light exercise are similar in low- and high-TA subjects, but subjects with high TA have a greater plasma NE response to the psychologic stress or homeostatic challenge, or both, of moderate exercise.

► Earlier Canadian research demonstrated that catecholamine secretion was greater during a game of hockey than during the development of an equivalent power output on a cycle ergometer, particularly if the comparison of the two types of activity was made in those involved in the higher levels of hockey competition (Blimkie, C.J., et al., in Lavallée, H., and Shephard, R.J. (eds.): *Frontiers of Activity and Child Health,* Québec City: Editions du Pélican, 1977, pp. 313–321). It is thus not surprising that subjects with a high trait anxiety show a greater response to laboratory exercise than do those with a low trait anxiety. It would be interesting to repeat this comparison when the exercise was associated with a stressful or exciting game; presumably, this would exacerbate the anxiety-related differences demonstrated by Peronnet and associates.—R.J. Shephard, M.D., Ph.D.

Altered Cardiovascular Responsiveness to Adrenaline in Endurance-Trained Subjects
J. Svedenhag, A. Martinsson, B. Ekblom, and P. Hjemdahl (Karolinska Inst., Stockholm)
Acta Physiol. Scand. 126:539–550, April 1986   1–34

It is well established that exercise of moderate to high intensity activates sympatho-adrenal mechanisms, as shown by increased levels of non-adrenaline and adrenaline in plasma. Furthermore, it is known that the exercise-induced changes in heart rate and contractility, as well as blood flow distribution and substrate and hormone levels are influenced by adrenergic receptor stimulation. However, it is not clear as to whether repeated activation of the sympatho-adrenal system by regular exercise training alters the responsiveness of different tissues to catecholamines. The effect of training on the cardiovascular sensitivity to adrenaline in men was examined further.

The authors measured responses of heart rate, systolic and diastolic blood pressures, and systolic time intervals and related these to plasma adrenaline concentrations attained during infusions of adrenaline in 10 well-trained runners (mean age, 35 years; $\dot{V}O_{2max}$, 61.9 ml/kg per minute) and in age-matched sedentary controls (mean age, 36 years; $\dot{V}O_{2max}$ 37.5 ml/kg per minute). In addition, the untrained subjects were reexamined

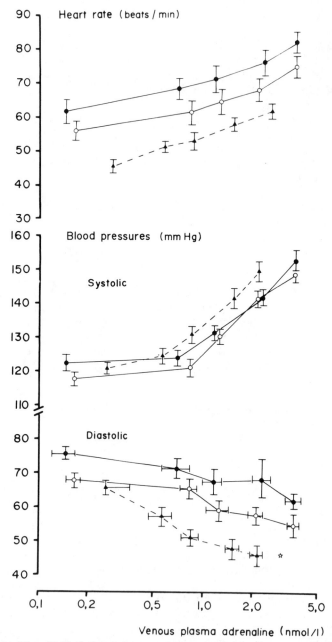

Fig 1–7.—Effect of infused adrenaline (venous plasma concentrations) on (**A**) the heart rate and (**B**) the systolic and diastolic blood pressures in the different training conditions. *Black dots with solid line* and *white dots with solid line* denote the untrained subjects before and after training, respectively. *Black triangles with broken line* represents the well-trained runners. *denotes a significant (*P* < .05) difference between the untrained and well-trained subjects. Values are means ± SE. (Courtesy of Svedenhag, J., et al.: Acta Physiol. Scand. 126:539–550, April 1986.)

after 4 months of endurance training which increased their $V_{O_{2max}}$ by 18%. Resting heart rate and diastolic blood pressure were signifiantly lower in the trained state (Fig 1–7). Furthermore, the venous plasma adrenaline concentrations attained during infusions were lower in the well-trained than in the untrained subjects. However, the adrenaline-induced increases in heart rate (see Fig 1–7) and in plasma cyclic AMP and decreases in preejection period (PEP) and PEP/LVET ratio were not dependent on the training state. The adrenaline-induced decrease in diastolic blood pressure was more marked in the well-trained than in the untrained group and tended to be enhanced by training in the later group. The increases in systolic blood pressure were greater in well-trained subjects, but training did not alter this response in the untrained subjects. The plasma noradrenaline response to maximal cycle ergometer exercise ($\dot{V}_{O_{2max}}$ test) was substantially greater in the well-trained than in the untrained subjects, although no difference was observed for adrenaline. The submaximal exercise systolic blood pressure was similar in all training conditions when it was related to the absolute rate of work.

Both vasodilator and systolic pressor responses to adrenaline are enhanced in endurance-trained subjects. However, the cardiac chronotropic and inotropic effects of adrenaline seem to be independent of the training state.

▶ In recent years, it has been increasingly recognized that there is not a single, fixed response to catecholamines, but that responses are substantially modified by periodic changes in receptor density and sensitivity to catecholamines.

The literature to date has presented somewhat conflicting findings. The present report shows that trained subjects produce more norepinephrine, and it might be thought that this would induce a "down-regulation" of the catecholamine receptors, lessening the response to a fixed dose of catecholamine. However, in practice, the heart rate response to epinephrine was unchanged, while the increase of systolic pressure and the decrease of diastolic pressure were actually greater in the trained subjects. Possibly, training induced an increased sensitivity of β_2 receptors in the vessels supplying skeletal muscle. Such a change could explain the greater circulatory clearance of epinephrine in trained subjects. However, any change of β_2 sensitivity was selective, since the receptors involved in the c-AMP response were unaffected. The increase of systolic pressure may arise from altered venous return or changes in geometry of the heart induced by training.—R.J. Shephard, M.D., Ph.D.

Plasma Renin Activity, Aldosterone and Catecholamine Levels When Swimming and Running
C.Y. Guezennec, G. Defer, G. Cazorla, C. Sabathier, and F. Lhoste (Research Ctr. for Aerospace Medicine, Paris, and Hosp. Henri Mondor Créteil, Créteil, France)
Eur. J. Appl. Physiol. 54:632–637, February 1986   1–35

Maximal exercise leads to increased plasma catecholamines (CA), plasma renin activity (PRA), and cortisol and plasma aldosterone (PAC) levels. It has been suggested that acute elevation of plasma catecholamines induces renin release from the kidney. This study investigates PRA, PAC,

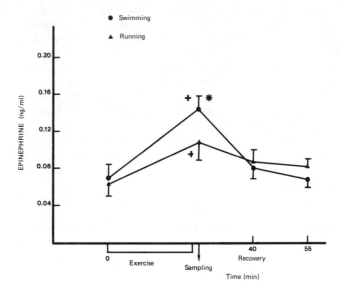

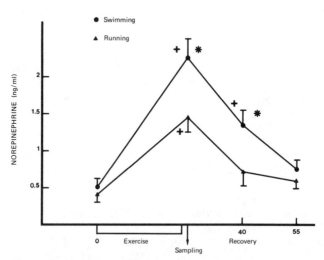

Fig 1–8.—Plasma catecholamine changes during maximal exercise tests when swimming and running and during recovery: [+] indicates that results differ significantly ($P < .05$) from rest values; [*] indicates that results differ significantly ($P < .05$) between swimming and running. (Courtesy of Guezennec, C.Y., et al.: Eur. J. Appl. Physiol. 54:632–637, February 1986.)

and CA responses to two different maximal exercises that differ in posture, environment and distribution of blood volume.

Seven men, aged 19 to 25 years, performed treadmill running and swimming tests that increased in severity every 5 minutes. Blood samples were taken before, during and after the exercises, exhaled air was collected, and heart rate was monitored continuously during the exercises.

Oxygen consumption, heart rate, and blood lactate were similar during both exercises. Levels of PRA, PAC, and CA rose in both groups, but PRA was significantly higher during running compared with swimming. The level of plasma CA was higher after the swimming test (Fig 1–8); the PAC level was not significantly different between exercise groups.

These data indicate that the PRA response during swimming was decreased by the volume shift induced by the water pressure and the supine position. The association of a decreased PRA with an increased CA in response to swimming negates a strict dependence of renin release on catecholamine levels. These results suggest that neural pathways play a major role in renin release during exercise.

▶ It is well known that a fluid shift toward the upper half of the body increases the stroke volume and cardiac output in swimming relative to other types of exercise such as running (Gauer, O.H., and Henry, J.P., in Guyton, A.C. and Cowley, A.W. (eds): *Cardiovascular Physiology II,* University Park, Md., vol. 9, pp. 145–190). The present article notes further that the humoral responses differ markedly between the two types of exercise. From the viewpoint of the practicing physician who is recommending exercise to a "coronary-prone" middle-aged adult, it is worth remarking that the blood level of norepinephrine immediately after exercise was almost twice as great in the swimming experiments as in running. The temperature of the pool (26 C) was not cold enough to stimulate catecholamine production. However, the authors admit that the subjects continued maximal exercise for longer while swimming, and it also remains to be checked whether the subjects perceived a progressive pool test with expired gas collection as more stressful than a progressive treadmill test.—R.J. Shephard, M.D., Ph.D.

Respiratory Physiology

Exercise-Induced Asthma
Jan I. Schulz and Allan E. Olha (McGill Univ. and St. Mary's Hosp., Montreal)
Physiother. Can. 38:208–213, July–August 1986   1–36

After strenuous exercise, patients with bronchial asthma often experience episodes of exercise-induced asthma (EIA), characterized by wheezing, coughing, and shortness of breath.

The mechanism that causes EIA has not yet been clearly defined. However, it is known that continuous exercise such as running, cross-country skiing, and cycling, when performed in cool and dry weather, provokes more severe attacks of EIA than intermittent exercise such as hockey or football. Bronchoconstriction is even more severe in persons with allergic

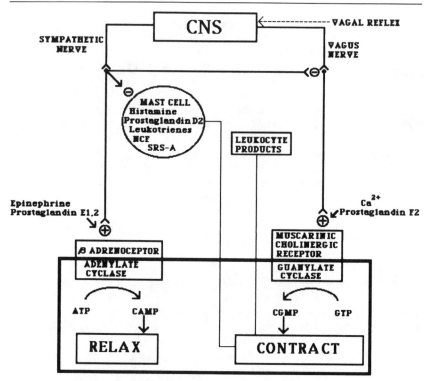

BRONCHIAL SMOOTH MUSCLE

Fig 1–9.—Factors modulating bronchial smooth muscle tone. *ATP*, adenosine triphosphate; *CAMP*, cyclic adenosine monophosphate; *GTP*, guanosine triphosphate; *CGMP*, cyclic guanosine monophosphate; *NCF*, neutrophil chemotactic factor; and *SRSA*, slow-releasing substance of anaphylaxis. (Courtesy of Schulz, J.I., and Olha, A.E.: Physiother. Can. 38:208–213, July–August 1986.)

asthma. Bronchial smooth muscle contractions are controlled by parasympathetic and sympathetic nerves, which regulate a complex enzyme system in the bronchial smooth muscles (Fig 1–9). The sequence of events leading to bronchoconstriction in response to exercise is presented in Figure 1–10.

Treatment of EIA includes the prophylactic use of drugs such as salbutamol, terbutaline, and fenoterol. Physical training has also been investigated as another treatment for EIA, but a 1982 study of endurance training in asthmatics showed that such training failed to improve the degree of EIA, despite observed improved maximal oxygen uptake.

Physiotherapists will play an increasingly important role in advising asthmatic patients on available treatments and possible precautions for prevention or attenuation of EIA.

▶ This is a common problem. It has been estimated that 90% of patients with asthma have bronchoconstriction with exercise and 40% of those with allergic

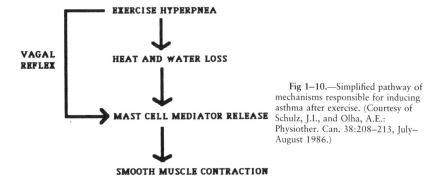

VAGAL
REFLEX

EXERCISE HYPERPNEA

↓

HEAT AND WATER LOSS

↓

MAST CELL MEDIATOR RELEASE

↓

SMOOTH MUSCLE CONTRACTION

Fig 1–10.—Simplified pathway of mechanisms responsible for inducing asthma after exercise. (Courtesy of Schulz, J.I., and Olha, A.E.: Physiother. Can. 38:208–213, July–August 1986.)

rhinitis likewise. The authors offer both pharmacologic and nonpharmacologic options for this condition. In fact most patients end up using preventive and acute drug measures to handle the severity of symptoms. If drugs are used, there is a general consensus that metered doses of the inhaled beta agonists such as metaproterenol, albuterol, or fenoterol (which is still investigational) are the most effective and with minimal side effects. Cromolyn, taken in prophylactic fashion five to 15 minutes before exercise, is often equally effective and with minimal side effects.

There is a standardized exercise protocol for younger people with six to 8 minutes of treadmill exercise at 75% to 85% of predicted maximum heart rate with pulmonary function testing performed before and at intervals after exercise. This is not without risk in the older patient as Owens has pointed out. This also lacks the sensitivity of the inhalation challenge with methacholine or with cold air. (Owens, G.R.: *Consultant,* vol. 27, No. 3, p. 25). The article of recent date is the most comprehensive updated summary I have seen.—L.J. Krakauer, M.D.

Prevention With and Without the Use of Medications for Exercise-Induced Asthma
Roger M. Katz (Univ. of California Los Angeles and Allergy Research Found., Los Angeles)
Med. Sci. Sports Exerc. 18:331–333, June 1986   1–37

Nearly 12% of the population suffer from exercise-induced asthma or bronchospasm. The author presents a review of the prevention of exercise-induced asthma, with or without the use of medication.

Exercise-induced asthma can be prevented with proper techniques of exercise and environmental exposure. Exercise-induced asthma classically occurs after a maximum work load extending 5 minutes or longer. Hence, exercising to less than full tolerance for less than 5-minute intervals or utilizing warm-up sessions timed within 1 hour of the event can prevent exercise-induced asthma. In some individuals, exercising in a warm, humidified environment is less asthmogenic than exercising in dry, cold air.

Many persons have learned to breathe through the nose, an organ that humidifies and warms the air, while others have learned to breathe deeply and slowly to counter the effects of bronchospasm associated with rapid breathing.

Bronchodilators, such as β_2-agonists and theophylline, are effective in preventing exercise-induced asthma. Beta$_2$-agonists appear to be the drugs of choice, while theophylline appears to be effective only in high, potentially toxic concentrations. Cromolyn sodium, which inhibits both immediate and late phase bronchospastic reactivity, is effective in the atopic or sulfite-exposed individual; its effectivity is maximal within 2 hours of therapy and often is dose related. For many patients, a combination of physiologic changes and medication may be needed to prevent further episodes of exercise-induced asthma.

▶ This is another view of a controversial subject that emphasizes that the non-pharmacologic approach can be important and, if not effective alone, can at least modulate the amount of medication needed. There will also be a difference in the age group that is being treated. Theophylline still has its proponents, but it would appear that the toxicity of this agent is much higher than that of some of the alternative aerosol preparations at this time.—L.J. Krakauer, M.D.

The U.S. Olympic Committee Experience With Exercise-Induced Bronchospasm, 1984

Robert O. Voy (U.S. Olympic Committee, Colorado Springs)
Med. Sci. Sports Exerc. 18:328–330, June 1986   1–38

Exercise-induced bronchospasm (EIB) is a handicap to an athlete's performance. The U.S. Olympic Committee has met the challenge of recognizing and dealing with this common yet unappreciated medical condition aggravated by athletic exertion. Prior to the 1984 Los Angeles Olympic games, the U.S. Olympic Committee devised a screening sequence to identify members of its Olympic team suffering from asthma or EIB. A self-administered questionnaire was developed to obtain information about the presence of EIB, the history of other allergic or untoward reactions related to exercise, and any medications used. The athletes underwent simple pulmonary evaluations as well, generally by Wright flow meter spirometry.

Of the 597 Olympic athletes, 67 (11.2%) had asthma or EIB. Coordination of medical care was achieved through members of the American Academy of Allergy and Immunology, the U.S. Olympic Committee Chief Medical Officer, the athlete's personal physician, and the athlete. Most athletes were controlled with cromolyn sodium, theophyllines, β_2-sympathomimetics, antihistamines, beclomethasone, atropine aerosol, and corticosteroids; these drugs were permitted by the International Olympic Committee (IOC) Medical Commission. Athletes with inadequate control were counseled to take cromolyn sodium daily or before exercise. Beta$_2$-

agonists such as albuterol or terbutaline were recommended for athletes unresponsive to cromolyn and those taking IOC-banned medications. Forty-one medals were won by this group of handicapped athletes.

Exercise-induced bronchospasm is a handicap that can be reversed. It need not be a deterrent to an individual's athletic performance.

▶ The official Olympic Committee position at the 1984 Los Angeles Olympic games. The flexibility in the use of medication for these handicapped individuals is commendable. The number of medals won by handicapped athletes using medication is cited above. The individualization of medication for given sports in future Olympic competition or the equivalent will be an ongoing problem and challenge, especially as it will interrelate with other drugs of more controversial nature.—L.J. Krakauer, M.D.

Plasma Gastrointestinal Regulatory Peptides in Exercise-Induced Asthma
D. Hvidsten, T.G. Jenssen, R. Bolle, and P.G. Burhol (Univ. Hosp. of Tromsø, Norway)
Eur. J. Respir. Dis. 68:326–331, May 1986   1–39

Earlier studies have shown that several gastrointestinal regulatory peptides play a regulatory role in the lung and influence airway activity. The authors studied the role of gastrointestinal regulatory peptides in patients with exercise-induced asthma (EIA) after they performed a short exercise bronchoprovocation test.

Fifteen subjects were divided into two study groups, based on the results of peak expiratory flow tests (PEF). Group A included seven known asthmatics who had a reduction in PEF of 12% or more; group B included three known asthmatics with no significant reduction in PEF and five control subjects. All participants performed a 6-minute exercise test on a bicycle ergometer. Blood samples were taken immediately before and 1, 2, 3, 5, 7, 9, 15, 30, and 60 minutes after the test. Plasma concentrations were determined by radioimmunoassay for vasoactive intestinal polypeptide (VIP), cholecystokinin (CCK), somatostatin, secretin, pancreatic polypeptide (PP), motilin, and insulin.

At 5 minutes the mean PEF showed maximum falls of 30% in the EIA group and 3% in the control group. Plasma VIP concentration rose significantly at 5 minutes and plasma CCK concentration at 0 and 20 minutes in the EIA group compared with values in the control group. The changes observed in somatostatin, secretin, PP, motilin, and insulin plasma concentrations after exercise did not differ significantly between the groups.

Plasma VIP concentrations followed inversely the variation in lung function as assessed by PEF in EIA patients and thus may play an ameliorating role in bronchial asthma. However, the relation of CCK to the lung is speculative and should be studied further.

▶ It is possible that VIP is derived from the lung in this instance. The rise of CCK may be failure of inactivation in the lung noting that this is also true of the hormone gastrin. The possibility that the rise in VIP ameliorates the symptoms of asthma and the bronchoconstriction involved at the physiologic level remains hypothetical at this point. It is a relatively new and fascinating observation. It is increasingly apparent that the lung is a rich neuroendocrine organ.—L.J. Krakauer, M.D.

Effects of Ozone Exposure on Four Consecutive Days on Work Performance and $\dot{V}_{O2max}$
William J. Foxcroft and William C. Adams (Univ. of California, Davis)
J. Appl. Physiol. 61:960–966, September 1986   1–40

Exposure to ozone in the laboratory produces lung dysfunction and symptoms of respiratory discomfort. Ozone adaptation in humans after several days of exposure suggests the possibility of improved exercise performance. The effects of 4 days of exposure for 1 hour at 0.35 ppm ozone

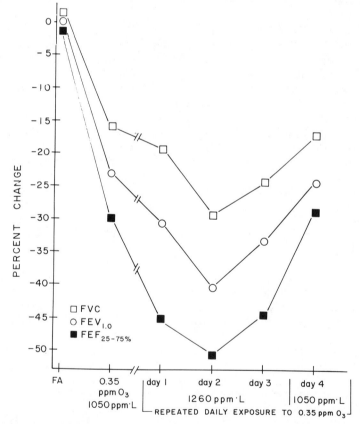

Fig 1–11.—Percent change in pulmonary function on initial exposure and as a result of 4 consecutive days exposure to 0.35 ppm O_3. (Courtesy of Foxcroft, W.J., and Adams, W.C.,: J. Appl. Physiol. 61:960–966, September 1986.)

on work performance and maximal oxygen uptake were examined in eight males who had actively participated in aerobic training for at least 6 months. Subjects were exposed to filtered air or ozone while exercising on a bicycle for 50 minutes at a work load eliciting minute ventilation of about 60 L per minute.

Acute ozone exposure led to a rise in respiratory frequency and a nearly reciprocal reduction in tidal volume. Decrements in pulmonary function were similar after all ozone exposures (Fig 1–11). Initial exposure led to significant reductions in peak oxygen uptake, maximal heart rate, and performance time, but improvement was seen in several parameters after repeated exposures. Subjective responses reflected this improvement with successive exposures to ozone during exercise.

Exercise performance and subjective symptoms both improved during successive ozone exposures in these normal subjects, but adaptation of pulmonary functional impairment was not noted. Increased exercise performance may reflect less subjective respiratory discomfort. The findings do not suggest that continued exposure to ozone is without adverse long-term effects.

▶ Earlier work from our laboratory (Folinsbee, L., et al.: *J. Appl. Physiol.* 38:996–1001, 1975) demonstrated respiratory disturbances and an impairment of maximum oxygen transport immediately following acute exposure of moderately exercising subjects to the levels of ozone encountered in large cities. However, concern over this observation was tempered to some extent by reports suggesting that repeated exposure to ozone led to a lessening of responses (Hackney, J.D., et al.: *Arch. Environ. Health* 32:110–116, 1977).

The present report shows the initial increase of breathing frequency and decrease of peak oxygen transport described previously in acute ozone exposure. While repeated exposure lessens the impact on oxygen transport, in contrast with earlier studies respiratory function remains impaired. The authors offer two possible explanations—first, their subjects may have been more sensitive to ozone, and second, the inhaled dose was larger. The latter seems the main explanation. In many of the earlier experiments, subjects performed intermittent rather than continuous exercise, and even during the exercise bouts ventilation was 20 to 25 L per minute, rather than 60 L per minute as in the present study. The modest exercise used in earlier work was appropriate for examining reactions of the general population, but a ventilation averaging 60 L per minute seems the minimum exposure that an endurance athlete will encounter. Continuing impairment of respiratory function may thus be anticipated if an athlete visits a smog-ridden city for a period of several days.—R.J. Shephard, M.D., Ph.D.

Air Ionization: Influence on Cardiorespiratory Variables and Attention Span
Peter Vogelaere, S. Bekaert, N. Depester, H. Malcorps, and F. De Meyer (Vrije Univ., Brussels)
Medisport 60:214–218, 1986   1–41

Since the early 1930s, many reports have appeared in the literature which claim that positive or negative ionization in the environment affects a wide variety of biologic and psychologic functions. Some studies claim that negative ionization has a positive influence on an individual's behavior and attention span. Other reports have stated the very opposite. Some authors have reported that changes in atmospheric ionization were found to affect blood pressure, aggravate angina, decrease or increase work capacity, and precipitate an asthma attack. However, none of these studies was done under properly controlled conditions. The authors studied the influence of positive, neutral, and negative ionization on cardiac variables during ergometric exercise and on attention span during psychologic testing.

The study was done with six normal, healthy, male volunteers, ranging in age from 18 to 20 years, each of whom took three identical tests to measure their attention span in a room with negative, neutral, and positive atmospheric ionization. Prior to taking each test, the subjects were acclimatized for 8 days during 1 hour each day to the ionic atmosphere to be tested. Each subject was also tested in the same room on an ergometric bicycle to assess how oxygen consumption and other cardiac variables were affected by changes in ionization.

Results show that high concentrations of negative, positive, or neutral ions in the air did not in any way affect a subject's attention span or his work capacity on an exercise bicycle.

▶ Many people hate working in the controlled atmospheres of modern highrise office buildings, and a variety of vague symptoms have been attributed to noxious changes in the inhaled air, including alterations in the ion content. Some buildings use electrostatic precipitators, in an attempt to scrub the air free of particles, an approach that is likely to increase the content of positive ions. Others have blamed symptoms upon an accumulation of negative ions.

Adverse reactions to certain winds, such as the Fohn in Switzerland and the Sharav in Israel have also been blamed upon alterations in atmospheric charge.

The present report tested positive and negative concentrations of 9.10^4 ions per milliliter. While there was no change of attention or heart rate during cycle ergometry, there was a suggestion that negative ions increased the oxygen cost of light ergometer work, a conclusion supported by J. Metadier (*L'ionisation de l'air et son utilisation*, Maloine Ed., Paris, 1981), but opposed by several other investigators; the response described by Vogelaere and associates would have been more convincing if it had extended to higher power outputs (which it did not).

Further work seems necessary before we can conclude either that highrises have an adverse effect on health, or that the situation would be helped by a change in the ionic balance of the inspired air.—R.J. Shephard, M.D., Ph.D.

Metabolism

Skeletal Muscle Damage: A Study of Isotope Uptake, Enzyme Efflux and Pain After Stepping

D.J. Newham, D.A. Jones, S.E.J. Tolfree, and R.H.T. Edwards (Univ. College, London, and Univ. of Liverpool)
Eur. J. Appl. Physiol. 55:106–112, April 1986   1–42

Previous studies showed that eccentric stretching exercise such as walking downhill can result in delayed postexercise pain and cause muscle cell injury, connective tissue damage, or both. Recent studies have shown that eccentric contractions can lead to a large loss of muscle creatine kinase (CK) into the circulation. Maximum enzyme release occurs about 3 to 6 days after exercise, and the magnitude of the release does not seem to be related to the extent of the ultrastructural damage. The authors studied the effects of stepping exercise on muscle groups in the legs and the occurrence of pain, release of CK, and uptake of ^{99m}Tc-pyrophosphate (Tc-PYP)in five normal subjects, aged 23 to 40 years, who were normally active, but not involved in regular physical training programs. In the stepping exercise one leg was used to step up, the other to step down a high bench.

Pain only developed in muscles used for stepping down, including the quadriceps, adductors, and gluteal muscles of one leg and the calf muscles of the other. In four subjects a large rise in plasma CK concentration was observed, and they showed increased radionuclide uptake in the thigh adductors that were used for stepping down. However, no increase in Tc-PYP muscle uptake was seen in the quadriceps. Muscle pain preceded, but was not well correlated with, the magnitude of CK release or the amount and distribution of increased muscle radionuclide uptake.

Delayed-onset muscle pain is a poor indicator of muscle damage. However, Tc-PYP skeletal muscle uptake can provide useful information about the site and time course of muscle damage.

▶ There is no simple relationship between pain, tenderness, enzyme elevation, and structural muscle damage. The authors suggest that if enzyme release and muscle fiber degeneration are inevitably linked, then this may involve macrophages which have been seen infiltrating damaged muscle in animals. Further morphological study is necessary to answer this question. Note also that this is a study of eccentric stretching exercise alone.—L.J. Krakauer, M.D.

The Pathophysiology of McArdle's Disease: Clues to Regulation in Exercise and Fatigue
Steven F. Lewis and Ronald G. Haller (Univ. of Texas and VA Med. Ctr., Dallas)
J. Appl. Physiol. 61:391–401, August 1986   1–43

McArdle's disease is a rare disorder, characterized by a deficiency of skeletal muscle phosphorylase. Symptoms may include exercise-induced muscle pain, cramping, and premature fatigue. Although clinical evidence strongly implicates an imbalance between muscle energy supply and demand, the exact metabolic mechanisms involved in this abnormal fatigability are unknown. McArdle's disease is considered to be a disorder of glycogenolysis, but its associated abnormality of oxidative metabolism has been mostly overlooked. The authors present evidence to support a hypothesis of oxidative metabolic impairment in McArdle's disease patients with the help of a model of physiologic regulation during exercise based on the pathophysiologic changes of such patients.

Muscle glycogen is normally the primary oxidative fuel for exercise workloads that require more than 75% to 80% of maximal oxygen uptake. The authors' evidence supports the hypothesis that a limited flux through the Embden-Myerhof pathway in McArdle's disease reduces the capacity to generate reduced nicotinamide adenine dinucleotide (NADH), which is needed to support a normal maximal oxygen uptake. It is thought that the extent of this oxidative defect is substrate dependent, and that it can be partially corrected by increasing the availability to working muscles of other oxidative substrates such as glucose and free fatty acids.

Experimental data suggest that the premature muscle fatigue and cramping in patients with McArdle's disease may be due to a pronounced decline in muscle phosphorylation potential. These abnormalities are apparently not the result of adenine triphosphate (ATP) depletion, but rather of an increased accumulation of inorganic phosphate, and probably of adenosine diphosphate (ADP), in skeletal muscle. It is known that accumulations of inorganic phosphate and ADP in skeletal muscle inhibit myofibrillar enzymatic reactions.

► In this metabolic muscle disease studied in over 100 papers to date, the authors present data that assess the basis of the oxidative impairment in this condition and the physiologic consequences for the regulatory mechanisms during exercise and fatigue. This is an alternative approach to exercise tolerance studies in normal skeletal muscle and can be of great value when used in that regard.—L.J. Krakauer, M.D.

Physiological Changes in Hemostasis Associated With Acute Exercise
M. Elyse Wheeler, Gerald L. Davis, W. Jay Gillespie, and Murray M. Bern (New England Deaconess Hosp., Boston)
J. Appl. Physiol. 60:986–990, February 1986   1–44

The effect of acute exercise on the hemostatic system is an increase in blood coagulability and fibrinolytic activity (FA). Exercise also alters oxygen uptake and blood lactate levels; however, the underlying mechanisms and the magnitude and direction of these changes are not known. The authors investigate the relationship of changes in metabolic variables with changes in blood coagulability and fibrinolytic activity in response to acute exercise. Nineteen healthy males were exercised to maximal exertion on a branching multistage treadmill protocol, following overnight fasting. Heart rate, ECG, heart rhythm, oxygen uptake, carbon dioxide production, ventilation rate and respiratory exchange rate were monitored. Blood was drawn before, immediately after, and 8 minutes after exercise. Samples were analyzed for serum cholesterol, triglyceride, glucose, high-density lipoprotein (HDL), fibrinolytic activity (FA), factor VIII coagulant activity, lactate and 2,3-diphosphoglycerate levels.

All hemostatic variables increased with exercise, with a significant correlation of factor VIII coagulant activity with lactate levels 8 minutes after exercise. Preexercise HDL levels increased the correlation between FA and blood lactate values. Peak fibrinolytic activity coincided with maximum heart rate, which occurred 8 minutes postexercise.

There is a positive correlation between exercise-enhanced blood FA and blood lactate levels with basal HDL concentrations. Although the mechanism behind these exercise-induced changes is unknown, their measurement may permit the identification of individuals with impaired fibrinolytic systems. Since such impairment is implicated in atherosclerosis, these measurements may help predict who is at risk for thrombotic episodes or atherogenesis.

▶ The present report shows the anticipated biphasic change in blood clotting associated with vigorous exercise. Although there is a substantial increase of Factor VIII coagulant activity, this is offset by a fourfold increase of fibrinolytic activity in the period immediately following exercise. The authors draw attention to previous reports that one factor in ischemic heart disease could be an imbalance between these two responses (Cash, J.D.: *Br. Med. J.* 2:502, 1966; Shaper, A.G., et al.: *Br. Med. J.* 3:571–573, 1975), and point out that such an imbalance is not revealed by resting data on blood clotting. They note that measurements of blood lactate concentration are correlated with exercise-induced fibrinolysis, and may thus provide a simple index of such activity.

It is difficult to see why there should be a direct correlation between these two variables, but it may be that exercise above the anaerobic threshold is needed to induce fibrinolysis.—R.J. Shephard, M.D., Ph.D.

Effect of Long-Term Anemia and Retransfusion on Central Circulation During Exercise
F. Celsing, J. Nyström, P. Pihlstedt, B. Werner, and B. Ekblom (Karolinska Inst., Stockholm)
J. Appl. Physiol. 61:1358–1362, October 1986   1–45

Hemoglobin concentration is recognized as one of the most important determinants of maximal aerobic power and thus of performance in many types of physical activities. The effects of acute and short-term anemia on the circulatory response to physical exercise are fairly well known and some specific aspects of longterm anemia have been studied. However, the effects of an artificially induced long-term anemia with subsequent retransfusion of erythrocytes and the adaptive response to exercise has not been established. It is also of interest to determine the interrelationship between heart rate and stroke volume as mediators of a compensatory increased cardiac output during submaximal exercise as well as the circulatory response to shortterm maximal exercise. The goal of the present study was to evaluate the effect of artificially induced long-term anemia and acute retransfusion on the central circulation during submaximal and maximal exercise.

The study population consisted of eight healthy male subjects in whom anemia was induced by repeated venesections. The stored blood was then retransfused after 9 weeks (range, 8 to 11 weeks). Exercise tests were carried out before venesection in the control state (C), in the anemic state (A) and 46 hours after retransfusion (R). It was found that hemoglobin concentrations levels were 146 ± 10 g/L in C, 110 ± 7 g/L in A, and 145 ± 9 g/L in R. The maximal O_2 uptake was found to be 4.55 ± 0.6 L per minute in C, 3.74 ± 0.7 L per minute in A, and 4.45 ± 0.6 L per minute in R. The authors detected a decrease in heart rate of seven beats per minute and in cardiac output of 2 L per minute at maximal exercise in the anemic state compared with control values. Surprisingly, these values were not reversed, but instead were further accentuated after retransfusion. The adaptive response to submaximal exercise (cycling at 150 to 175 W) in anemia was mediated to the amount of 50% by an increase in cardiac output and 50% was attributed to increased O_2 extraction in the peripheral tissue.

It is concluded that longterm anemia decreased heart rate and cardiac output at maximal exercise. In addition, the present data confirmed the close correlation between hemoglobin concentration and maximal O_2 uptake in humans.

▶ The effects of hemoglobin level upon human performance have been studied not only from the viewpoint of "blood doping," but (perhaps more importantly in a broad social context) in tropical environments where the populations have become grossly anemic through parasitic infections. In some countries, poor productivity is due not to the laziness of the local people, but rather to a decrease of physical working capacity induced by anemia, and in such situations correction of the anemia has allowed substantial gains of both maximum oxygen intake and working capacity (Davies, C.T.M.: *Acta Paediatr. Belg.* 28[suppl.]253–256, 1974).

The main effect of anemia upon oxygen transport is due to a reduction of the maximum arterio-venous oxygen difference; it is possible to compensate for the lesser oxygen carrying capacity of the blood during submaximum effort through an increase of heart rate and stroke volume, but such an adaptation is no longer possible once maximum heart rate and stroke volume have been attained. The five- to ten-beat decrease in maximum heart rate during anemia and the immediate retransfusion period is a little puzzling. The authors suggest a parallel to the decrease of maximum heart rate which occurs at high altitudes; there certainly is a substantial decrease of arterial oxygen content during anemia, but the post-retransfusion content is immediately restored to 192 ml/L. One might wonder about more long-term changes in tissue iron stores, but there were apparently no changes in the activity of iron-dependent enzymes (Celsing, F., et al.: *Med. Sci. Sports Exerc.* 18:156–161, 1986). Nor does there seem to have been any difference in the quality of maximal effort due to general "tiredness" in the anemic state; peak lactate levels, gas exchange ratios, and ventilatory equivalents were closely similar in the three experimental conditions. Further study of this question is needed.—R.J. Shephard, M.D., Ph.D.

The Anemias of Athletes
Edward R. Eichner (Univ. of Oklahoma)
Physician Sportsmed. 14:122–130, September 1986   1–46

Diagnosing anemia in athletes may be complicated since athletes normally have lower hemoglobin and serum ferritin concentrations than do nonathletes. The author discusses the hematologic adaptations to exercise and anemias in athletes.

Exercisers, particularly endurance athletes, normally have lower hemoglobin concentrations than do sedentary subjects as a result of the normal body adaptation to exercise to increase plasma volume. This dilutional pseudoanemia is not a true anemia, but it is a beneficial adaptation that enhances athletic performance. Red blood cell mass is also increased in elite athletes—a beneficial balance of increased red blood cell mass with decreased blood viscosity that improves performance by enhancing delivery of oxygen to the exercising muscles. Dilutional pseudoanemia in athletes requires no treatment.

True anemia can develop in athletes. According to Wintrobe, true anemia exists in athletes if the hemoglobin level is under 13 gm/100 ml in a man or 11 gm/100 ml in a woman. Iron deficiency is the most common cause of true anemia in athletes. The earliest symptoms include decreased athletic performance and ice-craving or other forms of pica. Performance in athletes with marginal iron stores but no anemia is probably not impaired, but even very mild iron deficiency anemia can impair maximal performance. Footstrike hemolysis can cause true anemia in athletes. Such hemolysis is recognized by the triad of mild macrocytosis, mild reticulocytosis, and subnormal plasma haptoglobin concentration. Footstrike hemolysis can limit the expansion of red blood cell mass that enables the athlete to reach peak performance, as well as drain the body iron and contribute to iron deficiency anemia. True anemia can be treated with iron supplements and diet modification to increase absorbable iron; foot hemolysis can be minimized by paying attention to body weight, gait, shoes, and terrain. Only by exclusion should iron deficiency anemia be ascribed to athleticism.

▶ Eichner suggests that athletes often have a slightly lower hemoglobin concentration, and commonly a lower serum ferritin concentration than the nonathlete group. He considers this a dilutional pseudoanemia that enhances performance and does not of itself require treatment. The problem is further compounded by footstrike hemolysis in the runner, but this is a fairly minor contribution to a true iron deficiency state or true anemic state. Footstrike anemia is a true anemia and is characterized by a macrocytosis in contrast to the microcytosis of iron deficiency. Gait, shoes, terrain, and body weight are all contributory factors to footstrike anemia and amenable to some correction. Iron deficiency anemia can be treated directly with iron, but this is not considered a panacea or ubiquitous therapy for athletic performers as a whole nor even the female half, unless confirmation iron deficiency is obtained. The complexity of the problem is further addressed in the following article of which Eichner is a coauthor.—L.J. Krakauer, M.D.

Endurance Swimming, Intravascular Hemolysis, Anemia, and Iron Depletion: New Perspective on Athlete's Anemia

George B. Selby and Edward R. Eichner (Univ. of Oklahoma and Oklahoma City VA Hosp.)

Am. J. Med. 81:791–794, November 1986   1–47

Endurance athletes such as marathon runners may develop an anemia in which the red blood cell mass is normal or increased, but the plasma volume is even more increased, causing a dilutional fall in hemoglobin concentration. Some intravascular hemolysis ascribed to the footstrike has also been shown to occur in runners. Since intravascular hemolysis has not been reported in nonimpact sports, the authors investigated whether swimming is associated with similar patterns of anemia.

Nine collegiate scholarship swimmers, aged 18 to 22 years, and 23 competitive Masters swimmers, aged 24 to 40 years, were evaluated before and after 1.5-km, 10-km, and 1-hour continuous swims. Blood samples were drawn 5 minutes before and 5 minutes after completion of the swims. In all samples, ferritin, haptoglobin, and hemoglobin concentrations were measured.

About 10% of the swimmers were found to have low hemoglobin concentrations. There was a steady decline in hemoglobin values in the collegiate swimmers, which rebounded about 2 weeks after the end of competition. A significant difference in hemoglobin concentrations was found between those swimming less and those swimming more than 10,000 yd per week. Intravascular hemolysis occurred during all the races, with the fastest swimmers in the longest races showing the greatest decreases in haptoglobin concentrations. Although 25% of the swimmers had low baseline haptoglobin concentrations, and 11% of the men and 57% of the women had iron depletion, their athletic performance was not notably impaired.

Since iron depletion, anemia, and intravascular hemolysis are present in athletes who participate in nonimpact sports, mechanisms other than footstrike must be responsible for athlete's hemolysis.

▶ The significance of anemia in competitive swimmers remains an enigma. Intravascular hemolysis may be a factor and seems to correlate with skill and speed as measured by the greatest decreases in haptoglobin. Some iron depletion is present in roughly half of the women and 11% of the men, but athletic performance is not impaired by this. In the authors' own words, "Swimmers share with runners an "anemia" that is probably mainly dilutional, but the mild effort-related intravascular hemolysis of swimmers must result from something other than footstrike. Mechanisms and implications of the anemia, hemolysis, and low ferritin levels of swimmers and runners remain intriguingly unknown."

It is encouraging to know that iron deficiency per se can be treated and that the intravascular hemolysis that occurs in both running and swimming is a self-limiting phenomenon.—L.J. Krakauer, M.D.

Osteoporosis and Physical Activity
Everett L. Smith and Diane M. Raab (Univ. of Wisconsin, Madison)
Acta Med. Scand. [Suppl.] 711:149–156, 1986   1–48

Bone involution is a common and increasing problem for older adults, especially women. Bone mass is affected by local and systemic homeostatic control mechanisms. Local forces acting on bone are due to gravity and muscular contraction. Systemic controls include parathyroid hormone, calcitonin, vitamin D, growth hormone, and gonadal hormones. The hormonal controls of bone act to maintain plasma calcium homeostasis.

Several theories exist concerning local bone mechanisms. When bent, bone functions as a piezoelectric crystal with calcium accumulation on the negatively charged concave surface. When a microscopic damage occurs due to bone stress, osteoclastic action is stimulated to remove the damaged structure. Osteoblastic activity deposits matrix and mineral along the osteoclast's path, when rate of damage is low. With a high rate of damage, osteoblastic activity lags, which can result in reduced bone mass and more susceptibility to fractures.

Studies on astronauts and immobilized subjects showed bone atrophy, despite adequate dietary calcium intake. The degree of bone loss is related to the difference in stress levels ordinarily applied and those at bed rest in the site studied. Greater bone mass has been demonstrated in athletes compared to the sedentary population. Also, the greatest hypertrophy was found in the areas most stressed. Studies on active adult women have shown increases in bone mass compared to inactive controls. With physical activity intervention programs, bone mass is increased, or the rate of bone loss reduced in middle-aged and older women.

From the literature reviewed, it is concluded that bone hypertrophies with adequate stimulus. While the interaction between local and hormonal action is not fully clear, the authors hypothesize that this increase is due to both local and systemic responses to activity.

Physical Activity and Bone Mineral Content in Women Aged 30 to 85 Years
Rachel J. Stillman, Timothy G. Lohman, Mary H. Slaughter, and Benjamin H. Massey (Univ. of Illinois, Urbana)
Med. Sci. Sports Exerc. 18:576–580, October 1986   1–49

The relationship of bone mineral content and levels of physical activity was studied in 83 white premenopausal and postmenopausal women, aged 30 to 85 years, to see if those more physically active have a significantly higher bone mineral content than do their less active counterparts. Physical activity questionnaires were independently evaluated by five physical education professionals. Subjects were assigned to low (N = 19), moderate (N = 36), and high (N = 28) activity groups. Anthropometric measurements were taken and percent fat estimated. Bone mineral content was measured by photon absorptiometry at a site one third the distance from the distal radius to the olecranon process.

Results showed that no woman over 60 years of age was in the high activity group. The high activity women were basically younger (mean, 42.2 years) than the moderate (mean, 52.9 years) and low activity (mean, 51.5 years) groups. While sitting and standing heights and weights and skeletal widths were not significantly different, the mean for all three groups showed slightly more height and less weight for those engaging in greater physical activity. Anthropometric measurements showed that the most active women were leaner than those who were less active. A lower level of fat percentage was seen in the most active group. No difference was observed between the two other groups.

A significant difference ($P < .05$) was observed in bone mineral content and in bone mineral content divided by bone width between the most active group and the two other groups, even with age and menstrual status as covariates. No difference was found between the moderate and low activity groups.

Thus results show that physical activity can be valuable in inhibiting bone loss, with significantly higher bone mineral content seen in women who maintain an active lifestyle especially during their premenopausal years. An alternative explanation is that changes do occur in bone with moderate activity and would be detected if more sensitive methods were used or if sites other than the radius were chosen for measurement.

▶ There is no question that exercise is a critical cofactor in the prevention of osteoporosis, and the earlier in one's life it becomes a habitual part of the lifestyle, the better. The role of hormonal adjuvants in the post-menopausal female may be even more critical. The importance of calcium supplementation is a third factor that remains unchanged in the equation. Smith (Abstract 1–48) has pointed out in discussion that the forces acting on the bone ideally should be transmitted to the bone. Weightlifting exercises and impact loading activities such as hitting a tennis ball or kicking a soccer ball appear to be very effective. Newer techniques have shown an increase in bone stress in one region will mobilize calcium from another less active region. This is an ongoing dynamic that is of importance to the immobilized patient and to the astronaut alike.—L.J. Krakauer, M.D.

Physical Fitness is a Major Determinant of Femoral Neck and Lumbar Spine Bone Mineral Density
Nicholas A. Pocock, John A. Eisman, Michael G. Yeates, Phillip N. Sambrook, and Stefan Eberl (Gorvan Inst. of Med. Research and St. Vincent's Hosp., Sydney, Australia)
J. Clin. Invest. 78:618–621, September 1986   1–50

Osteoporosis is a major health problem which affects up to half of the elderly female population in western countries. Although the postmenopausal state is thought to be a major factor, decreased physical activity has also been suggested to be related to the development of osteoporosis. It is well known that athletes have higher bone density than do age-matched sedentary controls, with the most dramatic effects seen in individuals participating in sports that place a large stress on the skeleton. On the basis of these studies in athletes, it has been hypothesized that physical activity is an important determinant of bone mass in the general population. However, evidence to support this claim has not been provided. The goal of the present study was to investigate the relationship between physical fitness, various life-style factors, and bone mass.

The study population consisted of 84 white women with no previous history of bone disease; age rage was 20 to 75 years, and 46 women were postmenopausal. Bone mineral density was determined in the femoral neck and lumbar vertebrae by absorptiometry, and bone mineral content was determined in the distal forearm using the same method. Fitness was assessed from predicted maximal oxygen uptake. It was found that femoral neck and lumbar bone mineral density was significantly correlated with fitness as well as with age and weight (Fig 1–12). In the 46 postmenopausal subjects, fitness was observed to be the only significant predictor of femoral neck bone mineral density, while both weight and fitness predicted the lumbar bone mineral density.

These data represent the first demonstration of a correlation between physical fitness and, by implication, habitual physical activity, and bone mass in the femoral neck. The data also support the previously reported correlation between lumbar bone mass and physical activity. It is suggested that increased physical fitness may increase bone mass at the sites of clinically important fractures in osteoporosis.

▶ Previous studies of exercise and osteoporosis have tended to look either at whole body calcium levels or local bone density measurements in the arms and the ankle regions. The present contribution is useful in that it examines the impact of activity (as assessed rather indirectly from the predicted maximal

Relationship between femoral neck bone density and fitness

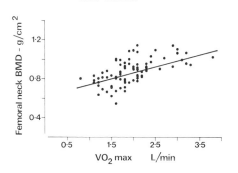

Fig 1–12.—Plot of femoral neck bone mineral density (BMD) against physical fitness ($\dot{V}O_2$ max) in 82 normal women. Equation for regression: femoral neck BMD = .61 + .13 ($\dot{V}O_2$ max). (Courtesy of Pocock, N.A., et al.: J. Clin. Invest. 78:618–621, September 1986. Reproduced from The Journal of Clinical Investigation, Copyright permission of The American Society for Clinical Investigation.)

oxygen intake) upon common sites of fracture in old age (especially the neck of the femur).

While moderate, weight-bearing activity undoubtedly has a positive effect in correcting osteoporosis, it is worth noting that in young female athletes who exercise to the point of inducing amenorrhea, there is a danger that the disturbance of menstrual function may lead to decalcification of the skeleton.—R.J. Shephard, M.D., Ph.D.

The Temporal Response of Bone to Unloading
Ruth K. Globus, Daniel D. Bikle, and Emily Morey-Holton (NASA-Ames Research Ctr., Moffett Field, Calif., Univ. of California and VA Med. Ctr., San Francisco)
Endocrinology 118:733–742, February 1986   1–51

Prolonged absence of skeletal loading results in osteopenia in both adult and growing animals. In adults, osteopenia results from inhibition of bone formation and stimulation of bone resorption. The authors investigated the effect of skeletal unloading on bone formation in growing rats.

Male rats were elevated by clipping the tail to a pulley so that their hindlimbs were not weightbearing. These experiments lasted from 2 days to 4 weeks during which the animals behaved normally. Following the period of hindlimb elevation, the animals were guillotined, and bones were removed for analysis of bone weight, uptake of ingested radioactive calcium and proline, and histomorphometry based on tetracycline labeling.

Bone growth in hindlimbs and lumbar vertebrae ceased 1 week after initiation of elevation. Bone formation was inhibited by day 5 and returned to normal by day 12 (Fig 1–13). Tetracycline-labeling of bone showed the same growth pattern. Cancellous bone incorporated more radioisotopes and had a greater absolute response to elevation than did cortical bone.

Weightlessness due to elevation results in an initial inhibition of bone formation in the unloaded limbs, followed by a cessation in the accretion of bone weight. Despite continued unloading, bone weight increases at the normal rate by 14 days. The authors suggest that this model may be useful for studying the hormonal and mechanical factors regulating bone formation during space flight, immobilization of limbs, or bed rest.

▶ A number of authors have drawn attention to the need for weight-bearing forms of exercise if osteoporosis is to be avoided in older adults. The present study was unfortunately in rats of unspecified age, rather than in humans. The main point of interest is that whereas unloading of the hind limbs initially led to an inhibition of bone formation, after 14 days in the experimental situation, a normal rate of increase in bone weight was resumed.

It is difficult to compare a 2-week period of weightlessness in a rat to the human time-scale, but nevertheless one might infer that the bone loss initially seen in groups such as astronauts and those confined to bed would be reversed with continuation of the exposure. There are two immediate limitations to this intriguing hypothesis—first, the present research was apparently with

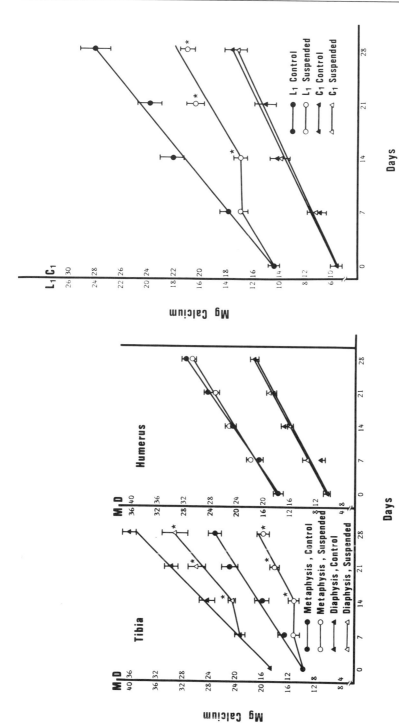

Fig 1–13.—Temporal effects of unloading on calcium content of bone during 4 weeks of hindlimb elevation. Bones were hydrolyzed and analyzed for calcium content. Data presented as mean ± SE. *, significant decrease in bone weight compared with control value; M, metaphyseal region; D, diaphyseal region. (Courtesy of Globus, R., et al.: Endocrinology 118:733–742, February 1986. Copyright 1986 by the Endocrine Society.)

growing rats, and second, even in the rats matrix formation was restored more completely than mineralization as the exposure to weightlessness continued.—R.J. Shephard, M.D., Ph.D.

Liberation of Muscle Carbonic Anhydrase Into Serum During Extensive Exercise

H.K. Väänänen, M. Leppilampi, J. Vuori, and T.E.S. Takala (Univ. of Oulu, and Deaconess Inst., Oulu, Finland)
J. Appl. Physiol. 61:561–564, August 1986   1–52

Carbonic anhydrase (CA) is known to catalyze the reaction between CO_2 and water to form carbonic acid. There are three isozymes of CA in mammalian tissue, but the recently discovered sulfonamide-resistant isozyme III of CA has only been found in type I (slow twitch or red) skeletal muscle fibers. Because CA III is a water-soluble enzyme located in the sarcoplasma, serum measurements could be utilized to monitor damage

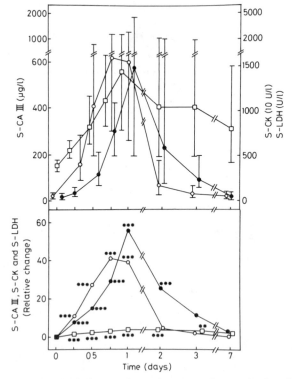

Fig 1–14.—Serum enzyme levels during 24 hours of running, and 2, 3, and 7 days after beginning of run: *open circles*, serum carbonic anhydrase III (S-CA III); *filled circles*, serum creatine kinase (S-CK); *open squares*, serum lactate dehydrogenase (S-LDH); n = 8. *Top*, geometric means of enzyme values ± SD *(vertical bars)*; bottom: relative change of geometric means of enzyme values. **$P < .01$ (vs. initial values); ***$P < .001$. (Courtesy of Väänänen, H.K., et al.: J. Appl. Physiol. 61(2):561–564, August 1986.)

to cell membranes in type I skeletal muscle. This measurement may be useful because prolonged physical exercise has been shown to result primarily in injury to red or slow twitch skeletal muscle cells. The goal of the present study was to assess the effect of prolonged physical exercise on the serum concentration of CA III in healthy long-distance runners participating in a competitive 24-hour run.

The authors established a sensitive radioimmunoassay for measurement of human CA III. The study population consisted of eight healthy male long-distance runners ranging in age from 32 to 41 years (mean, 36) who participated in a 24-hour race; five healthy male long-distance runners who were not participating in the race served as controls. It was found that serum CA III increased gradually during the first 18 hours to 410-fold above initial values, with no further increase during the last 6 hours of the race. One day after termination of the race, serum CA III was not found to be different from the initial value. Serum creatine kinase and serum lactate dehydrogenase, which are other indicators of damage to the skeletal muscle during exercise, were found to increase gradually throughout the run, and to be elevated 1 to 2 days later (Fig 1–14).

It is concluded that serum CA III increases as a consequence of physical exercise. The authors suggest that the lack of increase in CA III during the last hours of exercise, and the decrease after exercise which is more rapid than the decrease in serum creatine kinase and serum lactate dehydrogenase, may reflect differences in the rates of penetration through the sarcolemma and different degrees of injury in different fiber types or in the half-lives of these enzymes in serum.

▶ Electron microscopy has now shown categorically that excessive exercise can cause damage to skeletal muscle (Hikida, R. S., et al.: *J. Neurol. Sci.* 59:185–203, 1983). There is thus increasing interest in biochemical markers of "overtraining." The development of a radioimmunoassay procedure to detect the isozyme of carbonic anhydrase specific to slow-twitch fibers is a valuable contribution to this process. Previous authors have used less specific markers of muscle damage, such as serum creatine kinase and serum lactate dehydrogenase.

The report shows differences in the time course for the three markers, which the authors have linked to differences in their molecular weight (29,000, 82,000, and 130,000); presumably, this influences both the rate of leakage of the molecule from the muscle cell and also its subsequent clearance from the circulation.—R.J. Shephard, M.D., Ph.D.

Muscle Cell Leakage of Myoglobin After Long-Term Exercise and Relation to the Individual Performance
L.-E. Roxin, G. Hedin, and P. Venge (Univ. Hosp., Uppsala, Sweden)
Int. J. Sports Med. 7:259–263, October 1986   1–53

After severe or prolonged exercise, myoglobin is found at increased levels in blood. It is thought that untrained individuals are particularly sensitive and react to exercise with greatly increased myoglobin levels in the serum. It is also known that short-term exercise of the isokinetic type leads to increased levels of myoglobin, and again physical conditioning has been shown to reduce myoglobin leakage from muscles. However, little is known about the cause of the leakage of proteins over the muscle cell membrane in either shortterm or longterm exercise, although it is likely that insufficient energy production is partially responsible. The goal of the present study is to provide a detailed description of the kinetics of the occurrence in the circulation of myoglobin and other muscle proteins after prolonged exercise.

The study population consisted of three groups. The first group included 13 men and 1 woman who competed in an 89-km cross-country ski race; their mean age was 42 years (range, 29 to 65) and they completed the race in a mean time of 7 hours. The second group included 35 men who competed in an 89-km cross-country ski race; their mean age was 40 years (range, 20 to 63) and they completed the race in a mean time of 7.5 hours. The third group consisted of 11 male students with a mean age of 28 years (range, 23 to 42) who were subjected to 5 hours of bicycling. Muscle protein release was studied during and after prolonged exercise by means of serum myoglobin determinations. Increased serum myoglobin levels were regularly observed after performance of long-term exercise, and the correlations to muscle enzymes suggested nonselective release from muscle cells. Myoglobin measured after completed exercise was correlated to the

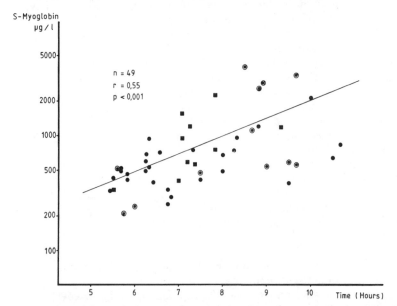

Fig 1–15.—S-myoglobin vs. finishing time in a group of 49 skiers after completion of an 89-km ski race. The following symbols were used: ■, skiers more than 49 years of age; ●, skiers between 20 and 49 years of age; ◉, individuals participating in the race for the first time. (Courtesy of Roxin, L.-E., et al.: Int. J. Sports Med. 7:259–263, October 1986.)

finishing time in a ski race, with the fast skiers exhibiting lower myoglobin levels than the slow skiers. In addition, inexperienced skiers and skiers older than 49 years were shown to have higher myoglobin levels than the others, although the mean finishing times were similar (Fig 1–15). When myoglobin was measured before and after 5 hours of bicycling, large interindividual differences were observed, even though the relative workload was identical to the ski exercise. The myoglobin level started to rise a median of 1.2 hours after the commencement of the bicycle exercise, and the time at which the myoglobin levels started to rise correlated with the myoglobin levels after completed exercise and was not related to the physical fitness of the individuals.

There are large individual differences with regard to muscle protein leakage during exercise. The leakage is not simply related to the individual's physical fitness status, but probably also to constitutional factors, such as age and metabolic capacity of the muscle cells.

▶ Myoglobin is quite a small protein molecule (molecular weight around 16,000), and it is thus not surprising that it leaks very readily from the muscle cell when the level of energy supply is inadequate to sustain the function of the sarcolemmal membrane.

The fact that myoglobin leakage was lowest in those with the best times in the Vasa ski race could reflect not only their shorter total time on the course, but also a much more efficient pattern of skiing than the slower entrants; the latter may have expended several times the amount of energy to cover the same 89 km distance, thus subjecting the muscle fibers to much more severe energy depletion.

Leakage of myoglobin during a cycle ergometer test (where there is much less variation in mechanical efficiency) was said to be unrelated to habitual activity or fitness; this is an interesting point and merits stronger documentation.—R.J. Shephard, M.D., Ph.D.

Ethanol Reduces Myoglobin Release During Isokinetic Muscle Exercise
Lennart Lundin, Roger Hällgren, Christer Lidell, Lars Eric Roxin, and Per Venge (Univ. Hosp., Uppsala, Sweden)
Acta Med. Scand. 219:415–419, 1986   1–54

It is well established that chronic excessive alcohol intake has an adverse effect on striated muscle, and chronic alcoholics often have increased serum myoglobin levels during their drinking periods, despite the absence of muscle symptoms. It is thought that an increase in circulating myoglobin reflects an enhanced release from affected striated muscle cells. Little is known about the acute effect of ethanol on muscle tissue in nonalcoholics, although signs of acute modest functional disturbance of heart muscle in healthy individuals after a single intake of ethanol have been reported. The goal of the study was to test the anticipated unfavorable acute effect of ethanol on muscles during work.

MAXIMAL MUSCLE POWER, POWER OF ENDURANCE, MAXIMAL HEART RATE, AND INCREASES
IN BLOOD LACTATE AND SERUM MYOGLOBIN ON THREE OCCASIONS: WITHOUT ALCOHOL
INTAKE (CONDITION I), DURING ALCOHOL INFLUENCE (CONDITION II), AND ON THE DAY
AFTER ALCOHOL INTAKE (CONDITION III) (MEAN ± SD)

	Condition I	Condition II	Condition III
Maximal muscle power (Nm)	405±62	402±57	391±60
Power of endurance (%) †	56.9±7.3	58.8±10.2	60.3±8.1
Maximal heart rate (beats/min)	151±28.9	147±24.8	152±23.2
Blood lactate increase (mmol/l)	6.1±2.7	5.4±2.5	6.1±1.9
Serum myoglobin increase (µg/l)	158±130	69±79*	86±87*

*Significantly lower increment ($P < .05$) compared with condition I and calculated on paired values.
†Residual muscle power after 2-minute muscle work.
(Courtesy of Lundin, L., et al.: Acta Med. Scand. 219:415–419, 1986.)

The authors studied myoglobin release in 12 healthy men (mean age, 37 years; range, 30 to 44) performing an intense 2-minute isokinetic muscle work. Measurements were carried out under three separate conditions: in the habitual state, during moderate ethanol intoxication, and 1 day after ethanol intake. Although the performed muscle work, maximal heart rate, and blood lactate levels did not differ between the three test occasions, the serum myoglobin increments after exercise were significantly reduced in the ethanol-intoxicated state, and also 10 to 15 hours after ethanol intake (table). The decrease in the exercise-induced myoglobin increment was not explained by increased elimination of the protein. Therefore, it is likely that the mechanism is a reduction of myoglobin release from skeletal muscle due to an ethanol-induced alteration of the muscle cell membrane, possibly by means of adenylate cyclase activation.

There is a reduction of the exercise-induced rise in serum myoglobin by ethanol. Since the reduced increments of serum myoglobin could not be explained by a change in the elimination of the protein, the cause of the changes observed after ethanol intake are probably due to a lower release from striated muscle.

▶ Disturbances of the muscle membrane cause a loss of myoglobin from muscles, both with excessive bouts of exercise and with chronic alcoholism. It is thus a little surprising that a substantial acute intake of ethanol (0.8 gm/kg) reduced the release of myoglobin associated with a 2 min bout of heavy isokinetic exercise.

The authors were inclined to attribute this phenomenon to an activation of membrane-bound adenylate cyclase by the alcohol (Rabin, R. A.: *J. Pharmacol. Exp. Ther.* 227:551–556, 1983). However, it is also possible that the energy supply to the muscle membrane was increased through the alcohol itself (some 1,850 kJ of energy), a stimulation of epinephrine release and thus glycogenolysis, or a local improvement of blood flow (a local vaso-dilator action of the alcohol, or a reduction of muscle tension thus offering less mechanical impedance to blood flow).—R.J. Shephard, M.D., Ph.D.

Effect of Alcohol Intake and Exercise on Plasma High-Density Lipoprotein Cholesterol Subfractions and Apolipoprotein A-I in Women

G. Harley Hartung, Rebecca S. Reeves, John P. Foreyt, Wolfgang Patsch, and Antonio M. Gotto, Jr. (Baylor College of Medicine, The Methodist Hosp., Houston)
Am. J. Cardiol. 58:148–151, July 1, 1986   1–55

The combined effect of regular aerobic exercise training and alcohol consumption on plasma high-density lipoprotein (HDL) cholesterol in women is not known. The effect of alcohol on plasma HDL cholesterol, its subfractions (HDL_2 and HDL_3 cholesterol), and apolipoprotein A-I (Apo A-I) was determined in 18 inactive and 18 physically active (runners) premenopausal women. All subjects abstained from alcohol for 3 weeks, then followed abstinence with 3 weeks of wine consumption. Mean ethanol intake was 32 gm per day and 30 gm per day for the inactive and active women, respectively. All active women ran or jogged at least 20 miles per week.

Compared with the inactive women, the runners weighed less and had higher plasma HDL cholesterol and lower low-density lipoprotein cholesterol. Plasma total cholesterol, triglyceride, and Apo A-I concentrations did not differ between groups. Plasma HDL_2 cholesterol values were higher in runners, whereas HDL_3 values were similar in both groups. Consumption of alcohol had no significant effect in any of the variables measured in either group.

The amount of exercise in premenopausal women appears to be a more important determinant of plasma lipoprotein and Apo A-I concentrations than alcohol consumption.

▶ Another article supporting the relationship of vigorous exercise and the beneficial HDL elevations and its significant subfraction HDL_2. If this one study can serve as a guide, there may be true sex difference. The level of HDL cholesterol was much higher in inactive women than inactive men and similar to that of male runners. Unlike the response of inactive men, there was no significant change with alcohol abstinence or reintroduction. Of incidental interest is that the triglyceride level did not change relative to alcohol consumption per se, but was significantly lower in the active population than in the inactive group.—L.J. Krakauer, M.D.

Chronic Low Level Physical Activity as a Determinant of High Density Lipoprotein Cholesterol and Subfractions

Timothy C. Cook, Ronald E. Laporte, Richard A. Washburn, Neal D. Traven, Charles W. Slemenda, and Kenneth F. Metz (Univ. of Pittsburgh)
Med. Sci. Sports Exerc. 18:653–657, December 1986   1–56

Intense activity is associated with elevated high-density lipoprotein cholesterol (HDL-C) and thereby a lowered risk of coronary heart disease, but the effects of lower-level exercise are unknown. The effects of chronic low-intensity exercise of long duration on HDL-C were studied in 35 male postal carriers over 1 year. There is epidemiologic evidence suggesting lower coronary mortality among walking postal carriers than in more sedentary persons. Subjects were studied four times during the year.

The study subjects walked more than 5 miles per day on average. Reported miles walked correlated significantly with the HDL_2-C, and the relationship with HDL-C approached significance. Both levels correlated with Large Scale Integrated measures, an activity monitor. Miles walked correlated with HDL_2-C after controlling for age, alcohol consumption, body mass index, and leisure time activity. The same was true of the relation between Large Scale Integrated readings and the HDL_2-C.

Exercise of low to moderate intensity may be necessary to significantly raise HDL-C levels. Chronic low-intensity activity as engaged in by mail carriers may have an important role in raising both HDL-C and HDL_2-C levels. It may be possible to reduce cardiovascular disease risk without large changes in cardiovascular fitness through participation in low intensity physical activity of long duration.

▶ Until recently, the threshold of activity for increase of HDL-cholesterol has been thought to be the attainment of a weekly jogging distance of 18 to 20 km (Wood, P. D., and Haskell, W. L.: *Lipids* 14:417–427, 1979; Kavanagh, T., et al.: *Arteriosclerosis* 3:249–259, 1983). While this presents no problem to the younger coronary-prone patient, it may seem an unattainable objective for the elderly patient. J. Arnold et al. (*J. Cardiac Rehabil.* 5:373–377, 1985) thus made an important contribution in showing that the sustained moderate walking of the postal carrier was also associated with high serum HDL-cholesterol readings.

Cook and associates have now confirmed these observations on U.S. mail carriers; their proof is a little more complete than that of Arnold and associates in that they measured the most important of the HDL subfractions (HDL_2), and demonstrated a correlation of this variable with the route mileage as estimated by an activity monitor. The report is particularly interesting in that it provides an example of the successful use of a simple electronic mercury switch to measure leg activity. The authors suggest that the mail carriers have a 35-lb mail pouch; however, I think this is the *maximum* permitted weight at the beginning of the mail route. On many days the initial loading of the pouch is much lighter, and of course its weight diminishes as the day progresses. Nevertheless, mail carrying is one of the heavier of current-day occupations.—R.J. Shephard, M.D., Ph.D.

Increased HDL-Cholesterol Following Eight Weeks of Progressive Endurance Training in Female Runners
Laurie J. Goodyear, Michael S. Fronsoe, David R. Van Houten, E. Victoria Dover, and J. Larry Durstine (Univ. of Vermont, Univ. of South Carolina, and Univ. of Cape Town, South Africa)
Ann. Sports Med. 3:33–38, 1986

Physically active persons have a favorable lipid profile. To determine whether a large increase in the number of miles run each week can have additional effects on blood lipid and lipoprotein profiles in moderately trained young women, the lipid profiles of five female runners were examined before and after 8 weeks of increased endurance training. Five sedentary women served as controls. The average number of miles added each week was four.

The number of miles run per week by the runners increased steadily over the training period, from 20 to 25 miles to 62 miles a week. Training resulted in a significant 2.6 mL/kg per minute increase in maximal oxygen consumption and decreased body fat, but did not affect total body weight. Although triglyceride levels were substantially lower in runners initially, increased training had no effect on plasma triglycerides as well as low-density lipoprotein-cholesterol or total cholesterol level. High-density lipoprotein-cholesterol level increased significantly from 59 ± 3 mg/dL to 76 ± 4 mg/dl during the training period. All variables remained unchanged pretest to posttest in the sedentary controls.

High-density lipoprotein cholesterol level can be increased dramatically over a short period of time when the number of miles run per week is increased.

▶ The HDL-C was not fractionated in this study in comparison with the previous one and therefore, although trends seem similar, direct comparison cannot be made. The level of HDL-C may indeed rise with training time, but many papers in the literature do not document that 8 weeks of training, even if intensive, are sufficient to do so. The plasma triglyceride data, lower in physically active women to a significant degree, may be as important if not more so in the long run, than changes in HDL fractions.—L.J. Krakauer, M.D.

Prolonged Exercise Augments Plasma Triglyceride Clearance
Stanley P. Sady, Paul D. Thompson, Eileen M. Cullinane, Mark A. Kantor, Evelyn Domagala, and Peter N. Herbert (Miriam Hosp., Providence, R.I.)
JAMA 256:2552–2555, Nov. 14, 1986   1–58

Previous studies have shown that a marathon run acutely lowers serum triglyceride concentrations and increases postheparin lipoprotein lipase (LPLA) activities for several days after the race. The ability of ten endurance athletes to clear fat emulsions before and after a marathon run was studied.

The healthy, nonsmoking, well-trained men participated in a 42-km foot race. All had been taking a normal diet before the race. Serum lipid and lipoprotein concentrations, intravenous fat clearance, and postheparin LPLA activities were measured 24 hours before and about 18 hours after completion of the race. After the initial samples were drawn, each runner received an intravenous infusion of a 10% soybean oil solution that contained a mixture of neutral triglycerides of mostly unsaturated fatty acids. Blood samples were obtained every 5 minutes for 40 minutes. Heparin

Mean ± SD Lipid and Lipoprotein Concentrations, Lipolytic Activity, and Intravenous Fat Clearance (K_2) Before and After Marathon Run (N = 10)

Variable	Prerace Value	Postrace Value	% Difference
Triglycerides, mg/dL (mmol/L)	80±32.8 (0.90±0.37)	56±12.3 (0.63±0.14)	−26±13.3*
Total cholesterol, mg/dL (mmol/L)	197±31.2 (5.10±0.81)	189±37.3 (4.90±0.97)	−4±7.1
LDL† cholesterol, mg/dL (mmol/L)	118±25.1 (3.06±0.65)	109±27.7 (2.82±0.72)	−8±8.1‡
HDL† cholesterol, mg/dL (mmol/L)	63±18.3 (1.63±0.47)	70±21.4 (1.81±0.55)	+10±8.4‡
HDL$_2$ cholesterol,§ mg/dL (mmol/L)	26±15.3 (0.67±0.40)	30±19.5 (0.78±0.51)	+19±16.6*
HDL$_3$ cholesterol, mg/dL (mmol/L)	38±4.2 (0.98±0.11)	39±3.7 (1.01±0.10)	+4±7.3
Apoprotein A-I, mg/dL (mmol/L)	156±23.3 (0.056±0.0083)	157±25.8 (0.056±0.0092)	+0±5.3
Apoprotein A-II, mg/dL (mmol/L)	32±4.7 (0.021±0.0031)	31±5.6 (0.021±0.0037)	−3±6.4
Lipoprotein lipase activity, μmol/mL/h	10.4±2.82	14.3±1.63	+46±35.1*
Hepatic triglyceride lipase activity, μmol/mL/h	12.2±2.46	11.5±2.03	−4±16.2
K_2, %/min	4.5±1.8	7.1±2.3	+76±63.9*

* $P < .01$.
† LDL: low-density lipoprotein; and HDL: high-density lipoprotein.
‡ $P < .05$.
§ Logarithmically transformed before analysis.
(Courtesy of Sady, S.P., et al.: JAMA 256:2552–2555, Nov. 14, 1986. Copyright 1986, American Medical Association.)

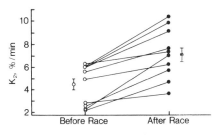

Fig 1–16.—Individual changes in intravenous fat clearance rate (K_2) before *(open circles)* and after *(solid circles)* marathon. Means ± SD are given. (Courtesy of Sady, S.P., et al.: JAMA 256:2552–2555, Nov. 14, 1986. Copyright 1986, American Medical Association.)

sodium was then injected, and a final blood sample was drawn 10 minutes later for determination of postheparin plasma lipase activities.

Lipid and lipoprotein concentrations were typical of endurance athletes before the race, but there were dramatic changes in the measures of triglyceride metabolism after the race (table). The mean clearance rate of exogenous fat increased 76%, mean postheparin LPLA activity increased 46%, and mean fasting triglyceride concentration decreased 26% after the race (Fig 1–16). The mean high-density lipoprotein (HDL) cholesterol concentration increased 10%, mostly because of a 19% increase in the HDL_2 subfraction. The change in the clearance rate of exogenous fat was directly related to the change in HDL cholesterol concentration and the HDL_2 subfraction.

The rise in HDL cholesterol concentration in athletes after prolonged exercise may be due to enhanced fat clearance.

▶ Changes in the clearance rate of exogenous fat were directly related to changes in HDL cholesterol level and the HDL_2 subfraction.

Elevated blood HDL concentration in endurance athletes has been attributed to two complementary mechanisms—HDL varying inversely with the activity of hepatic triglyceride lipase, which plays a role in HDL catabolism, and HDL positively related to the activity of lipoprotein lipase, which transfers lipids to HDL from VLDL and chylomicrons.—L.J. Krakauer, M.D.

The Influence of Exercise Training on Plasma Lipids and Lipoproteins in Health and Disease
William L. Haskell (Stanford Univ.)
Acta Med. Scand. [Suppl.] 711:25–37, 1986   1–59

It has been reported that men and women who lead a physically active life have a lower overall risk of coronary heart disease. They also display a lipoprotein profile commensurate with this lower risk. The results of numerous studies have shown decreased plasma triglyceride concentrations in trained athletes; however, few studies have shown an exercise effect in women and children, since they generally have low Tg concentrations. Exercise seems to have very little effect on total cholesterol circulating in the plasma or serum though plasma HDL-C concentrations in athletes are consistently higher than those of inactive peers. Of the two major subfractions of plasma HDL, higher HDL_2 levels occur in trained athletes but no difference in HDL$_3$ is observed. When LDL-C concentrations are compared in athletes and sedentary controls, a lower value is found about two thirds of the time in the athletes, but no difference and higher values have been found.

Very little is understood regarding the relationship of the content of the various LDL subfractions to CHD even though a positive association between LDL-C and CHD has been established. A sex difference exists as women have lower concentrations of small LDL and IDL and higher concentrations of large LDL than men. As with HDL-C subfractions, exercise training may alter LDL-C subfractions of men to resemble those of women. Regarding VLDL cholesterol, exercise training has resulted in either no change or decreased concentrations. Of the apoproteins, only apoprotein A-I and A-II have been investigated. Substantially higher apoprotein A-I but not A-II have been demonstrated in endurance athletes.

Our understanding of the changes in body chemistry produced by exercise training that lead to changes in lipoprotein metabolism will remain incomplete until regulatory mechanisms for synthesis, transport and catabolism of the specific lipoproteins become better defined. Though the causal link between low risk for coronary heart disease and the lipoprotein profile has not been established, there is sufficient evidence that increased physical activity may be warranted for the prevention of heart disease in high risk populations.

▶ Of all of the articles reviewed this year in the complex area of lipid metabolism, this stands, I think, as the best correlation of the questions relating to cholesterol, low density lipids, triglycerides, and HDL in different populations of age and sex. The bibliography is extensive. Knowledge about the basic regulatory mechanisms for the synthesis, transport, and catabolism of the specific lipoproteins remains incomplete, and this is the large unknown in the field at this time. A nice distinction is made between the different primary therapeutic goals of decreasing total cholesterol or LDL cholesterol which must call for dietary change or lipid lowering medication, with exercise strictly a secondary factor. On the other hand, in terms of the mass of HDL, exercise may have the most appeal, although it will be difficult to augment increased exercise in a sedentary population of long-term habit and of increasing age. A physically active life-style is strongly endorsed and I quote his final sentence: "The age-related rise in triglyceride concentrations seen in sedentary population of adults can virtually be eliminated by a physically active life-style." For those who seek precise numbers, an expenditure of 1,000 kcal per week is minimal to produce a favorable lipoprotein change. This can vary in a positive sense up to energy expenditures of 4,500 kcal per week. Another number worth commenting on: At exercise intensity requiring less than 40% of $Vo_{2\ max}$, it is unlikely that HDL will increase at any age.—L.J. Krakauer, M.D.

Effect of Physical Training in Humans on the Response of Isolated Fat Cells to Epinephrine

F. Crampes, M. Beauville, D. Riviere, and M. Garrigues (Faculté de Médecine

Toulouse-Purpan and Institut de Physiologie and Unité d'Enseignement et de Recherche en Education Physique et Sportive, Toulouse, France)
J. Appl. Physiol. 61:25–29, July 1986   1–60

During prolonged muscular exercise, the energy needed for adenosine triphosphate resynthesis is primarily derived from aerobic metabolism which uses lipids and carbohydrates simultaneously in proportions that depend on the intensity and duration of the exercise. Although the lipid reserves of the organism are practically inexhaustible, the carbohydrate reserves are very limited, and a close correlation exists between muscle glycogen decrease and duration of exercise. Because of this, depletion of muscle glycogen stores is one major limiting factor in the ability to perform long-term exercise. Endurance training helps muscle tissue oxidize lipids and therefore helps to conserve glycogen. The goal of the study was to determine whether in addition to this preferential use of fatty acids by muscle tissue in endurance trained individuals, there is an increase in the capacity of their adipose tissue to mobilize lipids.

The study population consisted of ten male marathon runners and ten male sedentary individuals of similar age. The authors determined the response to epinephrine of collagenase-isolated fat cells obtained after biopsies of fat from the periumbilical region. Adipocyte lipolysis was assessed using a bioluminescent glycerol release assay. Epinephrine caused

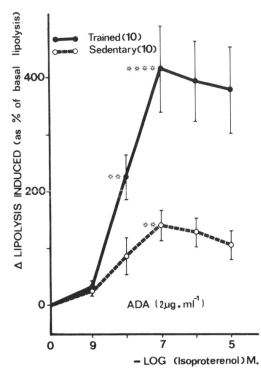

Fig 1–17.—Concentration-response curves to isoproterenol with 2 μg/ml of adenosine deaminase (ADA). Lipolysis responses as percent of basal lipolysis are plotted against negative logarithm of molar isoproterenol concentrations. Values are means ± SE. **P < .01; ***P < .001. (Courtesy of Crampes, F., et al.: J. Appl. Physiol. 61:25–29, July 1986.)

a significant increase in lipolysis only in the trained subjects. The dose response curves for epinephrine-induced lipolysis were significantly different for the trained and sedentary subjects at 10^{-6} M and above. To determine the modification mechanisms involved, lipolysis with isoproterenol and epinephrine plus propranolol were investigated. Isoproterenol markedly increased lipolysis in both groups and the dose-response curves were substantially different at 10^{-7} M and above (Fig 1–17). In both groups, epinephrine plus propranolol was observed to significantly decrease lipolysis without distinction between trained and sedentary subjects.

In male subjects, endurance training increases the sensitivity of subcutaneous abdominal adipose tissue to the lipolytic action of epinephrine; this effect seems to be related to an increased response of the β-adrenergic pathways.

▶ This article agrees with several other recent reports showing enhanced lipolysis in humans after training (Després, J. P., et al.: *J. Appl. Physiol.* 56:1157–1161, 1984; Martin, W. H., et al.: *J. Appl. Physiol.* 56:845–848, 1984). One would infer some increase in activity of the adenylate cyclase system within the fat cell, and the data thus stand in apparent contrast to that of J. Svedenhag (Abstract 1–34), who found no change in plasma cAMP activation by a standard dose of catecholamine after training.

One possible point of discussion is the method of expressing the data, all findings being expressed as a percent of resting lipolysis; however, if there is an effect of earlier activity upon resting lipolysis (Després, J. P., et al.: *Int. J. Obes.* 7:231–240, 1983), this would tend to enhance rather than diminish baseline values in the active subjects. A second possible variable is a decrease in size of the adipocytes (Bukowiecki, L., et al.: *Am. J. Physiol.* 239:E422–E429, 1980), although in humans lipolysis does not seem strictly related to adipocyte diameter. A final factor to consider is the increased clearance of catecholamines, as discussed by Svedenhag and associates.

By comparing responses to epinephrine plus propranolol and epinephrine plus isoproterenol, Crampes and associates argue that the pathway responsible for the enhanced lipolysis is β-adrenergic rather than α_2 adrenergic.—R.J. Shephard, M.D., Ph.D.

Effects of Ingesting Carbohydrate Beverages During Exercise in the Heat
Mallard D. Owen, Kevin C. Kregel, P. Tim Wall, and Carl V. Gisolfi (Univ. of Iowa)
Med. Sci. Sports. Exerc. 18:568–575, October 1986   1–61

During sustained exercise in the heat, profuse sweating occurs which can result in dehydration, reduction in plasma volume with accompanying impaired body heat dissipation and endurance performance, and an increase in core temperature. When dehydration is minimized by fluid replacement, individuals can work in the heat longer with smaller increases in core temperature. Because of these considerations, fluid replacement during prolonged exercise in the heat is important for maintaining endurance performance and preventing thermal injury.

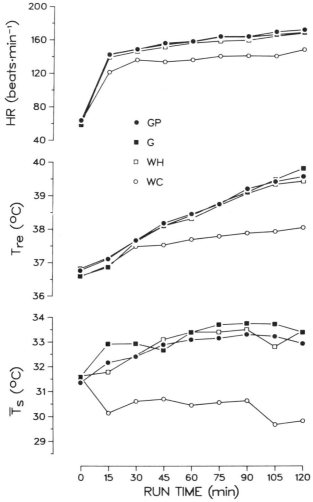

Fig 1–18.—Responses of HR, T_{re}, and T_s to four different 2-hr treadmill runs at 65% $\dot{V}O_{2\,max}$. Three runs were performed in the heat (T_{db} = 35 C) and included receiving 200 ml every 20 minutes of either a glucose polymer (GP), glucose (G), or water (WH) drink. The fourth run was performed in a cool environment (T_{db} = 25 C) and included receiving 200 ml every 20 minutes of a water drink (WC). (Courtesy of Owen, M.D., et al.: Med. Sci. Sports Exerc. 18:568–575, October 1986. Copyright 1986, the American College of Sports Medicine. Reprinted by permission.)

To enhance endurance performance, fluid replacement beverages often contain a simple sugar such as glucose as a supplementary energy source. It is thought that these sugars allow muscle glycogen to be spared. However, as the carbohydrate content of beverages increases, the gastric emptying time increases and the rate of fluid repletion is slowed. The goal of the present study was to test the hypothesis that ingesting a hypoosmotic glucose polymer beverage during prolonged exercise in the heat would minimize the decline in plasma volume and the rise in core temperature as effectively as drinking water and would also maintain blood glucose levels.

To determine the effect of osmotically different beverages on prolonged (2-hour) treadmill exercise in the heat (35 C), five male runners (aged 24 to 41 years) performed three separate runs, drinking 200 ml every 20 minutes of either 10% glucose polymer (GP), 10% glucose (G), or saccharin-sweetened water (WH). In addition, the subjects performed a fourth run in a cool (25 C) room and included drinking saccharin-sweetened water (WC). The drink osmolalities (Osm) for runs GP, G, WH and WC were 194, 586, 94 and 71 mmol/kg, respectively. There were no significant differences between runs in the heat for heart rate, rectal and mean skin temperatures, sweat rate, percent change in plasma volume, and gastric residue volume (Fig 1–18). However, when compared with the WC run, both the GP and G runs yielded greater declines in percent change in plasma volume, but only the G run had a greater gastric residue volume. Neither plasma osmolality, total protein, nor sodium concentration varied between runs, and plasma glucose, insulin, and respiratory exchange ratios were similar between the GP and G runs. However, the GP run exhibited the lowest plasma glycerol values.

Although gastric residue volume and final percent change in plasma volume were significantly correlated with drink osmolality, thermoregulation was similar between runs in the heat despite the beverage consumed.

▶ Various authors have suggested that the problem of delayed gastric emptying induced by concentrated glucose solutions can be overcome by ingesting newer glucose polymers such as Polycose, which provide the same amount of energy per unit volume of fluid despite a much lower osmotic pressure.

The present experiments, continued over a 2-hour run, show surprisingly little difference between trials using water, 10% glucose, or 10% Polycose in terms of such practical indices of performance as the exercise heart rate and the core temperature. Such findings can be interpreted in two ways. If the goal is to maintain plasma volume, then money can be saved by drinking water. If the goal is to provide the athlete with energy as well as water, then there may be some advantage in offering a Polycose solution. The lack of difference between the Polycose and the glucose probably reflects the choice of relatively high concentrations, where the energy content of the solution as well as the osmotic pressure influences the rate of gastric emptying (Foster, C., et al.: *Res. Q.* 51:299, 1980); more benefit might have been found from the Polymer preparation if both forms of carbohydrate had been offered as 5% solutions.— R.J. Shephard, M.D., Ph.D.

Factors Affecting Changes in Muscle Glycogen Concentration During and After Prolonged Exercise
Per C.S. Blom, Nina K. Vøllestad, and David L. Costill (Inst. of Muscle Physiology, Oslo, Norway, and Ball State Univ.)
Acta Physiol. Scand. 128(suppl. 556):67–74, 1986   1–62

When exercise intensity is increased, muscle glycogen breakdown increases as well. It has been observed that muscle glycogen concentration decreased continuously during exercise at about 75% of $\dot{V}O_2$ max until almost total depletion occurred at exhaustion or after approximately 90 minutes. Subjects with higher preexercise muscle glycogen concentrations could exercise for a longer period of time than could subjects with a lower initial concentration. From these observations, it is generally agreed that intramuscular store is one of the most important limiting factors of performance capacity during intensive exercise of 1 to 2 hours' duration. When individual muscle fibers types I and II were subjected to increasing exercise intensity, there was a gradual increase in the number of fibers where glycogen depletion occurred and the rate of glycogen breakdown in the individual fibers increased. The muscle, therefore, is able to generate sufficient force even though some fibers are depleted of glycogen and fatigued.

Resynthesis of glycogen stores is an important part of postexercise recovery. Studies suggest that, up to a certain limit, there is an increasing rate of postexercise glycogen resynthesis with increasing oral glucose intake regardless of the route of administration. Glucose infusion, however, induces a considerably higher rate of resynthesis. In trained athletes, continuous light training and a slightly higher than normal carbohydrate intake stimulate muscle glycogen synthesis enough to obtain levels which are almost twice as high as those found in untrained subjects. Therefore, a complete glycogen loading regimen that disturbs training and dietary habits undertaken for the purpose of attaining high glycogen levels and improved performance is unnecessary.

▶ The originally prescribed regimen for muscle glycogen supercompensation was relatively complicated, including a high-fat diet, a bout of exhausting exercise, and several days of high carbohydrate intake. The end result was usually a doubling of the initial glycogen stores, but at the expense of a dramatic disturbance of both diet and training. It is thus encouraging to note that similar benefit can be obtained from some lightening of the training program and provision of a moderate increase in carbohydrate intake.

The important comment is made that during the recovery period, glucose provides a more effective source of carbohydrate than fructose. This is probably because the fructose tends to be metabolized largely in the liver rather than the skeletal muscle (Zakim, D., et al.: *Biochem. Med.* 2:427–437, 1969).— R.J. Shephard, M.D., Ph.D.

Muscle Glycogen Utilization During Prolonged Strenuous Exercise When Fed Carbohydrate
Edward F. Coyle, Andrew R. Coggan, Mari K. Hemmert, and John L. Ivy (Univ. of Texas, Austin)
J. Appl. Physiol. 61:165–172, July 1986   1–63

The authors have previously reported that carbohydrate feedings during prolonged strenuous exercise (i.e., 74% of maximal O_2 uptake) can delay

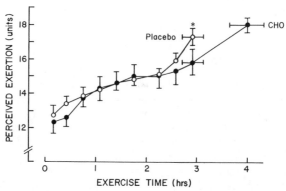

Fig 1–19.—Rating of perceived exertion during exercise with the placebo solution and when carbohydrate was ingested every 20 minutes (CHO). *Placebo significantly higher than carbohydrate; $P < .05$. (Courtesy of Coyle, E.F., et al.: J. Appl. Physiol. 61(1):165–172, July 1986.)

the development of fatigue. Although they did not obtain muscle glycogen data, they suggested that carbohydrate administration may result in increased utilization of blood glucose with a proportional slowing of muscle glycogen depletion. Muscle glycogen utilization was measured directly during strenuous exercise with and without carbohydrate feedings to determine whether muscle glycogen sparing can explain the postponement of fatigue.

The study population consisted of seven endurance-trained male cyclists (mean age, 28 ± 1 years). The subjects were exercised at $71 \pm 1\%$ of maximal O_2 consumption to fatigue, while ingesting a flavored water solution (placebo) during one trial and while ingesting a glucose polymer solution (i.e., 2.0 gm/kg at 20 minutes and 0.4 gm/kg every 20 minutes thereafter) during another trial. Fatigue during the placebo trial occurred after 3.02 ± 0.19 hours of exercise and was preceded by a decline in plasma glucose to 2.5 ± 0.5 mM and by a decline in the respiratory exchange ratio. Glycogen within the vastus lateralis muscle declined at an average rate of 51.5 ± 5.4 mmol glucosyl unit (GU)/kg per hour during the first 2 hours of exercise and at a slower rate of 23.0 ± 14.3 mmol GU/kg per hour during the third and final hour. When the subjects were fed carbohydrate, which maintained plasma glucose concentration (4.2 to 5.2 mM), the subjects were able to exercise for an additional hour before experiencing fatigue (Fig 1–19). However, the pattern of muscle glycogen utilization was not different during the first 3 hours of exercise with the placebo or the carbohydrate feedings. The additional hour of exercise performed when fed carbohydrate was carried out with little reliance on muscle glycogen and without compromising carbohydrate oxidation.

When they are fed carbohydrate, highly trained endurance athletes are capable of oxidizing carbohydrate at relatively high rates from sources other than muscle glycogen during the later stages of prolonged strenuous exercise, and this postpones fatigue.

▶ The present results are a little puzzling. The feeding of carbohydrate (a glucose polymer) decreases the rating of perceived exertion in the later phases of prolonged exercise and also postpones the onset of fatigue, but the rate of utilization of muscle glycogen is essentially unchanged.

The authors hypothesize that fatigue is occurring when the local muscular reserve of glycogen is depleted and there is insufficient glucose in the blood to make good the shortfall. The ingested carbohydrate thus postpones fatigue by sustaining blood glucose. Their data show that in the late stages of exercise the carbohydrate-fed subject is able to derive a substantial proportion of the total energy requirement from carbohydrate sources other than muscle glycogen. Perhaps because the subjects were athletes with a high proportion of slow twitch fibers and an enhanced muscle capillarization, they were able to use blood glucose at rates as high as 2 gm per minute.

The lack of sparing of glycogen by the glucose-polymer is at variance with earlier reports (Bjorkman, O., et al.: *Clin. Physiol.* 4:483–494, 1984; Shephard, R. J.: *Sports Medicine,* in press). Possibly, the discrepancy can be explained by differences in the type of feeding or the exercise protocol, but it is hard to understand why there was absolutely no benefit from the glucose polymer.—R.J. Shephard, M.D., Ph.D.

Remarkable Metabolic Availability of Oral Glucose During Long-Duration Exercise in Humans
N. Pallikarakis, B. Jandrain, F. Pirnay, F. Mosora, M. Lacroix, A.S. Luyckx, and P.J. Lefebvre (Univ. of Liège, Belgium)
J. Appl. Physiol. 60:1035–1042, April 1986   1–64

Recent studies indicate that an oral glucose load during moderate, long-duration exercise is a readily available metabolic substrate. This is true for glucose ingested early or late after initiation of exercise. This study investigates the extent to which repeated oral loads of glucose administered during exercise can be metabolized.

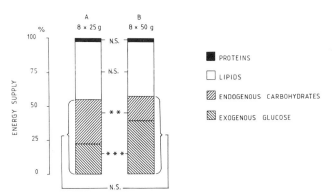

Fig 1–20.—Respective contributions of various energy fuels in two groups of four subjects receiving either 8 × 25 (group G 200) or 8 × 500 (group G 400) gm glucose during exercise. Asterisks, statistically significant differences between two groups: **, $P < .02$; ****, $P < .001$. NS, not statistically significant difference. (Courtesy of Pallikarakis, N., et. al.: J. Appl. Physiol. 60:1035–1042, April 1986.)

Healthy male volunteers exercised on a 10% uphill treadmill at 45% of their maximal oxygen uptake for 285 minutes. After 15 minutes, they received eight doses totaling either 200 or 400 gm of oral glucose every 30 minutes. Carbohydrate and lipid oxidation were measured by indirect calorimetry. Oxidation of exogenous glucose was followed by carbon-13-labeled glucose.

Total carbohydrate and lipid oxidation were similar for both groups. Exogenous glucose oxidation was significantly lower and endogenous glucose oxidation was significantly higher in the group ingesting 200 gm of glucose, compared with the group receiving 400 gm (Fig 1–20). Exogenous glucose oxidation represented 55.3% and 87.5% of total carbohydrate utilization during the last hour in the low and high glucose groups, respectively.

Glucose ingested at the rate of 50 gm per 30 minutes can cover 85% to 90% of total carbohydrate utilization during the last 60 minutes of 285 minutes of moderate exercise. This allows significant sparing of endogenous carbohydrates. However, whether glucose ingestion improves performance is not known.

▶ The glucose used in these experiments was given in the form of a 25% solution (25 gm/100 ml), a mixture with a relatively high osmotic pressure, which would slow gastric emptying below the usual exercise rate of 600 to 1,000 ml per hour; in fact, the doses of glucose used corresponded to fluid ingestions of 200 and 400 ml per hour.

The authors are not quite correct in suggesting that the influence of such treatment upon performance is unknown. Saltin (cited by Astrand and Rodahl, *Textbook of Work Physiology,* McGraw Hill, 1977) demonstrated that in situations where water balance was not a problem, glucose concentrations as high as 30% to 40% were helpful in preventing a fading of performance toward the end of a long race.

In North America, correction of fluid depletion is usually more critical than the treatment of glycogen exhaustion, and the use of high concentrations of glucose is then an inappropriate method of treatment.—R.J. Shephard, M.D., Ph.D.

A Controlled Randomized Study on the Effect of Long-Term Physical Exercise on the Metabolic Control in Type 2 Diabetic Patients
Tapani Rönnemaa, Kari Mattila, Aapo Lehtonen, and Veikko Kallio (Turku Municipal Hosp., Turku, Finland)
Acta Med. Scand. 220:219–224, 1986   1–65

Physical activity is an important treatment for patients with non–insulin-dependent (type 2) diabetes. The effects of long-term exercise on metabolic control were examined in a randomized trial of 30 patients having type 2 diabetes, 20 males and 10 females with a mean age of 52.5 years, who had had diabetes for a mean of 7 years. Two patients were managed with diet alone. Three patients had mild hypertension, but none were receiving treatment for cardiovascular disease. Comparable groups of 15 patients were entered into an exercise program and control condition. Five to seven weekly sessions of walking, jogging, or skiing were held over 4 months, maintaining the pulse at about 70% of peak aerobic capacity.

Maximum aerobic capacity rose by nearly 10% in the exercise group. Metabolic control improved significantly, although the decline in fasting plasma glucose was not significant. The insulin response to oral glucose increased significantly in the exercise group. None of these parameters changed significantly in control patients. Improved metabolic control in exercising patients correlated with the rise in peak aerobic capacity. The fall in plasma insulin on acute exercise correlated with the increase in plasma insulin response to oral glucose in exercising patients.

Long-term physical exercise improves metabolic control in most type 2 diabetics, but no benefit should be expected if initial control is poor or insulin reserves are weak. The favorable effects of exercise in this setting relate to increased pancreatic sensitivity to oral glucose.

Effects of Exercise on Glucose Tolerance and Insulin Resistance: Brief Review and Some Preliminary Results
John O. Holloszy, Joan Schultz, Judith Kusnierkiewicz, James M. Hagberg, and Ali A. Ehsani (Washington Univ., St. Louis)
Acta Med. Scand. [Suppl.] 711:55–65, 1986   1–66

Previous studies have shown that glucose tolerance (GT) declines with aging. The decline is usually associated with the development of hyperinsulinemia, which is partly the result of stimulation of insulin secretion by the higher glucose concentration. More recent studies suggest that impaired insulin clearance may also be implicated in the process. There is evidence that this decline in GT and insulin sensitivity can be prevented by regular vigorous exercise. The authors investigated whether prolonged and vigorous exercise by nonathletic, middle-aged and elderly persons can normalize GT by decreasing resistance to insulin in patients with mild, non–insulin-dependent diabetes mellitus (NIDDM) or with impaired GT.

Forty-nine patients were studied. They had completed 12 months of exercise training in a cardiac rehabilitation program and included five men with NIDDM, eight with impaired GT, and eight with high-normal plasma glucose concentrations and moderate hyperinsulinemia on oral glucose tolerance testing.

Three of the five men with NIDDM had completely normal GT after 12 months of exercise training; the other two had markedly improved GT. Test results in normal men and men with mild NIDDM are compared in Figures 1–21 and 1–22. All 8 patients with impaired GT had completely normal GT despite a marked blunting of the insulin response to the glucose load when they were retested after 12 months of exercise training. All

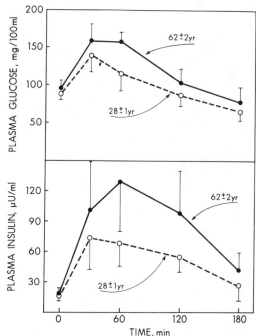

Fig 1–21.—Plasma glucose and insulin responses to 100-gm oral glucose tolerance test. Values are means ± SD for 26 healthy, sedentary, nonoverweight men, aged 61 to 68 years, and for 30 healthy, sedentary, nonoverweight men, aged 25 to 29 years. (Courtesy of Holloszy, J.O., et al.: Acta Med. Scand., Suppl. 771, pp. 55–65, 1986.)

eight men with high-normal plasma glucose concentrations and mild hyperinsulinemia had improved GT and a markedly reduced insulin response on retesting after 12 months of exercise training.

Exercise training can normalize GT by reducing insulin resistance in some patients with mild NIDDM if they are not severely insulin deficient and in some patients with impaired GT. However, because of the relatively small number of patients in this study, these preliminary results should be confirmed in a larger group.

▶ Both of these patients (Abstracts 1–65 and 1–66) deal with the non–insulin-dependent type 2 diabetic, and in this group there is no question and no disagreement among investigators that diet and exercise are critical in the control of the diabetes. Moreover, in many instances abnormal glucose tolerance tests can revert to normal with vigorous regular exercise. In the Finnish study, it was clear that the patients with the poorest metabolic control were not able to improve physical fitness and in turn did not show significant improvement in metabolic control. The Washington University group states further that exercise seems to be effective in normalizing glucose tolerance only in those patients with an adequate capacity to secrete insulin and in whom insulin resistance is the major cause for abnormal glucose tolerance. When feasible, exercise must be of a significant order of magnitude—25 to 35 km per week of running or equivalents on a regular basis. This is not an easy prescription if other diseases coexist. On the other hand, in those capable of meeting this

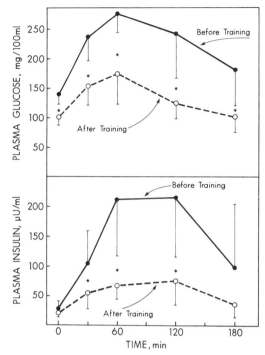

Fig 1–22.—Plasma glucose and insulin responses to 100-gm oral glucose tolerance test in patients with mild NIDDM before and after 12 months of intense endurance exercise training. After-training oral glucose tolerance test was performed about 18 hours after patients' most recent bout of exercise. Values are means ± SD for five patients. Asterisks indicate P < .01. (Courtesy of Holloszy, J.O., et al.: Acta Med. Scand., Suppl. 711, pp. 55–65, 1986.)

challenge, it has tremendous preventive implications for the ravages of diabetes and atherogenic disease.—L.J. Krakauer, M.D.

Haemodynamic and Hormonal Responses to Exercise: Studies in Patients With Diabetes Mellitus and Adrenomedullary Deficiency
A. Barnett, A. Maslowski, J. Livesey, G. Nicholls, H. Ikram, and E. Espiner (Princess Margaret Hosp., Christchurch, New Zealand)
Eur. J. Clin. Invest. 16:5–10, Feburary 1986   1–67

It is well known that the hemodynamic response to a change in posture or to sustained exercise is mediated by increased sympathetic nervous activity, increased catecholamine concentrations, and the associated activation of the renin angiotensin system. In diabetics with autonomic neuropathy the hemodynamic response and renin and adrenergic hormonal responses are often diminished. The hemodynamic response to a change in posture and to exercise was studied in patients with autonomic neuropathy and in patients with adrenomedullary deficiency. For comparison, patients with mild essential hypertension or uncomplicated diabetes were also studied.

The 21 subjects in the study were divided into four groups: group I included 5 insulin-dependent diabetics without autonomic neuropathy; group II, 5 insulin-dependent patients with autonomic neuropathy; group

III, 5 patients who had undergone adrenalectomy because of Cushing's disease or pheochromocytoma; and group IV, 6 mildly hypertensive subjects. Hemodynamic and hormonal responses were measured during standard exercise and postural maneuvers. Continuous arterial blood pressure monitoring was performed.

There was no significant difference in blood pressure and heart rate after exercise among any of the groups. Patients with autonomic neuropathy had normal blood pressures and heart rates in response to posture and sustained exercise, but they had a significant rise in plasma cortisol concentration after exercise. Adrenalectomized subjects had significantly lower epinephrine concentrations than controls after exercise, but those receiving conventional corticosteroid replacement therapy had normal hemodynamic responses to posture and exercise.

Diabetics, including those with mild autonomic neuropathy, have normal blood pressure and pulse responses to posture and sustained exercise. Similar normal responses in adrenalectomized patients suggest that circulating epinephrine is not obligatory for a normal hemodynamic response to exercise.

▶ One is constantly impressed with the "fail-safe" design of the human body. This article provides one more example of this phenomenon. While one might anticipate an adverse response to changes of posture and to sustained exercise where neuropathy has affected adrenal function, in fact apparently normal hemodynamic adjustments are achieved via alternative pathways.—R.J. Shephard, M.D., Ph.D.

Influence of the Degree of Metabolic Control on Physical Fitness in Type I Diabetic Adolescents

J.R. Poortmans, Ph. Saerens, R. Edelman, F. Vertongen, and H. Dorchy (Hôp. Univ. Saint-Pierre, Brussels)
Int. J. Sports Med. 7:232–235, August 1986   1–68

Although for many years physical exercise was recommended in the management of diabetes, more recent reports have warned against exercise. The authors showed in earlier reports that exercise does have a beneficial effect on glucose assimilation in diabetic adolescents, provided adequate insulin therapy and a normal diet are adhered to. Since there is considerable controversy over the state of physical fitness in juvenile diabetics, the authors studied physical fitness in diabetic and matched normal adolescents in order to determine whether there is any relationship between physical fitness and the degree of metabolic control as measured by glycosylated hemoglobin (HbA_1).

The study comprised 17 type 1 male diabetic adolescents and 17 control subjects matched for sex, age, height, and weight. All subjects led sedentary lives. The diabetic group included seven patients who were carriers of incipient retinopathy and four patients with subclinical peripheral neuropathy. The diabetic subjects were divided into two groups according to their base levels of HbA_1: group I included nine diabetics with HbA_1 levels lower than 8.5% and Group II included eight diabetics with HbA_1 levels higher than 8.5%. All subjects underwent bicycle ergometric testing. Oxygen uptake, pulmonary ventilation, and heart rate were recorded at rest and at maximal load. Glucose, lactate, and free fatty acid levels were also determined before and after exercise.

The maximal work load and oxygen uptake were significantly lower in both groups of diabetic adolescents than in the healthy volunteers. In addition, there was an inverse relationship between HbA_1 levels and maximal workload.

Diabetic adolescents need to obtain the best possible degree of metabolic control if they wish to increase their physical fitness levels to those matching a healthy population.

▶ In the type 1 insulin-dependent diabetic, the picture is quite different. The prior prescription for almost ubiquitous exercise is no longer granted. Rather, there is a prerequisite of maintaining free fatty acids within normal range and keeping such individuals free of ketosis. Otherwise exercise will actually induce increased hyperglycemia. Maximal work load and oxygen uptake are significantly lower in the diabetic groups whether under good or poor control with insulin dependency, and the diabetic groups cannot match the healthy control in either situation irrespective of the exercise prescription or interdiction. An inverse relationship was observed between hemoglobin A_1 concentration and maximal work load. The point is reemphasized that there is a striking physiologic difference between insulin-dependent diabetes and the type 2 non–insulin-dependent diabetic group and milder variants of glucose intolerance.—L.J. Krakauer, M.D.

TSH and Prolactin Responses to TRH in a Treated Hypothyroid Athlete: Effect of Activity and Rest
D.C. Cumming, J.A. Grainger, L.G. Campbell, and S.R. Wall (Univ. of Alberta, Edmonton)
J. Sports Med. 25:243–245, December 1985   1–69

It has been shown that endurance training over a 6-month period increases responses of TSH and PRL to thyrotropin-releasing hormone (TRH) in women. However, it is unclear what physiologic events led to the changes observed in the response of TSH. Although levels of thyroid hormones were reduced after increased training, they were within normal range and the response of TSH to TRH was increased but was also within normal levels. Thus, it seems difficult to accept that the observed changes are other than physiologic adjustments. The authors have investigated whether training that was not designed to increase endurance in a treated hypothyroid athlete induced changes similar to those described in endurance-trained women.

Woman, 21, was a high jumper whose training consisted of repetitive anaerobic and resistance training for 2 hours per day, 5 days each week. She had been hypothyroid for 1 year prior to the study and was treated with replacement of 0.05 mg of synthetic thyroxine. Baseline levels of thyroid hormones, together with responses of TSH and PRL to TRH, were determined during a period of intensive training and again 1 month later after 10 days of rest without training. Baseline levels of thyroid hormones were normal and identical at rest and in a training situation (table). The responses of TSH and PRL to TRH were substantially increased during heavy physical work, compared to responses after 10 days of rest.

Any heavy training load can enhance the responses to TRH, and the mechanism is an adjustment in thyroid physiology rather than an impairment of thyroid function.

▶ While baseline thyroid hormones were normal and identical in the rest and training situations, as the table indicates, there was a marked response of TSH and PRL to TRH when tested during the heavy physical work interval after 10 days of rest. These responses were similar to those in women undergoing training for the marathon, but without change in baseline thyroid hormone levels. Enhanced responses are not specific to endurance training. Earlier papers in the literature have considered TSH response to exercise in general to be minimal.

Incidental note is made that in measuring thyroid function on replacement dosage of T4 (Synthroid), a false-positive elevation may be suggested by the Synthroid formulation, and T3 (triiodothyronine) may play a more important role in regulating the serum thyrotropin concentration. (Fish, L., et al.: *N. Engl. J. Med.* 316:764–770, 1987).—L.J. Krakauer, M.D.

Stress Hormonal Response to Exercise After Sleep Loss
Bruce J. Martin, Paul R. Bender, and Hsiun-ing Chen (Indiana Univ.)
Eur. J. Appl. Physiol. 55:210–214, April 1986   1–70

Stress is defined as a factor to which a person fails to make a satisfactory adaptation. Sleep deprivation is considered to be a stressful event. However, it is unclear whether prolonged loss of sleep fulfills the definition of physiologic stress, i.e., provocation of excessive cortisol and β-endorphin secretion. Results of recent studies assessing the influence of sleep deprivation on cortisol excretion have been inconclusive. The authors studied the effect of prolonged sleep deprivation on the physiologic stress imposed by subsequent exercise.

The study was performed with eight healthy volunteers who participated in two series of experiments. In the first series, volunteers were subjected to two fragmented nights of sleep before performing 30 minutes of heavy treadmill walking exercise. In the second series, they performed light treadmill walking exercise for 3 hours after 36 sleepless hours. Oxygen uptake, minute ventilation, and heart rate were recorded before, during, and after exercise. Concentrations of cortisol and β-endorphin were determined within 1 minute after completion of the exercises.

In the first series of experiments, plasma cortisol and β-endorphin concentrations were identical with control values after the heavy treadmill walking exercise, although sleep loss did disturb the mood of the participants before and during exercise walking, as verified by psychologic testing. Results of the second series were similar in that there was no change in plasma cortisol or β-endorphin concentration and in that the volunteers experienced mood disturbance before and during exercise walking. Sleeplessness left heart rate, oxygen uptake, minute ventilation, and body core temperature unchanged during exercise walking.

Sleep loss provokes psychologic but no physiologic changes during subsequent exercise walking.

▶ Interest in sleep deprivation has been stimulated not only by the ever-increasing need for shift work in modern industry, but also by a NATO requirement that ground forces be capable of operating for several days with minimal sleep while reinforcements are sought. The athlete who must switch time zones may also pass one or more sleepless nights during the period of adjustment of circadian rhythms to the new environment.

Martin and colleagues examine the possibility that excessive secretions of cortisol and β-endorphin, induced by the stress of sleeplessness, may influence subsequent exercise responses. While their findings in this regard are negative, it is not altogether fair to say that there is no change in physiologic responses to exercise after sleep deprivation. Our own studies, for example, have shown a significant decrease of maximum oxygen intake, albeit after a longer period of sleep deprivation (Plyley, M. J., Shephard, R. J., Angus, R.: *Proceedings of International Conference on Occupational Ergonomics,* Toronto: Human Factors Association of Canada, 1984, pp. 223–227).—R.J. Shephard, M.D., Ph.D.

Effects of Human Menstrual Cycle on Thermoregulatory Vasodilation During Exercise
K. Hirata, T. Nagasaka, A. Hirai, M. Hirashita, T. Takahata, and T. Nunomura (Kanazawa Univ., Kanazawa, Ishikawa, Japan)
Eur. J. Appl. Physiol. 54:559–565, February 1986   1–71

During exercise, skin blood flow (SBF) rises in proportion to the increase in core temperature (T_c). Many factors affect this thermoregulatory response of cutaneous vessels. In females, periodic changes in T_c are associated with the menstrual cycle. However, the relation of SBF to T_c during exercise at different stages of the menstrual cycle has not been fully studied.

The subjects were four healthy sedentary females with normal menstrual cycles. At rest and during semisupine cycle ergometer exercise, finger blood flow, skin temperatures, esophageal temperatures, heart rate, oxygen consumption, and carbon dioxide production were measured. These measurements were taken twice each in the follicular and luteal phases of the menstrual cycle.

Resting esophageal temperature was higher in the luteal phase, but there were no differences between the phases in finger blood flow, oxygen consumption, carbon dioxide production, heart rate, or minute ventilation at

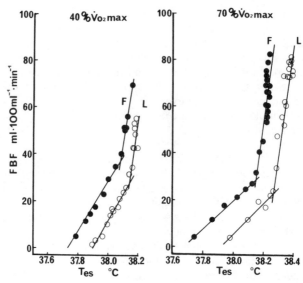

Fig 1–23.—Effects of the follicular and luteal phases during the menstrual cycle on the individual relationship between finger blood flow (FBF) and esophageal temperature (T_es) at 40% (**left**) and 70% $\dot{V}_{O_{2max}}$ (**right**) in one subject. (Courtesy of Hirata, K., et al.: Eur. J. Appl. Physiol. 54:559–565, February 1986.)

rest and during exercise. The relation of finger blood flow to T_c was characterized by two slopes. The slope was shallow below the threshold for vasodilation, and steep above this threshold. This threshold temperature was shifted higher in the luteal phase and with more intense exercise. The slopes of finger blood flow versus esophageal temperature for both luteal and follicular phases were similar (Fig 1–23).

This study demonstrates that in women, setpoint temperatures may be higher with exercise during the luteal phase. As in men, increasing exercise-induced vasoconstrictor tone in proportion to exercise intensity decreases the thermoregulatory vasodilator response. This is true of both phases of the menstrual cycle when heat storage is insufficient in women.

▶ The changes in resting core temperature with the menstrual cycle are well recognized, and some impact on thermoregulation during exercise might thus be anticipated. Hirata and associates show rather nicely that during the luteal phase of the menstrual cycle the threshold temperature where a steep increase of finger blood flow begins is displaced upward. This is true during both moderate and more vigorous work. Comparison with earlier experiments on male subjects (Hirata, K., et al.: *J. Therm. Biol.* 9:117–120, 1984) further suggests that at any given intensity of effort women develop a two- to three-fold greater finger blood flow than men; this may possibly reflect differences in heat acclimatization or training, always a problem when making cross-sectional comparisons of exercise responses between the two sexes.—R.J. Shephard, M.D., Ph.D.

Vitamin E Deficiency and Vitamin C Supplements: Exercise and Mitochondrial Oxidation

K. Gohil, L. Packer, B. de Lumen, G.A. Brooks, and S.E. Terblanche (Univ. of California, Berkeley)

J. Appl. Physiol. 60:1986–1991, June 1986   1–72

Studies in rats have shown that tissue stores of vitamin E are depleted in skeletal muscle and liver after endurance training, and that the resulting vitamin E deficiency increases susceptibility to oxygen toxicity. The effects of vitamin E deficiency and the increased oxygen metabolism imposed by exhaustive exercise on mitochondrial oxidative capacity of gastrocnemius muscle, heart, liver, and brown adipose tissue were studied. Since previous in vitro studies showed that vitamin C can interact with vitamin E, the effect of dietary vitamin C supplementation in vitamin E-deficient rats was also examined.

Forty-eight female Sprague-Dawley rats were randomly divided into three groups. Group I was fed a normal diet, group II was given a vitamin E-deficient diet, and Group III was fed the same diet as group III with the addition of vitamin C. Weekly blood samples were taken to monitor vitamin E concentrations. Endurance capacity was measured by running the rats to exhaustion.

Endurance capacity was decreased 38.1% in group II and 33.6% in group III rats, compared with controls. Despite an 82% increase in the blood concentration of vitamin C in group III, there was no effect on the increased peroxide-induced hemolysis that accompanies dietary vitamin E deficiency.

Vitamin C supplementation cannot counteract the detrimental effects associated with vitamin E deficiency.

▶ There is a tendency for toxic peroxides to be formed by metabolism. Adverse effects of these substances on the body, such as the oxidation of structural lipids, can be countered by antioxidant substances such as vitamins E and C. It is but a short step from this basic hypothesis to the concept that when metabolism is greatly increased by endurance training the body needs an increased intake of vitamins E and C (Aikawa, K. M., et al.: *Biol. Sci. Rep.* 4:253, 1984).

Some animal experiments, such as those reported here, apparently support such a view. However, it is important to recognize that the experimental animals were kept on a diet totally deficient in vitamin E. The normal mixed diet of the athletic competitor bears little resemblance to this experimental regimen. Attempts to test the benefit from vitamins in humans are plagued by subjects who deliberately break double-blind coding. Our own experiments found little advantage from three months of vitamin E supplementation in distance swimmers (Shephard, R. J., et al.: *Eur. J. Appl. Physiol.* 33:119–126, 1974); swimming performance was unchanged, although the experimental subjects tended to less loss of muscle strength in the inactive muscles than that seen in the controls.—R.J. Shephard, M.D., Ph.D.

Laboratory Evaluation of Lactic Anaerobic Capacity: Development of a Test

J.M. Crielaard, Ph. Ledent, M. Grosjean, F. Pirnay, and P. Franchimont (Hôpital de Bavière, Liège, Belgium)
Medisport 60:66–71, 1986

1–73

Measurement of blood lactate levels after maximal exercise provides a clear indication of anaerobic energy expenditure in athletes. However, previous laboratory studies to measure anaerobic performance were complex and have provided inconclusive data. The authors present a simple method for the assessment of lactic anaerobic capacity that is sufficiently sensitive and reliable to be used on a routine basis.

The study was done with five physical education students who were accustomed to participating in laboratory experiments. Each subject was tested a total of three times on an ergometric bicycle at 1-week intervals. Each subject warmed up for 10 to 15 minutes and rested for 5 minutes prior to starting the test, which involved working on a cycle ergometer until exhaustion. Ventilation, oxygen consumption, and CO_2 excretion were determined at rest, during the test, and during the first 10 minutes of recuperation. Peak lactic acid levels were measured at 7 minutes and 40 seconds into the recovery period.

Results show that the test lasted between 45 seconds and 1 minute and 45 seconds when the cycle was set at speeds between 90 and 100 revolutions per minute and at a resistance of 0.555 kg of force per kilogram of body weight. Reproducibility of the test was rated good, with a highly significant correlation of test parameters, including maximal duration of the test, lactic anaerobic capacity, and peak lactic acid concentrations.

In another part of the study, the correlation between lactic anaerobic capacity, measured in the laboratory, and the personal records of 60 subjects over courses of 100, 400, and 1,500 m were also studied. The results of that study show that there is a highly significant correlation between performance over a 400-m course and measured lactic anaerobic capacity. However, the correlation between lactic anaerobic capacity and performance over a 100-m course is much weaker, which confirms the highly specific nature of this test.

▶ The method most widely used for the evaluation of anaerobic capacity in North American subjects at present is probably the Bar-Or test. In this procedure, the subject is required to maximize the work performed on a cycle ergometer over a 30-second interval. Inevitably, scores depend somewhat on the subject's experience of the test and knowledge of an appropriate pace of cycling which will induce total exhaustion in 30 seconds.

The present authors argue for a test where there is some latitude in total test duration; anaerobic capacity is assessed from the total work performed, in joules. With the population tested, they argue for a loading of 0.055 kg of force per kilogram of body mass; under these conditions, a suitable test duration of about 90 seconds is obtained with a pedal frequency of about 90 revolutions per minute. In terms of validity, the test predicts track performance best over distances of 400 m. Over this running distance, the correlation between track times and ergometer test score is 0.80; in other words, the laboratory test is accounting for about two thirds of the variation in track performance. The main difficulty with Crielaard's test, as with the Bar-Or procedure, is that the optimal pedal loading varies with the condition of the subject, and a nice judgment must be shown if maximal anaerobic capacity is to be revealed by means of a single test.—R.J. Shephard, M.D., Ph.D.

Effect of Hyperoxia on Substrate Utilization During Intense Submaximal Exercise
R.P. Adams, P.A. Cashman, and J.C. Young (Boston Univ.)
J. Appl. Physiol. 61:523–529, August 1986   1–74

There is controversy regarding the measurement of maximal O_2 uptake ($\dot{V}O_{2max}$) for exercise during hyperoxia. Some investigators have indicated as much as a 13% increase in $\dot{V}O_{2max}$, whereas others report no change or insignificant increases. In addition, theoretical problems arise because concurrently, CO_2 output ($\dot{V}CO_2$) is found to either remain unchanged or slightly decrease. It is well known that performance is improved with hyperoxia. In view of the findings that O_2 delivery to the working muscle may not be increased during hyperoxia and that $\dot{V}O_2$ may not be increased, it is important to provide an explanation for the performance enhancement outside the realm of O_2 utilization. The authors tested the hypothesis that with hyperoxia, there is a substrate shift toward greater fat utilization with a concurrent depression of glycolysis.

The study population consisted of six physically fit male subjects ($\dot{V}O_{2max}$ = 66 ml/kg per minute) who performed 30 minutes of cycling during normoxia ($21.35 \pm 0.16\% \ O_2$) and hyperoxia ($61.34 \pm 1.0\% \ O_2$). Values for $\dot{V}O_2$, CO_2 output, minute ventilation, respiratory exchange ratio, venous lactate, glycerol, free fatty acids, glucose, and alanine were obtained before, during, and after exercise. It was found that $\dot{V}O_2$, free fatty acids, glucose, and alanine values were not significantly different in hyperoxia compared with normoxia. However, CO_2 output, respiratory exchange ratio, minute ventilation, glycerol, and lactate levels were all discovered to be lower during hyperoxia (Fig 1–24).

There may be a substrate shift during hyperoxia, and this may be the mechanism responsible for the observed improvement in exercise tolerance seen with hyperoxia. Although the results do not indicate a specific mechanism, they suggest that the occurrence of a substrate shift to greater fat utilization may be accompanied by relative increases not only in splanchnic and nonexercising muscle blood flow but also by increases in blood and muscle pH. This concept of interacting mechanisms would explain the results of the study as well as the enhanced exercise tolerance and respiratory exchange ratio observed with hyperoxia.

▶ Although the authors have neglected to cite this classic reference, early

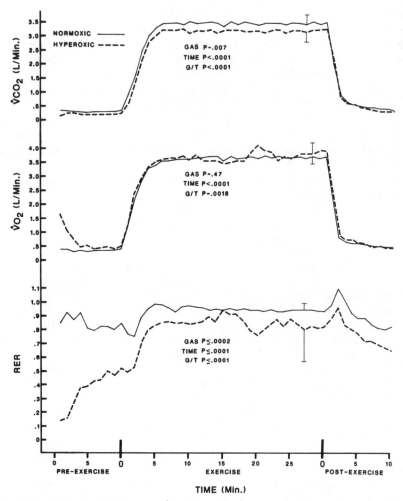

Fig 1–24.—Mean values for CO_2 output ($\dot{V}CO_2$), O_2 uptake ($\dot{V}O_2$), and respiratory exchange ratio (RER) before, during, and after exercise at 77% of maximal $\dot{V}O_2$ during inspiration of normoxic *(solid lines)* and hyperoxic *(broken lines)* gases. One average SD is shown on each curve. The *P* values are shown for differences between conditions (gas), over time (time), and for interaction (G/T). (Courtesy of Adams, R.P., et al.: J. Appl. Physiol. 61(2):523–529, August 1986.)

studies on the beneficial effects of oxygen go back to the period when Roger Bannister, as a young physiologist, was preparing himself for the 4-minute mile (Bannister, R. G., et al.: *J. Physiol.* 125:118–137, 1954).

The present report concerns longer (30-minute) periods of submaximal exercise at an intensity near the anaerobic threshold (76.8% maximum oxygen intake). The decrease of respiratory exchange ratio apparently supports the idea of a metabolic shift toward fat during oxygen inhalation; however, the failure to demonstrate an increase of blood glycerol levels is somewhat against this, and it may be that even over a period as long as 30 minutes the adverse effects of an increased pressure of oxygen upon carbon dioxide transport are leading to an increase of CO_2 storage, invalidating the respiratory gas exchange ratio as an indicator of muscle metabolism.

This is an important issue to resolve, for if oxygen administration did spare glycogen, it could be a useful ergogenic aid in prolonged, glycogen-depleting types of activity.—R.J. Shephard, M.D., Ph.D.

Exercise-Induced Anaphylactic Syndromes: Insights Into Diagnostic and Pathophysiologic Features
Thomas B. Casale, Thomas M. Keahey, and Michael Kaliner (Univ. of Iowa and Natl. Inst. of Allergy and Infectious Diseases, Bethesda, Md.)
JAMA 255:2049–2053, April 18, 1986   1–75

Exercise-induced anaphylaxis comprises various manifestations of physical allergy including pruritus, urticaria, and hypotension and/or upper airway obstruction. Cholinergic urticaria also can be precipitated by exercise. Provocative challenges were developed in two patients, one with cholinergic urticaria and one with exercise-induced anaphylaxis, with the goal of reliably distinguishing between these disorders.

Both patients had pruritus, urticaria, light-headedness, and angioedema following exercise. Symptoms were reproduced, with rises in plasma histamine during jogging under controlled conditions to raise the core body temperature by at least 1.1 C. On passive heat challenge, increasing the core temperature by more than 0.7 C, only the patient with cholinergic urticaria had anaphylactic symptoms and a rise in plasma histamine. Neither patient had anaphylactic symptoms when core temperature was raised by intravenous endotoxin; *Escherichia coli* RE-2 endotoxin was utilized. The temperature increased by more than 1.7 C in these studies.

Cholinergic urticaria appears related to effector mechanisms involved in compensatory responses in thermoregulation, sweating and/or vasodilation. Exercise-induced anaphylaxis, in contrast, is unrelated to core temperature and seems to be due either to abnormal release of a mast cell-degranulating factor or to an exaggerated response to a factor usually released on exercise which can induce mast cell degranulation. Passive heat challenge is a useful means of distinguishing between these syndromes.

▶ As this subject receives more study, it is apparent that there are two separate syndromes: an exercise-induced anaphylaxis and cholinergic urticaria–anaphylaxis. These two distinct but clinically similar syndromes can be distinguished by passive heat challenges which will reproduce symptoms in the cholinergic-urticaria group and which will bring about a rise in plasma histamine levels in that group. This cholinergic urticaria subgroup therefore may relate to thermoregulation patterns and compensatory responses involved therewith either sweating or vasodilatation.—L.J. Krakauer, M.D.

Heat Stroke at the Mekkah Pilgrimage: Clinical Characteristics and Course of 30 Patients

Basim A. Yaqub, Saed S. Al-Harthi, Ibrahim O. Al-Orainey, Mohammed A. Laajam, and Mahommed T. Obeid (King Khalid Univ. Hosp., Riyadh, Saudi Arabia)

Q. J. Med. (New Series) 59:523–530, May 1986   1–76

Heat stroke is a medical emergency caused by excessive storage of heat when high ambient temperatures prevent dissipation by radiation or convection and when evaporation of sweat is limited by ambient humidity. Individuals who are particularly susceptible to heat stroke include alcoholics, the elderly, those with cardiovascular disease, joggers or marathon runners, psychiatric patients who are taking antipsychotic drugs, patients who are taking combinations of medications, and infants who are wrapped too warmly during febrile illness.

The Mekkah pilgrimage occurs every year and may take place during the summer months when ambient temperatures may reach 48 C. During this occasion overcrowding, lack of sleep, strenuous exercise, and insufficient water and sanitation may contribute to heat stroke.

To analyze the clinical and biochemical observations of heat stroke the authors studied 20 men and 10 women aged 32 to 80 years who were diagnosed as suffering from heat stroke. All had a rectal temperature of 40 C or more, hot, dry skin, and disturbances of the CNS. Rapid cooling by the "evaporative method" was achieved in a mean time of 59 minutes (range, 15 to 135 minutes).

Prognosis was poor if the initial temperature was above 42 C and the cooling time was greater than 1 hour. In three patients (10%) fatal complications included acute hepatic failure, adult respiratory distress syndrome, and decerebrate convulsions. Two patients recovered, but 1 developed myocardial infarction and 1 developed cerebellar ataxia, 25 patients (83%) made an uncomplicated recovery.

Under the conditions of the Mekkah pilgrimage, heat stroke is unlikely to be completely preventable, but prompt recognition of the syndrome and early treatment do reduce the risk of high morbidity and mortality.

▶ This subject has been commented on extensively in our prior YEAR BOOKS, and comment is directed to 1985, p. 203, referring in that instance primarily to football players. "The point is made and now broadly accepted that sweating is desirable, that the mechanism should not be inhibited by rubber clothing or by any other means, and that hydration is the key to all heat syndromes."

With our parochial concerns, we forget that this is a worldwide problem and this particular report of 30 patients in Saudi Arabia is very vivid indeed. One has to be impressed that the mortality in this 30-patient group, unacclimatized and exposed to very significant heat environment, was no more than 10%. In their environment, treatment was by the evaporative method alone, and the observation, for what it's worth, was that prolonged cooling of longer than 1 hour resulted in a poorer final outcome. In patients who came to postmortem, the cause of coma in this particular group was due to cerebral edema and hemorrhage.—L.J. Krakauer, M.D.

Makkah Hajj: Heat Stroke and Endocrine Responses
O. Appenzeller, M. Khogali, D.B. Carr, K. Gumaa, M.K.Y. Mustafa, A. Jamjoom, and B. Skipper (Univ. of New Mexico, Albuquerque, Kuwait Univ., Kuwait, Saudi Arabia, Mass. Gen. Hosp., Boston, and Ministry of Health, Kingdom of Saudi Arabia)
Ann. Sports Med. 3:30–32, 1986   1–77

The Makkah Hajj is the traditional 7-day pilgrimage to Mecca. Participants in this event are squeezed into a small area at high ambient temperatures, and the rites of the pilgrimage involve extraordinary exertion. In 1982, 1,119 pilgrims were treated successfully for heat stroke, and several hundred others died before they could reach heat illness treatment centers.

It is well established that both exogenous and endogenous opiates modulate thermoregulation; consequently, a study was conducted to characterize endocrine responses associated with heat stroke by measuring "stress hormones," including immunoreactive beta-endorphin secreted by the pituitary and adrenal glands during heat stroke and after recovery in previously healthy pilgrims.

The study population consisted of 34 patients in heat stroke (15 females and 19 males). Stress hormones were measured by radioimmunoassay and included immunoactive β-endorphin, cortisol, prolactin, and growth hormone. Significant increases were found in circulating β-endorphin/lipotropin, cortisol, prolactin, and growth hormone in the heat stroke patients; the levels returned to normal after recovery (table).

PLASMA LEVELS OF STRESS HORMONES			
	Heat stroke patients	Convalescents	Change (%)
Cortisol (ng/dL) (n = 18)			
Mean ± SEM	36.2 ± 2.5	21.8 ± 2.7*	−39 ± 6
Median (range)	33.4 (17.6–54.7)	20.8 (9.0–53.1)	−42 (−68 to +24)
Prolactin (ng/mL) (n = 18)			
Mean ± SEM	42.5 ± 6.8	10.8 ± 1.7**	−59 ± 9
Median (range)	35.8 (5.3–119.7)	7.9 (5.0–30.6)	−76 (−96 to +17)
Growth hormone (ng/mL) (n = 16)			
Mean ± SEM	6.5 ± 1.2	1.6 ± 0.2*	−50 ± 15
Median (range)	3.6 (1.0–13.8)	1.2 (1.0–4.3)	−68 (−90 to +138)
Beta-lipotropin (pg/mL) (n = 18)			
Mean ± SEM	1,073 ± 428	25.1 ± 8.0**	−86 ± 5
Median (range)	303 (58–5,000)	6.6 (0.0–123.7)	−100 (−100 to −28)

*P < .01, **p < .001, Wilcoxon matched-pairs signed-ranks test. Convalescents vs. heat-stroke patients.
(Courtesy of Appenzeller, O., et al.: Ann. Sports Med. 3:30–32, 1986.)

Opioids are thus important in thermoregulation; moreover, their antagonists might help in the management of heat stroke victims.

▶ Some authors interested in heat stress have looked at participants in marathon races, but the clinical material derived from the pilgrimage to Mecca is much more extensive, partly because the ambient temperatures in Mecca are patently unsuitable to vigorous exercise (35 to 50 C), and partly because emotional excitement is combined with sustained exercise (7 days) undertaken by those who are poorly prepared for such a stress.

Earlier studies in saunas noted increases in blood concentrations of growth hormone, prolactin, and cortisol during intensive thermal stress (Leppaluoto, J., et al.: *Horm. Metab. Res.* 7:439–440, 1975). However, this seems the first report of an increased output of β-endorphins induced by hyperthermia.

The rise of β-endorphin levels is very dramatic, and this observation may be linked to a report of K. DeMeirleir and associates (*Br. Med. J.* 290:739–740, 1985) that naloxone administration can abolish the normal rise of core temperature induced by vigorous exercise. The possible role of opioid antagonists in the treatment of heat stress victims merits further examination.—R.J. Shephard, M.D., Ph.D.

Sauna Effects on Hemorrheology and Other Variables
E. Ernst, P. Strziga, Ch. Schmidlechner, and I. Magyarosy (Univ. of Munich)
Arch. Phys. Med. Rehabil. 67:526–529, August 1986   1–78

Sauna bathing is an increasingly popular pastime in Scandanavia, Europe, and the United States. Saunas are subjectively stimulating and have been proposed to induce beneficial effects on several body functions and to enhance overall health by strengthing the defense systems and activating cardiovascular function. Although objective measurements have been car-

Parameter and abbreviation	Unit	% of baseline
BV_1 Native blood viscosity $\tau = 0.84$ dyn/cm^2	mPa's	140±0.7
BV_2 Native blood viscosity $\tau = 16.68$ dyn/cm^2	mPa's	114±0.2
Hematocrit (hct)	%	106±0.1
$StBV_1$ Blood viscosity hct=45%, $\tau = 0.84$ dyn/cm^2	mPa's	113±0.6
$StBV_2$ Blood viscosity hct=45%, $\tau = 16.86$ dyn/cm^2	mPa's	107±0.1
Plasma viscosity(PV)	mPa's	106±0.04
Leucocyte count	$10^3 \mu l$	147±0.2
Heart rate	min^{-1}	134±0.2
Systolic blood pressure	mmHg	135±0.1

RELATIVE CHANGES IN PERCENT OF BASELINE VALUES AFTER ACUTE SAUNA*

*Only parameters showing a significant change are presented.
(Courtesy of Ernst, E., et al.: Arch. Phys. Med. Rehabil. 67:526–529, August 1986.)

ried out on a number of variables, little is known about the sauna's hemorrheologic effects. The goal of the present study was to clarify whether sauna, either acutely or chronically, leads to significant effects on blood fluidity and related factors.

The study population consisted of two groups of subjects. In the acute group there were five healthy female and ten healthy male subjects (mean age, 26.5 years; range, 25 to 34). In the chronic group there were two healthy female and nine healthy male subjects (mean age, 29.5 years; range, 21 to 53). Sauna bathing involved three 10-minute sessions in the sauna at 90 to 95 C and absolute humidity of 10 to 30 gm/cu m, interrupted by 10-minute rests in ambient temperature as well as cold water treatments ad libitum.

Acute sauna induced decreased blood fluidity, as quantified by measurements of blood and plasma viscosity, hematocrit, red cell filterability, and aggregation (table). This effect was observed to be far less prominent when sauna treatment was continued regularly for 8 weeks. In the case of long-term treatment, there were only minor changes in native blood viscosity and hematocrit together with slight variations in hematologic measurements, calcium, and serum protein pattern.

Sauna leads to predominantly acute adverse effects, while longterm effects appear to be negligible. The authors suggest considering such effects in patients with high cardiovascular risks and marked hypoperfusion. They recommend further studies to elucidate the biologic relevance of the described phenomena.

▶ The beneficial effects of sauna therapy were proposed by another senior German sports physiologist, Walter Hollmann (*ZFA* [Stuttgart] 59:55–58, 1983) quite recently. The long-term beneficial effects of the sauna are mainly attributable to heat acclimatization, which does interact to some extent with exercise training.

In an acute sense, the plasma loss from sweating and increased capillary filtration cause very substantial increases of blood viscosity (up to 40% in the present experiments). This could have serious consequences in subjects with a marginal blood flow, either in the coronary circulation or in the peripheral blood vessels.—R.J. Shephard, M.D., Ph.D.

Some Cardiovascular and Metabolic Effects of Repeated Sauna Bathing
J. Leppäluoto, M. Tuominen, A. Väänänen, J. Karpakka, and J. Vuori (Univ. of Oulu and Deaconess Inst., Oulu, Finland)
Acta Physiol. Scand. 128:77–81, September 1986   1–79

Sauna bath is an increasingly popular form of dry heat exposure. Although the physiologic responses are well described in the literature, little is known about the effects of repeated sauna exposures on the human body. Investigators have shown that long-term sauna exposures can reduce blood pressure in hypertensive subjects, and others have reported that increase in pulse rate declines in response to frequent sauna. Recently, in

EFFECT OF REPEATED SAUNA EXPOSURE ON VARIOUS SERUM CONSTITUENTS AND LEUKOCYTES

After sauna (2 × 1 h daily at +80 °C)

Parameter	Before sauna	Day 1	Day 3	Day 7
Serum Na (mmol l⁻¹)	141 ± 3	139 ± 5	141 ± 2	138 ± 4*
Serum K (mmol l⁻¹)	4.3 ± 0.1	4.5 ± 1.9	4.0 ± 0.2†	3.7 ± 0.3†
Serum Fe (μmol l⁻¹)	24 ± 6	27 ± 9	19 ± 10*	18 ± 5*
Serum total proteins (g l⁻¹)	76 ± 4	90 ± 26	83 ± 7*	79 ± 3
Hb (g l⁻¹)	152 ± 9	170 ± 10†	165 ± 13†	152 ± 10
Htc	0.46 ± 0.02	0.48 ± 0.3†	0.46 ± 0.03	0.46 ± 0.02
Leucocytes (10⁹ l⁻¹)	5.5 ± 1.2	7.4 ± 1.1†	7.6 ± 1.5†	6.1 ± 1.4
Serum urate (μmol l⁻¹)	367 ± 50	380 ± 49	358 ± 40*	360 ± 52*
Serum creatine (μmol l⁻¹)	97 ± 8	103 ± 8	99 ± 9	97 ± 9
Serum cholesterol (mmol l⁻¹)	4.6 ± 0.5	4.9 ± 0.6	4.8 ± 0.7	4.5 ± 0.6
Serum triglyserides (mmol l⁻¹)	1.0 ± 0.3	1.0 ± 0.4	1.3 ± 0.5	1.1 ± 0.6
Serum FFA (mmol l⁻¹)	0.4 ± 0.2	0.6 ± 0.2	0.4 ± 0.2	0.3 ± 0.1
Serum lactate (mmol l⁻¹)	1.0 ± 0.4	1.4 ± 0.3*	1.3 ± 0.3	1.4 ± 0.4

Mean ± SD is given; n = 9–10.
*P < .05.
†P < .01 "before" vs. "after" values.
(Courtesy of Leppäluoto, J., et al.: Acta. Physiol. Scand. 128:77–81, September 1986.)

healthy individuals, repeated hyperthermia has been demonstrated to increase serum levels of total proteins, α-antitrypsin, and transferrin, and to decrease serum levels of zinc and copper. Some basic physiologic parameters were investigated in subjects who participated in 2 hours of sauna bath daily over a period of 7 days.

The study population consisted of ten healthy male students aged 19 to 22 years. The subjects were exposed to the dry heat of a Finnish sauna (80 C) for 1 hour twice daily for 7 days. After each exposure, rectal temperature rose by 0.8 to 1.1 C and body weight dropped by 0.7 to 0.9 kg. The systolic blood pressure recorded 3 to 5 minutes after sauna was not observed to vary during the experiment, but the diastolic blood pressure was noted to drop by 7 to 37 mm Hg. The subjects' pulse rate rose from 75–80 to 106–116 beats per minute after the sauna. The increased responses of pulse and temperature adapted to heat exposures so that they were markedly lower after the third day (rectal temperature) or after the sixth day (pulse).

The metabolic rate was found to increase by 25–33% after the first day. Serum total proteins, Hb and Htc, were substantially elevated on the first and third days but not later (table), although the dehydration in response to sauna was unchanged as assessed by weight losses. The serum potassium, sodium, and iron levels were markedly decreased on the third and seventh days. No ECG changes were noted in recordings taken on the seventh day.

Physiologic responses to intense repeated heat stimuli change in some days, with the signs of acute hemoconcentration disappearing and signs of serum electrolyte loss developing. In addition, the increased responses of pulse and rectal temperature to heat exposure become less prominent. Although the authors did not observe any harmful cardiovascular effects in these young and healthy subjects, they recommend paying special attention to electrolyte balance during long-lasting and physiologically maximal heat exposure.

▶ The present results provide some quantitative data on the heat load imposed by a typical sauna exposure. Both in terms of the rise of core temperature and the volume of sweat production, the effect seems only about a half of what would be anticipated with running a marathon race on a warm day.

It is surprising that the preexposure serum potassium changes with just three days of sauna exposure; the cumulative potassium loss cannot have been more than about 15 mE, compared with a store of 80 mE in extracellular fluid and 3,500 mE in the tissues. Although the authors seem inclined to attribute the decrease in serum potassium concentrations to sweat losses, it may be that acclimatization to the heat stimulus with an altered secretion of aldosterone is also involved.

The changes in serum mineral ion concentrations could alter myocardial function, and while there were no long-lasting ECG changes in the present group of young subjects, persistent ST abnormalities have been described in older adults following sauna exposure (Sohar, E., et al.: *Isr. J. Med. Sci.* 12:1275, 1976); patients with ischemic heart disease should adopt a cautious approach to repeated and prolonged use of the sauna.—R.J. Shephard, M.D., Ph.D.

Endocrine Effects of Repeated Sauna Bathing
J. Leppäluoto, P. Huttunen, J. Hirovonen, A. Väänänen, M. Tuominen, and J. Vuori (Univ. of Oulu and the Deaconess Inst., Oulu, Finland)
Acta Physiol. Scand. 128:467–470, November 1986   1–80

Previously, the authors have shown that during intense long-term sauna exposure, some physiologic parameters, such as the pulse generating system and core temperature, adapt to the heat stimulus but that the metabolic rate increases along with the stimulus. However, less is known about the endocrine responses to repeated heat exposures in human subjects. The goal of the present study was to determine the responses of the pituitary, adrenal, and thyroid hormones to heat exposure taken daily for 2 hours over a period of 7 days.

The study population consisted of ten healthy male and seven healthy female students aged 19 to 22 years who were exposed in a sitting position while in the sauna bath. Before the experiment and on the first, third, and seventh days of the study, the levels of ACTH in plasma, cortisol, TSH, thyroid hormones, testosterone, gonadotropins, prolactin and GH in serum, and urinary excretion of catecholamines were assayed. There were no statistically significant changes in serum thyroid hormones, or in TSH, testosterone, FSH, and LH levels. However, serum cortisol and plasma ACTH levels dropped while urinary catecholamines increased slightly at the end of the experiment. In men, serum GH and prolactin exhibited 16- and 2.3-fold increases, and in women serum prolactin levels rose more than four-fold. The GH rise in response to hyperthermia declined after the third day but the prolactin level remained elevated in men at the end

Hormone	Before sauna	After sauna (2 h daily at +80 °C)		
		Day 1	Day 3	Day 7
ACTH (ng l⁻¹)	48 ± 45	70 ± 52	55 ± 48	48 ± 40
Cortisol (μmol l⁻¹)	0.48 ± 0.11	0.55 ± 0.12	$0.46 \pm 0.13^*$	$0.41 \pm 0.12^*$
TSH (mU l⁻¹)	2.5 ± 0.8	3.2 ± 0.7	2.9 ± 0.7	3.2 ± 0.9
T_4 (nmol l⁻¹)	115 ± 15	130 ± 14	134 ± 19	124 ± 16
T_3 (nmol l⁻¹)	1.7 ± 0.2	1.8 ± 0.1	2.0 ± 0.2	1.9 ± 0.2
FSH (U l⁻¹)	2.1 ± 0.4	2.2 ± 0.3	2.2 ± 0.3	2.2 ± 0.4
LH (U l⁻¹)	9.5 ± 5.4	10.0 ± 7.7	9.4 ± 5.3	9.4 ± 3.7
Testosterone (nmol l⁻¹)	32 ± 20	32 ± 16	31 ± 8	27 ± 7
Prolactin (μg l⁻¹)	14 ± 6	$32 \pm 14^{**}$	$29 \pm 21^*$	$24 \pm 12^*$
GH (μg l⁻¹)	0.6 ± 0.3	$10 \pm 4^{**}$	$3 \pm 1^*$	2 ± 2
Prolactin (μg l⁻¹) (females)	24 ± 10	11 ± 6	$106 \pm 22^{**}$	—

Mean ± SD is given (n = 7–10). *$P < .05$, and **$P < .01$ from the "before" values.
(Courtesy of Leppäluoto, J., et al.: Acta Physiol. Scand. 128:467–470, November 1986.)

of the experiments (table). It is thought that the release of prolactin in women was associated with the transient amenorrhea that occurred in five of seven subjects after the experiment.

Increased release of prolactin and perhaps of GH may be associated with the heat exposure-induced dehydration.

▶ It is a little unclear from the text whether subjects in this experiment undertook four ½-hour or two 1-hour sauna exposures per day. However, the increased output of prolactin and temporary amenorrhea draws further interesting parallels with an endurance exercise exposure.—R.J. Shephard, M.D., Ph.D.

Effects of Body Mass and Morphology on Thermal Responses in Water
Michael M. Toner, Michael N. Sawka, Michael E. Foley, and Kent B. Pandolf (U.S. Army Research Inst., Natick, Mass.)
J. Appl. Physiol. 60:521–525, February 1986   1–81

The surface area-to-mass ratio plays a role in the thermoregulation of human beings exposed either to high or to low temperatures. Thermal responses vary among individuals based on morphological and body mass characteristics. This study examines the role of these factors on the thermal and metabolic responses of persons immersed in water.

Ten healthy males were divided into two groups, to maximize differences in body mass and to minimize differences in subcutaneous and total body fat. All subjects were immersed in 26 C stirred water during rest and intense exercise. Oxygen uptake, rectal and esophageal temperatures, and skin temperatures were monitored constantly.

During resting exposures to water, metabolic rate and rectal temperature were similar between large- and small-body-mass groups. Esophageal temperature was higher and tissue insulation was lower in the low-mass group. During exercise, measurements of temperature and oxygen uptake were the same between groups.

At rest, large body mass increases overall tissue insulation, probably due to the large muscle volume. Exercise causes increased perfusion of the muscle mass, leading to lowered insulative properties, so that the thermal response is identical in large- and small-body-mass groups.

▶ It is increasingly recognized that insulation against a cold environment can be provided not only by fat but also by lightly perfused muscle (Sloan, R.E.G., and Keatinge, W.R.: *J. Appl. Physiol.* 35:371–375, 1973). For any given amount of body fat, a heavy person who falls into cold water thus has the dual advantage of a larger initial heat store and a greater potential muscular insulation.

The important practical lesson is that attempts to swim to safety increase heat loss, not only by stirring water flow over the body surface, but also by increasing muscle flow; the latter change dramatically reduces the insulation of the body. Unless the shore is close at hand, the optimum tactic for the capsized sailor is to crouch in the fetal position and await rescue (Hayward, J.S., et al.: *Can. J. Physiol. Pharmacol.* 53:21–32, 1975).—R.J. Shephard, M.D., Ph.D.

Energetics of Wet-Suit Diving in Japanese Male Breath-Hold Divers

K. Shiraki, S. Sagawa, N. Konda, Y.S. Park, and T. Komatsu, and S.K. Hong (Univ. of Occupational and Environmental Health, Kitakyushu, Japan, Kosin Medical College, Busan, Korea, and State Univ. of New York at Buffalo)
J. Appl. Physiol. 61:1475–1480, October 1986   1–82

Previous studies of professional breath-hold divers in Japan and Korea have focused primarily on female divers. However, in Japan the relative role of male divers in harvesting the ocean floor has become increasingly important. The diving pattern, respiratory function, and energy metabolism of Japanese male breath-hold divers were characterized, and these values were compared with those obtained in female divers of Korea.

The study population consisted of ten professional male breath-hold divers. The authors measured rectal and mean skin temperatures and rate of O_2 consumption during diving work in the summer (27 C water) and winter (14 C water), and thermal insulation and energy costs of diving work were estimated. In summer, comparisons were carried out on subjects who were clad either in wet suits (protected) or in swimming trunks (unprotected); in winter all divers wore wet suits. The average rectal temperature in unprotected divers decreased to 36.4 ± 0.2 C at the end of

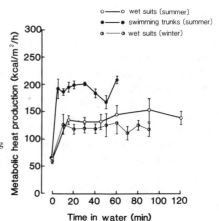

Fig 1–25.—Metabolic heat production during diving work in male divers. *Points* and *vertical bars,* means ± SE of four subjects. (Courtesy of Shiraki, K., et al.: J. Appl. Physiol. 61:1475– 1480, October 1980.)

1-hour diving work, but the average rectal temperature of protected divers decreased to 37.2 ± 0.3 C in 2 hours in the summer and to 36.9 ± 0.1 C in 1.5 hours in the winter. The average skin temperature of unprotected divers decreased to 28.0 ± 0.6 C in summer and that of protected divers decreased to 32.9 ± 0.5 C in summer and to 28.0 ± 0.3 C in winter. The average rate of O_2 consumption was observed to increase 190% (from 370 ml per minute before diving to 1,070 ml per minute) in unprotected divers in summer, but in protected divers it rose 120% (from 360 to 780 ml per minute in summer) and 110% (from 330 to 690 ml per minute) in winter. The increase in metabolic heat production was approximately 130% in protected divers and 220% in unprotected divers, with changes in protected divers in winter similar to those measured in summer (Fig 1– 25). The overall thermal insulation (tissue and wet suit) calculated for the protected divers was determined to be 0.065 ± 0.006 C/kcal/m^2 per hour in summer and 0.135 ± 0.019 C/kcal/m^2 per hour in winter. It was estimated that the total daily thermal cost of diving work was 425 kcal/ m^2 in summer (276 minutes of work) and 482 kcal/m^2 in winter (240 minutes of work).

When the present data were compared with similar data obtained for Korean female breath-holding divers, several differences were noted. The thermal balance during diving work was substantially different between male and female divers, with male divers having a significantly greater amount of extra heat production and a smaller reduction in body heat. The intensity of exercise during breath-hold diving was greater in male than in female divers. There was also a marked seasonal variation of thermal insulation in wet suit divers, with an increase in thermal insulation provided by the wet suit in winter; this phenomenon had not been observed in the Korean divers. Both studies suggested that the use of wet suits enabled divers to improve the thermal economy remarkably during diving work.

▶ One aspect of women's liberation has been an increasing influx of men into traditional female jobs. In Korea, the task of pearl diving was traditionally assigned to women, but is now increasingly undertaken by men. The other interesting development over the past few years has been adoption of the wet suit by divers of both sexes (Park, Y.S., et al.: *Undersea Biomed. Res.* 10:203–215, 1983). Earlier generations had pursued their occupation without such protection, even in winter, with a considerable exposure to cold stress. The availability of wet suits has greatly reduced the severity of cold exposure, with a substantial diminution in the energy requirements of diving. It has also led to a loss of cold adaptation, including nonshivering thermogenesis, which previously had been a marked feature of the diving women.—R.J. Shephard, M.D., Ph.D.

The Effects of Rapid Weight Loss and Rehydration on a Wrestling Performance Test
James E. Klinzing and William Karpowicz (Cleveland St. Univ. and Women's General Hosp., Cleveland)
J. Sports Med. 26:149–156, June 1986   1–83

It has been suggested that rapid weight loss is detrimental to physiologic function and individual performance requirements of wrestling. Despite this claim, many wrestlers lose from 8 to 20 pounds over a brief period in order to make a lower weight class. Weight loss is accomplished by exercise in rubber sweat suits, sitting in saunas or steam rooms, restricting fluid intake and use of laxative or diuretic drugs to accelerate fluid losses. As a result of this rapid weight loss, wrestlers are often dehydrated at the time of weigh-in and immediately prior to competition. Dehydration has been shown to cause substantial decreases in strength and muscular endurance, both of which are important factors in wrestling. The effects of a rapid 5% weight loss on wrestling performance were assessed.

WRESTLING PERFORMANCE SCORES: TIME AFTER WEIGH-IN				
	X̄ (sec)	SD	F-ratio *	p
First trial score - A				
1. No wt. loss	120.4	9.2	2.01	NS
2. 0-hour	123.1	7.1		
3. 1-hour	122.1	9.8		
4. 5-hour	118.9	7.9		
Second trial score - B				
1. No wt. loss	131.7	10.7	4.91	0.05 (2>1)
2. 0-hour	138.8	12.5		0.05 (2>4)
3. 1-hour	134.7	5.4		
4. 5-hour	129.4	9.0		
Total score				
1. No wt. loss	252.1	18.6	6.25	0.01 (2>4)
2. 0-hour	261.9	18.9		0.05 (2>1)
3. 1-hour	256.8	13.7		0.05 (3>4)
4. 5-hour	248.3	15.6		

*F-ratio at $P < .05$ = 3.16, and at $P < .01$ = 5.09 df trials -3; df experimental error = -18.
(Courtesy of Klinzing, J.E., and Karpowicz, W.: J. Sports Med. 26:149–156, June 1986.)

The study population consisted of seven healthy male subjects who were required to lose 5% of body weight by means of self-restricted fluid and food intake, dehydration, and exercise in 50 hours, immediately prior to a test which required the same performance factors as wrestling. Seven of the subjects were administered the test four times, including: after no weight loss, immediately after weight loss, 1 hour after weight loss, and 5 hours after weight loss. For the 1- and 5-hour tests, the subjects regained 22% and 44% of the lost weight. Performance was markedly slower when the test was taken immediately after making weight, somewhat improved at 1 hour but still significantly slower than the 5-hour performance test. After 5 hours of ad libitum fluid and/or food consumption, performance scores returned to baseline (table).

Wrestlers who lose up to 5% of their weight a few days before making weight at a lower weight class and then partially or fully regain their lost weight over a 5-hour period are not harming their performance.

▶ It is a sad commentary on U.S. sportsmanship that even at the high school level competitors are prepared to undergo a major weight loss in order to gain an unfair edge over their competitors (Tipton, C.M., and Tcheng, T.K.: *JAMA* 214:1269, 1969).

Some previous reports have suggested that muscular strength is not fully restored even after several hours of fluid replenishment. It is difficult to obtain an unequivocal answer to this question, since most of the tests of muscular strength and performance require voluntary effort on the part of the subject, and scores can be influenced by the individual's beliefs concerning the effects of dehydration upon performance. However, there seems little argument that the short-term effect of massive dehydration on performance is deleterious; thus, in regions where unsportsmanlike weight loss is endemic, the extent of the abuse could be minimized if weights were checked immediately before competition.—R.J. Shephard, M.D., Ph.D.

Fluid Balance in Exercise Dehydration and Rehydration With Different Glucose-Electrolyte Drinks
Bodil Nielsen, Gisela Sjøgaard, Jacob Ugelvig, Bo Knudsen, and Bengt Dohlmann (Univ. of Copenhagen)
Eur. J. Appl. Physiol. 55:318–325, June 1986   1–84

Large amounts of water may be lost from the body during prolonged exercise. This water loss results from thermoregulatory sweating and an increase in the water content of exercising muscles. Both of these events contribute to a reduction in plasma volume and to an increased plasma osmolality; the reduced plasma volume is thought to be the cause of the higher heart rate and core temperature observed after prolonged exercise. Much attention has been focused on the restoration of plasma volume as a main factor involved in the restoration of exercise performance; nevertheless, the composition of the fluid is also likely to be of significance for the recovery of plasma volume after exercise. Recently tested was the

MUSCLE POTASSIUM, SODIUM, GLYCOGEN, GLUCOSE, AND LACTATE IN MMOL · KG^{-1} DRY
WEIGHT AND WATER IN 1 · KG^{-1} DRY WEIGHT MEASURED BEFORE AND AFTER EXERCISE
DEHYDRATION, AND AFTER 2 H REHYDRATION WITH THE FOUR DRINKS,
MEAN VALUES ± 1 SD

Dry weight values		Rest			After dehydration		After rehydration			
K	C	404	± 18		389	± 39	411	± 16	⎫	
mmol · kg^{-1}	K	415	± 15		407	± 60	426	± 22	⎬	n = 6
	Na	400	± 19		388	± 42	415	± 26	⎭	
	S	433			372		401			n = 2
Na	C	87	± 29		94	± 26	75	± 14	⎫	
mmol · kg^{-1}	K	72	± 26		103	± 31	95	± 30	⎬	n = 6
	Na	84	± 37		117	± 53	77	± 19	⎭	
	S	76			144		72			n = 2
glycogen	C	392	± 43		233	± 103	259	± 47	⎫	
mmol · kg^{-1}	K	427	± 47		251	± 88	244	± 120	⎬	n = 6
	Na	429	± 121		245	± 79	319 *	± 38	⎭	
	S	335			223		286			n = 2
glucose	C	0.70±	0.46		1.25±	1.04	0.65±	0.53	⎫	
mmol · kg^{-1}	K	1.34±	1.02		0.70±	0.55	2.19±	1.90	⎬	n = 6
	Na	0.67±	0.36		1.37±	0.96	1.33±	1.04	⎭	
	S	1.51			1.67		1.52			n = 2
lactate	C	63	± 36		88	± 41	79	± 26	⎫	
mmol · kg^{-1}	K	66	± 40		84	± 49	77	± 60	⎬	n = 6
	Na	68	± 41		86	± 83	71	± 51	⎭	
	S	60			116		78			n = 2
H$_2$O	C	3.18±	0.02		3.31±	0.03	317 *±	0.02	⎫	
1 · kg^{-1}	K	3.17±	0.02		3.26±	0.03	3.20 ±	0.03	⎬	n = 6
	Na	3.17±	0.04		3.42±	0.02	3.12*±	0.02	⎭	
	S	3.24			3.31		3.22			n = 2

*Differed significantly from after dehydration.
(Courtesy of Nielsen, B., et al.: Eur. J. Appl. Physiol. 55:318–325, June 1986.)

hypothesis that drinks with a high osmolality after absorption produce
the greatest plasma volume expansion and best restore physical work
capacity.

The study population consisted of six male subjects, mean age 24 years
(range, 18 to 32 years). Restoration of water and electrolyte balance was
followed after exercise dehydration (3% of body weight). During a 2-hour
rest period after exercise, the subjects were given 9 × 300-ml portions of
a drink at 15-minute intervals. The drinks included control (C-drink), high
potassium (K-drink), high sodium (Na-drink), or high sugar (S-drink). The
subjects performed an exercise test before dehydration and after rehydration. Dehydration reduced the plasma volume by 16%; this process was
reversed on resting even before fluid ingestion began, as a result of release
of water accumulated in muscle during exercise. After 2 hours of rehydration, plasma volume was noted to be above initial resting value with
all four drinks. Nevertheless, the final plasma volumes after the Na-drink
(+14%) and C-drink (+9%) were markedly higher than after the K- and
S-drinks (table).

The Na-drink favored filling of the extracellular compartment, while
the K- and S-drinks favored intracellular rehydration. Despite the higher
than normal plasma volume following rehydration, mean heart rate was

found to be 10 bpm higher after rest and rehydration than during the initial test. Furthermore, the amount of work that could be performed in the supramaximal test (105% Vo_{2max}) was 20% less after exercise dehydration and subsequent rest and rehydration than before. This reduction is similar for all drinks and may be the result of decreased muscle glycogen content.

▶ Most authors who have looked at exercise dehydration have considered replacement fluids to be given during competition, and it is thus useful to have an article that considers the process of rehydration after the competition is over.

While the constancy of plasma composition during exercise is best assured by the drinking of unadulterated water, there is plainly a need to replace lost minerals and sugar during the first few hours following vigorous activity. I have argued that a normal intake of fluids with some extra salting of meals is probably adequate treatment during recovery, but a great deal will depend on the interval prior to further exercise. If one is anticipating a further bout of prolonged exercise within a few hours, then there could theoretically be some advantage in a more controlled replacement of the missing mineral elements. The present report offers the competitor four alternative drinks, all of which fail to restore work tolerance completely; unfortunately, there is no control group who are left to follow a more "natural" recovery regimen.—R.J. Shephard, M.D., Ph.D.

Factors Affecting the Gastric Emptying of Athletic Drinks
Gary Lee Harrelson (Univ. of Southern Mississippi at Hattiesburg)
Athletic Training 21:20–21, Spring 1986   1–85

It is well established that one of the most efficient ways to prevent heat illness is by unlimited consumption of water. This is because the human body consists of 40% to 60% water by weight, and water plays a vital role in the transfer of heat from internal to external environment. Athletes who exercise in the heat have been shown to lose between 4,000 and 6,000 ml of water daily, and this must be replaced in order to avoid dehydration. When replacing fluid orally, one must consider gastric emptying into the intestine where the fluid can be absorbed. Gastric emptying is known to be affected by the volume and osmolality of the solution consumed; the type and concentrations of solute in the solution; the temperature of the solution and exercise; and criteria for selecting a drink. The goal of the present study was to examine fluid replacement through commercially available drinks.

A high osmolality of the solution, which is incurred by adding sugar and electrolytes sufficient to produce a solution osmolality greater than 210 mOsm/L, will slow gastric emptying. Furthermore, the ingestion of solutions with volumes greater than 600 ml will slow gastric emptying, but gastric emptying can be enhanced with a cold solution of approximately 5 C. Exercise has little effect on gastric emptying so long as the workload is not greater than 70% of the individual's aerobic capacity.

The author recommends that commercial drinks not be used at full strength but rather should be diluted with two times the amount of water. He further points out that the needs of athletes vary depending on the sport in which they are engaged. Athletes who participate in events that require the rapid replacement of water should avoid solutions diluted with sugar.

▶ The most important section of my lecture on "Nutrition and the Athlete" is the fluid replacement section. Athletes and coaches continue to have some very strange ideas on this subject. Withholding water is no way to build mental toughness in an athlete. Performance can be improved and deaths can be prevented by providing unlimited consumption of water. Thirst is not a good indicator of the body's need to replace fluid. In some instances athletes playing in hot, humid conditions should be forced to drink water prior to, during, and after the contest. In a 2½-hour practice on a hot and humid day I would expect a 100-man football squad to go through more than 100 gallons of chilled water. It takes a concerted effort on the part of the trainers, managers, and coaches to provide the water and the time to drink the water. It is a very important part of our practice on hot days. We have found that the easiest way to provide this water is through a number of strategically placed, portable water pumps. We use as many as eight pumps for a 100-man squad. They are moved from individual groups to team groups and are refilled as needed.—F. George, A.T.C., P.T.

Physiology of Specific Sports

The Enigma of the Collapsed Marathon Runner
Mark D. Altschule (Harvard Univ.)
Chest 89:291, February 1986   1–86

Sudden death is well documented in trained long distance runners, skiers, and swimmers. However, the etiology of collapse at or near the end of a race in marathon runners remains obscure.

Although spontaneous pneumothorax can be easily excluded by physical examination, the diagnosis of myocardial infarction as a cause of collapse in marathon runners remains an enigma. Obtaining an ECG is not reliable under the circumstances. Levels of serum creatine kinase activity or MB isoenzyme, enzymes that are specific in the diagnosis of myocardial infarction, have been shown to be increased as well in endurance athletes after a race. These increases in healthy but exhausted athletes and patients with myocardial infarction are not significantly different as a whole, but the rate of clearance seems to be more rapid in exhausted athletes. There is yet no proof that the enzymes do not originate from the myocardium of normal exhausted athletes. Except for the signs of tissue damage in the myocardial infarction, such as fever, leukocytosis, and elevated sedimentation rate, clinical judgment at the time of clinical presentation remains the main diagnostic recourse.

As one Nobel recipient said, "One has to be a good clinician to interpret laboratory data." Biochemical tests describe biologic phenomena and do not have specificity required for clinical diagnosis. As yet, one has to rely on clinical judgment in the assessment of the collapsed marathon runner.

▶ A legendary clinician deals with the problem of marathon collapse. His comments are of value on the common false positivity of the cardiogram in this situation, the frequent unreliability of allegedly muscle and cardiac-specific enzymes, and the absence of any reliable laboratory tests short of fever, leukocytosis, and sedimentation rate elevation. A case is made for clinical judgment at the time of clinical presentation as the main diagnostic recourse. This may be a relatively rare quality and stands against rapidly increasing technological testing and ever-increasing numbers of entrants in any given race, local or national.—L.J. Krakauer, M.D.

The Immediate and Delayed Effects of Marathon Running on Renal Function
R.A. Irving, T.D. Noakes, G.A. Irving, and R. Van Zyl-Smit (Univ. of Cape Town, South Africa)
J. Urol. 136:1176–1180, December 1986   1–87

Acute renal failure associated with rhabdomyolysis, myoglobinemia, and hyperuricemia in marathon runners has been previously reported. However, the renal response to marathon running has not yet been clearly defined, partly because all previous studies to that effect have been of short duration and did not include analysis of 24-hour urine collections. The authors studied renal function in marathon runners before and after the event.

The study was done in six healthy male runners who had no history of renal disease. Daily blood samples and 24-hour urine specimens were collected for 2 days before and for 5 days following participation in a 42-km marathon which was run over a hilly course in South Africa under cool and rainy conditions.

Renal function was well maintained and creatine levels were normal during the marathon. However, marked changes were noted during the recovery period, including sodium retention during the first 24 to 48 hours following the race, followed by sustained diuresis of a more dilute urine. Glomerular proteinuria was present only on the first day after the marathon. All racers experienced muscle damage as shown by increased postrace serum creatine clearance and increased C-reactive protein levels.

The observed postrace changes in renal function are probably the result of catabolic, followed by anabolic processes which take place in muscles after prolonged exercise.

▶ We are provided with more data on the kidney in the extreme of marathon running thanks to the more elaborate 24-hour urine collection techniques. Previously unrecognized delayed effects of prolonged exercise on renal function may be substantial. This reflects catabolic processes followed by anabolic processes in muscle, and changes that may relate to excess sodium retention and the related fluid compartment shifts. The postrace interval of several days may be critical in the study of physiologic change in multiple systems.—L.J. Krakauer, M.D.

Changes in Adrenal and Testicular Activity Monitored by Salivary Sampling in Males Throughout Marathon Runs

N.J. Cook, G.F. Read, R.F. Walker, B. Harris, and D. Riad-Fahmy (Tenovus Inst. for Cancer Research, and Univ. of Wales, Cardiff)
Eur. J. Appl. Physiol. 55:634–638, November 1986   1–88

Increased cortisol and lower testosterone concentrations have been described in distance runners. The fall in testosterone could reflect a catecholamine-mediated reduction in testicular blood flow, or a direct inhibitory effect of a high cortisol level on the testis. Noninvasive salivary

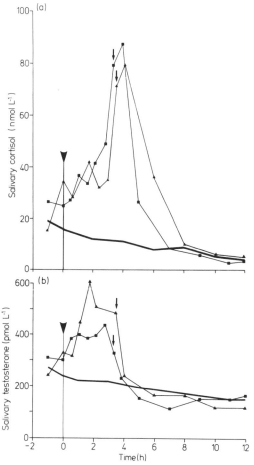

Fig 1–26.—A, mean salivary cortisol concentrations in runners during the Cardiff and Bristol marathons. B, mean salivary testosterone concentrations during the Cardiff and Bristol marathons. ▲, Bristol marathon; ■, Cardiff marathon; —, baseline on rest days; ▼, start; ↓, finish. (Courtesy of Cook, N.J., et al.: Eur. J. Appl. Physiol. 55:634–638, November 1986.)

sampling was used to monitor changes in adrenal and testicular activity during competition in nonelite marathon runners. Eight healthy men with a mean age of 35 years participated in the study. The mean training distance was 47 miles per week for several weeks before the marathon run. Samples were collected six times during the run and at intervals afterwards.

The rate of missed samples was lower than 10%. Both cortisol and testosterone levels were elevated just before the marathon began, compared with nonrun days. Levels of both steroids increased during the run. Testosterone levels peaked at 21 miles into the 26-mile run, while cortisol levels peaked 30 minutes after the end of the run. Comparison of hormone values with those from another marathon for four runners showed similar results (Fig 1–26).

Salivary sampling is a useful approach to monitoring acute and cyclical changes in endocrine function in distance runners. The temporal relation between changes in salivary cortisol and testosterone levels is consistent with direct inhibition of testicular secretion by a high cortisol concentration.

▶ Athletes are understandably reluctant to allow multiple blood-sampling in either monitoring or treatment, and the development of a method of assaying hormones in saliva is thus a valuable innovation.

The actual data provide one more piece of evidence concerning a depression of male testicular function by prolonged running.—R.J. Shephard, M.D., Ph.D.

Decreased Hypothalamic Gonadotropin-Releasing Hormone Secretion in Male Marathon Runners

Susan E. MacConnie, Ariel Barkan, Richard M. Lampman, M. Anthony Schork, and Inese Z. Beitins (Univ. of Michigan)
N. Engl. J. Med. 315:411–417, Aug. 14, 1986   1–89

Although it is known that long distance running has beneficial effects on the cardiovascular and musculoskeletal systems and on the metabolic control of diabetes and obesity, information about possible untoward effects is incomplete. For example, strenuous physical exercise alters the integrity of various neuroendocrine systems, and in women, an exercise-induced deficiency of the hypothalamic secretion of gonadotropin-releasing hormone results in the syndrome "hypothalamic amenorrhea." However, the signs of hypogonadism in men may be clinically inapparent. The goal of this study was to determine whether a phenomenon comparable to hypothalamic amenorrhea also occurs in male athletes.

The study population consisted of six male marathon runners who were running 125 to 200 km per week. The authors investigated the integrity of the hypothalamic-pituitary-gonadal axis in these subjects. The mean frequency of spontaneous luteinizing hormone pulses was diminished in the runners, as compared with healthy controls (2.2 ± 0.48 vs. 3.6 ± 0.24 pulses per 8 hours). In addition, the amplitude of the pulses was also low in the runners (0.9 ± 0.24 vs. 1.6 ± 0.15 mIU/ml), and the responses

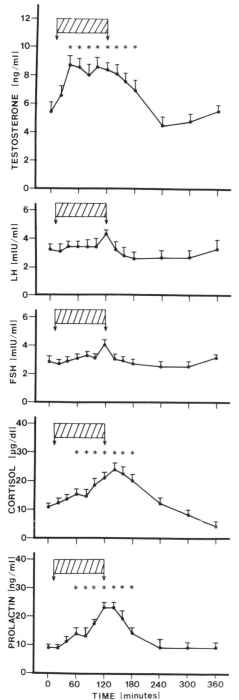

Fig 1–27.—Plasma hormone concentrations in male marathon runners before, during, and after a 2-hour treadmill run at 72 percent of maximum oxygen consumption. The exercise period is denoted by the striped rectangle; LH denotes luteinizing hormone, and FSH denotes follicle-stimulating hormone. Basal values (0 minutes) were calculated as the means ± SE of all measurements during the 6-hour period before the exercise. The asterisks denote hormone levels for which $P < .01$ vs. basal values. (Courtesy of MacConnie, S.E., et al.: N. Engl. J. Med. 315:411–417, Aug. 14, 1986. Reprinted by permission of The New England Journal of Medicine.

of luteinizing hormone to gradually increasing doses of exogenous gonadotropin-releasing hormone were decreased. Plasma testosterone levels were similar in the two groups and increased equally in response to an intramuscular injection of 2,000 units of human chorionic gonadotropin. During short-term intense physical exercise, the plasma gonadotropin levels in the athletes were found to be stable, but marked elevations in plasma levels of cortisol, prolactin, and testosterone occurred (Fig 1–27).

Highly trained male athletes, like their female counterparts, may have a deficiency of hypothalamic gonadotropin-releasing hormone. This condition may be due to the prolonged repetitive elevations of gonadal steroids and other hormones known to suppress gonadotropin-releasing hormone secretion that are elicited by their daily exercise.

▶ It is well recognized that vigorous exercise reduces the secretion of hypothalamic gonadotropin-releasing hormone in women, but evidence is now accumulating that there is a similar response in male athletes.

In the present study, testosterone levels were normal, suggesting that levels of gonadotropin are less critical to normal function in men than in women. However, other authors have described suppression of both testosterone production and spermatogenesis in men undergoing intensive physical training (Ayers, J.Y., et al.: *Fertil. Steril.* 43:917–921, 1985; Wheeler, G.D., et al.: *JAMA* 252:514–516, 1984). The long-term implications for fertility have yet to be worked out, but it is probable that as in women the condition is reversible once very strenuous exercise is halted.—R.J. Shephard, M.D., Ph.D.

Gastrointestinal Blood Loss Associated With Running a Marathon
Marshall E. McCabe III, David A. Peura, Shailesh C. Kadakia, Zdenek Bocek, and Lawrence F. Johnson (Walter Reed Army Med. Ctr. and Uniformed Services Univ. of the Health Sciences, Bethesda, Md.)
Dig. Dis. Sci. 31:1229–1232, November 1986   1–90

Long-distance running can be associated with a number of nonorthopedic problems, including gastrointestinal tract bleeding. A large, prospective study was conducted among runners of all ages with a wide range of ability levels to assess the risk of gastrointestinal bleeding in marathon races.

A total of 600 questionnaires were sent to subjects who had participated in a marathon race. The questionnaire contained questions about age, sex, whether the race had been completed, and elapsed time for the 26-mile course and questions about premarathon, intramarathon, and postmarathon gastrointestinal symptoms. The participants were also questioned about the use of aspirin and vitamin C before the race, and about whether they had eaten steak within 24 hours before the marathon. Each participant also received a set of six Hemoccult cards to test for occult fecal blood.

Of the 600 runners with whom contact was made, 125 (21%) (68 males) returned the questionnaire and stool specimens within 12 days of the first stool collection. Of 125 respondents, 120 had finished the marathon, and

117 (94%) reported their race time. In 29 participants (23%), stool specimens converted from Hemoccult negative to positive, which indicated that running the marathon was associated with gastrointestinal blood loss. Gastrointestinal bleeding did not appear to be associated with age, race time, abdominal symptoms, or recent ingestion of aspirin, vitamin C, or steak. Twenty-seven runners (22%) reported gastrointestinal symptoms during or after the race, and 21 participants (17%) reported previous hematochezia associated with running.

▶ Stool specimens converted from Hemoccult negative to positive in 29 (23%) of 125 participants, suggesting GI blood loss without question and noting that the test used is fairly insensitive. Whether this is due to traumatic jarring or ischemia is not known. Hemoglobin levels were not obtained in this series to correlate with the documented GI blood loss. Reference is made to the discussion of anemia and its complex causation in the athlete by Eichner et al. in the previous section.—L.J. Krakauer, M.D.

Gastrointestinal Bleeding in Competitive Runners
Rosemarie L. Fisher, Laurence F. McMahon, Jr., Michael J. Ryan, Daniel Larson, and Myron Brand (Yale Univ.)
Dig. Dis. Sci. 31:1226–1228, November 1986   1–91

Four cases are presented of runners with iron deficiency anemia and with guaiac positivity and/or rectal bleeding.

CASE 1.—Woman, 20, was referred for evaluation of an iron deficiency anemia and guaiac-positive stools. She was found to be of excellent health except for infrequent episodes of hemorrhoidal bleeding. No gastrointestinal pathologic findings were observed despite extensive examination, and iron replacement was begun for a low reticulocyte count and hematocrit reading. She experienced several more guaiac-positive stools, which temporally were related to periods of heavy running. After stopping running, no further guaiac-positive stools or anemia were present.

CASE 2.—A woman runner, 22, suffered from anemia and guaiac-positive stools. Colonoscopic examination demonstrated a 2-mm red spot in the cecum that was not thought to be responsible for her gastrointestinal tract bleeding. After stopping long distance running, stool guaiacs were negative, her hematocrit reading was stable, and she no longer needed iron supplements.

CASE 3.—Woman, 37, who had been a runner for more than 5 years, experienced lower abdominal pain and passed bright red blood rectally while jogging. A second episode occurred 3 weeks later while jogging again. Findings on colonoscopic and sigmoidoscopic examination were negative.

CASE 4.—A female marathon runner, 33, experienced maroon diarrhea with midabdominal cramping while racing. She took six to eight aspirins a day, but her bleeding time was normal. While gastrointestinal tests did not yield any positive diagnosis, this condition periodically reexhibited itself.

It is thus suggested that gastrointestinal tract blood loss in competitive runners is not unusual, nor is the inability to locate a fixed organic cause for the latter.

Possible causes could include stress, gastritis, drug-induced lesions, and ischemic injury. In prior literature on exercise physiology, marked decreases in visceral blood flow are seen as exercised subjects approach their maximum oxygen consumption. The clinical implications of iron depletion are unclear at present. Further studies are recommended.

▶ This validates the former study in terms of general incidence and the lack of a precise etiology for the bleeding phenomenon. The case reports provided are not sufficient to make the conclusion that ischemia is the most likely cause, nor that iron store deficiency without frank anemia is responsible for decreased performance.

Note that we have four possible causes for anemia in the runner: dilutional, iron deficiency, footstrike hemolysis, and now gastrointestinal blood loss. The last is not likely to be a significant contributory factor, but that too remains an unknown and will be highly individualized.—L.J. Krakauer, M.D.

Blood Platelet Activation and Increase in Thrombin Activity Following a Marathon Race
L. Röcker, W.K. Drygas, and B. Heyduck (Free Univ. of Berlin and Med. Academy of Lodz, Poland)
Eur. J. Appl. Physiol. 55:374–380, August 1986   1–92

There is general consensus that persons of all ages should try to be as physically active as possible to prevent disease and promote general well-being. However, strenuous physical activity may not be totally beneficial, as indicated by recent reports of sudden cardiovascular deaths connected with strenuous physical exertion. Some data suggest that intracoronary platelet aggregates and coronary spasm due to thromboxane release from aggregating platelets may be responsible for myocardial infarction or sudden death after strenuous exercise, but little is known about the mechanisms involved. Hemostatic changes were studied in 16 healthy, well-trained male amateur runners, aged 16 to 48 years. Blood samples were drawn 15 minutes before a marathon, within 1 minute of the end of the run, and 60 minutes and 22 hours later. Prothrombin, thrombin, reptilase, and partial thromboplastin times and β-thromboglobulin (β-TG), platelet factor 4 (PF_4), fibrinopeptide A (FPA), factor VIII, fibrinogen, antithrombin III, and α_2-antiplasmin values were measured.

After the marathon race, there was a significant increase in all runners in plasma β-TG, PF_4, FPA, and factor VIII values. The β-TG concentration and factor VIII activity were still significantly elevated 60 minutes after the race. The FPA concentration, which had continued to rise after completion of the run, reached a peak at 60 minutes after the race. At 22 hours, the factor VIII concentration was still significantly elevated.

Although no conclusions can be drawn as to the relation between marathon race-induced hemostatic changes and sudden cardiovascular complications, it seems prudent to warn persons at special risk of myocardial infarction or sudden death during exercise because of changes in their clotting mechanisms to abstain from strenuous exercise.

▶ For a long time, Dr. Tom Bassler propagated the myth that participation in marathon races would grant absolute protection against myocardial infarction. T. D. Noakes et al. (*N. Engl. J. Med.* 301:86–89, 1979) provided convincing proof that this protection was no more than a myth, and the present report indicates that in some men running over a marathon distance can cause adverse changes in clotting mechanisms. In general, vigorous exercise seems to cause an immediate increase in clotting tendency through thromboxane release from the platelets, with a longer lasting increase of thrombolysis (a combined reaction to prostacyclin and plasminogen activator release from the endothelial wall, and secretion of antithrombin III and protein C); whether exercise is helpful or disadvantageous to the coronary-prone subject depends on the relative balance of these various processes. In some people, the effect of prolonged exercise upon the clotting tendency seems to outweigh fibrinolysis, and such individuals might well be warned against marathon participation.—R.J. Shephard, M.D., Ph.D.

The Mean Red Cell Volume in Long Distance Runners
M. Staübli and B. Roessler (Inselspital, Berne, Switzerland)
Eur. J. Appl. Physiol. 55:49–53, April 1986   1–93

Some, but not all, studies demonstrate changes in mean red cell volume (MCV) and mean corpuscular hemoglobin concentration (MCHC) in response to exercise. The lack of agreement may be due to the use of two different methods of measurement. These authors studied various red blood cell (RBC) indices in long-distance runners using Coulter Counter determinations and centrifuged hematocrit, RBC count, and hemoglobin measurements.

Six long-distance runners with more than 7 years' experience trained daily for a 100-km race. Following each training session before and after the race, blood was drawn and analyzed. Hemoglobin, RBC count, MCV, and MCHC were determined by Coulter Counter (CC) and from calculated values from centrifuged (ctrf) hematocrit, RBC count, and hemoglobin measurements. Urine hemoglobin concentrations were also measured.

Following the race, MCV (ctrf) decreased by 4.9% and MCV (CC) increased by 1.9%. MCHC (ctrf) increased by 4% and MCHC (CC) decreased by 3% (table). Low urine hemoglobin levels showed that hemolysis had not occurred. Hematocrit values and plasma volume were stable throughout the observation period.

The decrease in MCV (ctrf) and the increase in plasma osmolality immediately after the race are not correlated, suggesting that plasma osmolality alone is not the predominant factor in regulation of red cell volume. The body might use changes in MCV (ctrf), which contribute to the stability of the hematocrit value and plasma volume, to maintain a

CHANGES OF HEMATOLOGIC VARIABLES (n = 6)

Day of sampling	Hct (ctrf) %	Hct (ctrf) %Δ	Hct (CC) %	Hct (CC) %Δ	Hemoglobin g·dl⁻¹	Hemoglobin %Δ	Plasma-volume %Δ	RBC X 10⁶·μl⁻¹	RBC %Δ	Reticulocytes %
-3d	42.0±2.6		42.8±2.7		14.6±1.0			4.67±0.44		0.7±0.5
-1d	41.2±2.5[c]	-2.0±1.8	43.4±2.6[c]	+1.4±1.2[b]	14.6±0.9	0±1.4	+1.1±2.0	4.72±0.41	+1.2±1.7	1.2±0.4
imm. post	41.3±3.1	-1.6±3.4	45.0±3.8	+5.0±4.5[b]	14.9±1.2	+2.2±3.3	-1.0±5.1	4.82±0.55	+3.1±3.9	0.9±0.3
+6½ d	42.5±2.0	+1.3±4.0	44.5±2.6[a]	+2.9±4.8[b,a]	14.7±1.0	+0.2±4.5	-0.6±6.4	4.76±0.46[a]	+3.4±5.5[a]	0.8±0.6
+20½ d	42.7±3.1	+1.6±2.0	42.4±2.8	-0.9±2.2[b]	14.7±1.0	+0.8±1.1	-1.6±1.5	4.59±0.42	-1.6±2.9	0.7±0.2

Day of sampling	MCV (ctrf) fl	MCV (ctrf) %Δ	MCV (CC) fl	MCV (CC) %Δ	MCHC (ctrf) fl	MCHC (ctrf) %Δ	MCHC (CC) %	MCHC (CC) %Δ	Osmolality mosM	Osmolality %Δ
-3d	90.4±6.6		92.1±6.6		34.4±0.8		33.8±0.4		299±2.8	
-1d	87.2±4.9[c]	-3.4±2.4	92.1±5.6	0±1.4[b]	35.1±0.6	+2.1±2.1	33.3±0.4	-1.4±1.5[b]		
imm. post	86.0±5.7[c]	-4.9±2.2	93.7±5.4[c]	+1.9±1.6[b]	35.8±1.0[c]	+4.0±1.5[c]	32.7±0.4[c]	-3.0±1.8[b]	305±3.9[c]	+2.1±1.6
+6½ d	90.1±4.8[c,a]	-2.4±1.3[a]	91.8±5.9	-0.2±1.0[b]	34.0±1.1	-1.2±2.4	33.0±0.4[c,a]	-2.2±1.7[b,a]		
+20½ d	94.7±5.7[c]	+3.3±2.2	92.6±5.9	+0.6±1.4[b]	34.1±1.2	-0.8±2.4	34.3±0.7	+1.7±2.1[b]		

a, n = 5.

b, significant difference between percent changes of Coulter Counter values (CC) vs. values derived from hematocrit centrifugation (ctrf).

c, significant difference vs. the value on day −3; % Δ values refer to values on day −3. Values are means ± SD. Differences considered significant at $P < .05$ as calculated by analysis of paired data.

(Courtesy of Stäubli, M., and Roessler, B.: Eur. J. Appl. Physiol. 55:49–53, April, 1986.)

favorable blood viscosity. Coulter Counter MCV determination does not appear to reflect in vivo changes in MCV due to training and competition.

▶ The Coulter Counter is widely used to allow automated determinations of mean red cell volume, and it is thus important to note that this instrument can yield erroneous values during exercise (the Coulter instrument dilutes the blood in a buffer of constant pH and osmolality, compensating for exercise-induced changes and allowing the red cells a chance to return to their preexercise dimensions).

The decrease of cell size following prolonged endurance exercise is one more example of the adaptability of the body; although plasma volume is decreased by a combination of sweating and extravasation of fluid into the active tissues, the viscosity of the blood is held relatively constant, so that the heart of the exercising subject is not working against an excessive blood viscosity.—R.J. Shephard, M.D., Ph.D.

Blood Lead Levels of South African Long-Distance Road-Runners
Sias R. Grobler, Leon S. Maresky, and Roelof J. Rossouw (Univ. of Stellenbosch, Tygerberg, South Africa)
Arch. Environ. Health 41:155–158, May–June 1986   1–94

Average blood lead concentrations in the United States dropped by about 37% after the lead content of gasoline was significantly reduced in the late 1970s. In South Africa, the presence of the antiknock additive tetraalkyl lead caused lead waste deposits in the atmosphere and in the soil. There has been a large increase in road running by persons of all ages who, when running in urban areas, expose themselves to increased lead inhalation and the danger of lead intoxication due to sustained elevated blood lead concentrations. The authors measured blood lead concentrations in South African marathon road runners and determined to what extent the training environment influenced the concentrations.

The study was performed in long-distance road runners who had par-

WHOLE BLOOD LEAD CONCENTRATIONS ($\mu g/dl$) OF RURAL AND URBAN AREA TRAINERS FOR THE COMRADES MARATHON

	Rural trainers ($N^* = 29$)	Urban trainers ($N = 51$)
Mean	20.1	51.9
Standard deviation	10.6	16.7
Median	17.7	55.5
Range	4.2-42.8	19.9-77.7

*Number of samples.

ticipated in either of the two major marathons held in Capetown each year. Blood samples were obtained before and after a marathon was run, and lead concentrations were determined by absorption spectrophotometry. Control samples were obtained from selected urban nonrunning subjects and from runners living in remote rural areas.

Urban runners had significantly higher blood lead concentrations than the control subjects, and rural runners had the lowest values (table). There was also a significant difference in blood lead concentrations in samples taken before and after the marathons were run, with postmarathon samples showing the highest values.

Road runners are exposed to increased lead inhalation. Atmospheric lead concentrations differ significantly between urban and rural areas of South Africa.

▶ The elevated blood lead levels in South African runners is disquieting and perhaps only the tip of the iceberg. To be sure, in this country much less leaded gasoline is used, but the volume of travel and the lack of total catalytic conversion in automobiles remain a problem. That there are multiple other pollutants in the atmosphere and that many runs are carried out in a polluted atmosphere is an unspoken problem of athletic performance in urban centers at least, and along highways that are well traveled. At its simplest level, this is a significant concern for urban South African runners in terms of lead concentration alone.—L.J. Krakauer, M.D.

Hypertension in the Runner
Arthur Dodek (Univ. of British Columbia)
Primary Cardiol. 12:14–26, July 1986   1–95

As a result of the increased popularity of running and other forms of exercise, many hypertensive patients are already participating in, or are planning to start, a running or exercise program. The author discusses the medical management of hypertensive patients involved in running or other physical activities.

Earlier studies have shown that physical training reduces resting heart rate and increases stroke volume without changing resting cardiac output. Although the role of sustained exercise in reducing cardiovascular mortality is controversial, it has been shown that exercise can reduce uncomplicated essential hypertension.

Data from diagnostic exercise testing with a treadmill or an upright bicycle ergometer may be used for early prediction of hypertension. Studies have shown that subjects with treadmill exercise blood pressures (BP) of more than 225/90 mm Hg are at increased risk of developing hypertension. Maximal exercise tests can be applied to hypertensive adolescents to identify those who have dangerously high BP responses to exercise. Such patients should be excluded from isometric exercise, but they need not be restricted from isotonic exercise, which may reduce their BP.

Although one diuretic or a combination of agents is often used to reduce

BP in mildly hypertensive patients, such agents are not appropriate for the treatment of runners because of potential volume depletion, natriuresis, hypokalemia, and metabolic side effects. β-Blockers are much more effective in the treatment of hypertensive athletes, since they reduce exercise heart rate and cardiac output for a given oxygen uptake.

Essential hypertension is not per se a contraindication to exercise training. Such training may even be beneficial in lowering of BP, provided proper diagnostic stress testing is performed.

▶ This article is presented in this section rather than in the general discussion of hypertension because so many individuals with mild hypertension are using running as a therapy, many quite successfully. In these people, it is all the more imperative that a thorough physical workup and laboratory workup be carried out before a commitment to running seriously is made, and before any commitment to specific therapy. Diuretics should be relatively contraindicated because of volume depletion and electrolyte loss. If β-blockers are selected, the long-term use of selective agents has been shown to be without diminished cardiac output or diminished maximal O_2 uptake in prior study (1986 YEAR BOOK OF SPORTS MEDICINE, p. 34). Note also that muscle fatigue may present in persons taking β-blocking agents, especially if the nonselective broader agents such as propranolol are used. This may be via slower heart rate and a delay in transfer of lactate from the muscular to the vascular compartment, as Shephard has suggested (1986 YEAR BOOK OF SPORTS MEDICINE, p. 35).—L.J. Krakauer, M.D.

Is Running Associated With Degenerative Joint Disease?

Richard S. Panush, Carolyn Schmidt, Jacques R. Caldwell, N. Lawrence Edwards, Selden Longley, Richard Yonker, Ella Webster, Janet Nauman, John Stork, Holger Pettersson (Univ. of Florida and VA Med. Ctr., Gainesville)
JAMA 255:1152–1154, March 7, 1986   1–96

The long-term consequences of regular recreational exercise are unknown. Populations of male runners and nonrunners were compared to determine whether long-term relatively high-mileage running was associated with premature degenerative joint disease in the lower extremities. Seventeen runners who ran a minimum of 20 miles weekly for at least the past 5 consecutive years and 18 nonrunners who did not run daily were included in the study. All subjects were at least 50 years of age. Subjects filled out a questionnaire regarding medical and exercise history, were examined by a rheumatologist, and underwent roentgenographic analysis of the hips, knees, and feet.

Musculoskeletal histories and physical findings were comparable between the two groups. There were no significant differences between the two groups with regard to osteophytes, cartilage thickness, or degenerative changes in the lower extremity joints. Reasonably long duration high-mileage running need not be associated with premature degenerative joint disease of the lower extremities.

Long-Distance Running, Bone Density, and Osteoarthritis

Nancy E. Lane, Daniel A. Bloch, Henry H. Jones, William H. Marshall, Jr., Peter D. Wood, and James F. Fries (Stanford Univ.)

JAMA 255:1147–1151, March 7, 1986   1–97

Strong data link increased physical activity to decreased risk of cardio-vascular disease, assistance in weight reduction, reduction of blood pressure, and improved mood. Hence, running has become a national phenomenon of importance, with nearly 15 million Americans participating. Concerns have been raised that this form of physical activity may accelerate the development of osteoarthritis in the weight-bearing joints, leading to increased prevalence. The effect of running on the development of osteoarthritis was studied in running and control subjects aged 50 to 72 years.

Forty-one long-distance runners aged 50 to 72 years were compared with 41 matched community controls to examine associations of repetitive longterm physical impact (running) with osteoarthritis and osteoporosis. Roentgenograms of hands, lateral lumbar spine, and knees were assessed without knowledge of running status. A computed tomographic scan of the first lumbar vertebra was performed to quantitate bone mineral content. It was found that runners, both male and female, have approximately 40% more bone mineral than do matched controls. Female (but not male) runners appear to have somewhat more sclerosis and spur formation in spine and weight bearing knee x-ray films, but not in hand x-ray films. There were no differences between groups in joint space narrowing, crepitation, joint stability, or symptomatic osteoarthritis.

Running is associated with increased bone mineral but not, in this cross-sectional study, with clinical osteoarthritis.

▶ These two studies (Abstracts 1–96 and 1–97) indicate that long-duration and high-mileage running is not associated with premature degenerative joint disease in the lower extremities. It should be noted that McDermott and Freyne (*Br. J. Sports Med.* 17:84–87, June 1983), in a study of 20 male middle-distance and long-distance runners, concluded that a third of long-distance runners with knee pain had degenerative changes in the joint. However, they also indicated that the frequent occurrence of both acute trauma and genu varum in the affected runners suggested that running itself is not necessarily the chief causative factor. The point is that although long-distance running does not cause degenerative disease, the runner with knee pain and degenerative disease cannot assume that continued running will not adversely affect the existing osteoarthritis. Thus, the question is whether long-distance running on preexisting osteoarthritis will adversely affect the degenerative process.—J.S. Torg, M.D.

Injuries in Elite Orienteers

Christer Johansson (Univ. of Umeå, Sweden)

Am. J. Sports Med. 14:410–415, Sept./Oct. 1986   1–98

The sport of orienteering requires the athlete to run 11 to 15 k at top speed over unknown and rough terrain, using only a map and compass for guidance to find the checkpoints. Elite orienteers are subject to injuries that affect both their training and performance during competitions. This study analyzes the incidence, type, and cause of orienteering injuries, with the aim of injury prevention.

The subjects of this prospective study were 33 women and 56 men of mean age 17.5 years, all students at an orienteering college. At the start of the study, all subjects were injury free. They kept complete training diaries, including occurrence of injuries, which were classed as minor, moderate, or major, depending on how long the athlete had to suspend training.

The rate of injuries was 3 per 1,000 training hours for both sexes. Men lost 20 days and women lost 19 days from training per year as a result of injury. The vast majority of the accidents occurred during training and affected the lower extremities. About 60% of the injuries were moderate, with approximately 20% major and 20% minor injuries. Preseason injuries tended to result from overuse, whereas incidence of overuse and traumatic injuries were equal during the season. Overuse injuries often involved the knee, and traumatic injuries usually were sprains occurring while the athlete ran over uneven ground.

Orienteering is a relatively safe sport, but prevention of unnecessary injuries is needed. The standard shoe lacks adequate stability and comfort and should be further developed. Prevention of sprains is best done by taping the ankles during competitions and by rehabilitating and strengthening the ankle muscles. Contusions in the knee can be prevented by inserting knee pads into the competition trousers. If injuries should occur, rehabilitation rather than rest is more effective in encouraging healing.

Injuries in Orienteering
F. Linde (Univ. of Åarhus, Denmark)
Br. J. Sports Med. 20:125–127, September 1986   1–99

Orienteering is a sport that requires training similar to that of long-distance running. As expected, overuse injuries occur. However, some acute injuries are associated with the rough terrain where the athletes run. This prospective study investigates the frequency and injury pattern in experienced orienteers.

Forty-two runners, 28 men and 14 women (average age, 24 years), completed questionnaires on injuries once monthly. Injuries were classed as acute if they were of sudden onset and resulted from physical violence or sprains, and as overuse if they were due to overuse of tissues subjected to normal loads. Only injuries lasting a minimum of 3 days were used.

Seventy-three injuries occurred during the 1-year study, of which 52% were acute and 48% were due to overuse. Of the acute injuries, 37% were sprains and 63% were contusions from falls or bumps against rocks and branches. Overuse injuries consisted of medial shin pain, Achilles peritendinitis, peroneal tenosynovitis, and iliotibial band friction syndrome. Overuse injuries were located in the lower extremities, whereas 18% of acute injuries occurred elsewhere.

Orienteers suffer no more injuries than joggers, and the injuries are of minor severity. Although more acute injuries occur among orienteers, the pattern of overuse injuries is similar to that of other long distance runners. Medial shin pain, Achilles peritendinitis, and iliotibial band friction syndrome are the dominant overuse injuries in orienteers and other long-distance runners.

▶ These two articles (Abstracts 1–98 and 1–99) conclude that orienteering is not a dangerous sport. However, they point out the need for prevention of unnecessary injuries. The Johansson study indicated that the frequency was greatest during training. It did not include competition injuries, which according to Folin (*Br. J. Sports Med.* 4:236–240, 1982) are mostly traumatic and need further analysis since they are rarely investigated.—J.S. Torg, M.D.

Influence of Water Temperature and Meals on the Outcome of Swimming Accidents
Mireille Laisney (Caen, France)
Médicine du Sport 60:53-277, 1986   1–100

There are 3,000 to 4,000 drowning deaths per year in France, and more than half occur in the course of swimming, either in the ocean or in a swimming pool.

Although most swimming accidents occur because of insufficient swimming skills, many are caused by "hydrocution" or "thermodifferential shock." For a long time such hydrocutions were thought to be linked to the postmeal digestive period. However, it has become apparent that meals play only a minimal role in swimming accidents, and in most countries swimming is allowed 1 to 2 hours after meals. Alcohol, however, even in small amounts, is a contributory factor to hydrocution.

Water temperature in itself is not a direct cause of swimming accidents, but rather the thermal gradient between skin and water causes thermodifferential shock. Yet, in many countries authors do not recommend exposure to temperatures lower than 16 to 20 C.

▶ This is a brief reference to an interesting French doctoral thesis. I have memories of myself as a teenager sitting on a sunny boat, feeling a little overheated, and plunging into an icy cold river to experience a similar type of shock. In my case, the problem was compounded by a relatively recent meal and the aspiration of some water, with attendant vomiting. Fortunately, I was able to retain sufficient consciousness to grasp the stays of the boat until the worst of the attack had passed. However, the incident could easily have ended in a fatality. This is an important hazard to stress to boating enthusiasts in the spring, before the lakes have reached a comfortable water temperature. Precooling of the skin by river or lake water is a wise precaution in this type of situation.—R.J. Shephard, M.D., Ph.D.

Inner Ear Trauma Caused by Decompression Accidents Following Deep-Sea Diving
P. Renon, D. Lory, R. Belliato, and M. Casanova (Hôp. d'Instruction des Armées Ste-Anne, Toulon Naval, France)
Ann. Otolaryngol. (Paris) 103:259–264, 1986   1–101

Barotrauma of the inner ear secondary to decompression accidents occurs about ten times less often than barotrauma of the middle ear, but inner ear barotrauma is much more serious, because the damage is often irreversible. Inner ear barotrauma is difficult to diagnose, but when immediate, proper, emergency treatment is provided, the outcome may be favorable.

For correct diagnosis of inner ear barotrauma in divers, an extremely detailed history is mandatory and should include persistent questioning about recent and past events such as the number of dives made on previous days, state of fatigue when diving, sensation of cold experienced, and sense of effort during the dive. It is particularly important to learn the maximum depth attained during the dive, since most accidents seem to occur at depths of more than 35 m. Diagnostic procedures should also include a thorough otorhinolaryngologic examination to verify nasal integrity, so as to exclude tubal impairment as the cause of symptoms, and tympanic integrity, so as to eliminate barotrauma incurred during descent as a cause of symptoms. Complete cochleovestibular and neurologic examinations should also be performed immediately.

Treatment of inner ear barotrauma includes therapeutic recompression, hyperbaric oxygen therapy, and perfusion with vasodilators and corticosteroids. Using this treatment regimen in ten patients, the authors obtained very good or good results in eight, a moderately good result in one, and a fair result in another.

Divers must be alert to the risk factors associated with deep-sea diving and impressed with the importance of seeking treatment immediately when decompression accidents occur.

▶ The pathologic condition under discussion in this article is decompression sickness, rather than traditional forms of otitic barotrauma. The authors argue that symptoms are due to the development of gas bubbles in the blood vessels supplying the inner ear; evidence to support their hypothesis includes the depth of dive associated with the symptoms (35 to 40 m), in some instances signs of decompression sickness elsewhere in the body, and regression of symptoms with recompression of the affected diver to the equivalent of 28 m. In most cases, the impact is on the vestibular system, with symptoms of vertigo, and in only a very few instances is there evidence of reduced auditory acuity; it remains unclear why the cochlea is spared in this situation.—R.J. Shephard, M.D., Ph.D.

Progressive Ulnar Palsy as a Late Complication of Decompression Sickness

Frank K. Butler and Carmen V. Pinto (Naval Experimental Diving Unit, Panama City, Fla.)

Ann. Emerg. Med. 15:738–741, June 1986   1–102

Decompression sickness is caused by a sudden reduction in the ambient pressure to which the body is exposed. Initial signs and symptoms are produced by the direct mechanical effects of a gas phase (bubbles) in the tissues of the body; later signs and symptoms include the localized hypoxia and ischemia which result from secondary microcirculatory effects of the bubbles. The authors describe an unusual case of decompression sickness, and the difficulties that may ensue when prompt and thorough treatment is not obtained.

Man, 23, who was right handed, made an uneventful sport scuba dive at 110 feet for 15 minutes. He did not require any decompression stops and had no symptoms that were suggestive of decompression sickness. He felt well throughout the day and evening. However, the next morning he noticed a numbness and a "pins and needles" tingling sensation on the palmar aspect of his left little finger. He did not seek medical attention and the symptom did not change throughout the day. On waking 2 days after the dive he noticed that the numbness and paresthesias had spread to include the palmar surface of his left ring finger and the medial aspect of his palm. When the symptoms continued essentially unchanged for 6 days after the dive, the patient went to a recompression facility. Examination revealed no objective signs of neurologic dysfunction. After recompression he reported 70% relief of his symptoms. Over the next 10 days the symptoms returned and he again had recompression. Eight days later weakness developed in his left hand. He was then thought to be suffering from neurologic decompression sickness and underwent a series of recompression treatments. The symptoms gradually improved and recompression therapy was discontinued after 11 days.

Because of the unusual features of this case, neurologic consultation was obtained and the clinical impression was a lower brachial plexopathy or ulnar neuropathy. Findings at electrodiagnostic studies were consistent with those of a left ulnar neuropathy with a conduction block that was fairly well localized to the level of the ulnar groove. The remaining symptoms gradually resolved and at 2-month follow-up he had been free from muscle weakness for 2 weeks and had had no paresthesias for 1 week. Four months after treatment findings at neurologic examination were normal.

It is concluded that a progressive ulnar nerve palsy occurred as a late complication of neurologic decompression sickness. The failure to conduct follow-up hyperbaric oxygen treatments for the residual symptoms after initial treatment may have contributed to the subsequent development of this unusual complication.

▶ To be sure, ulnar palsy is not a common complication of decompression sickness. The point of this article is that we should think in terms of late complications presenting in neurologic fashion once the patient has been exposed to decompression sickness. In practical terms, therapy can be effective (in this instance, hyperbaric chamber).—L.J. Krakauer, M.D.

Minimal Change Nephrotic Syndrome Presenting After Acute Decompression
P. D. Yin, K. W. Chan, and M. K. Chan (Univ. of Hong Kong)
Br. Med. J. 292:445–446, Feb. 15, 1986   1–103

A case is reported of a patient who, after decompression, had nephrotic syndrome due to minimal change glomerulonephritis.

Male diver, 19, experienced mild decompression sickness consisting of substernal pain, dizziness, headache, abdominal cramps, and increased bowel movements, after a rapid ascent from a depth of roughly 30.5 m. Puffy eyelids and swollen ankles were noted the following day. Recompression was started 3 days after decompression, but the patient defaulted after the first session of treatment. Six days later he was readmitted with shortness of breath and generalized anasarca. Ascites and bilateral pleural effusion were present. Urinalysis showed proteinuria (urine protein excretion over 24 hours = 18.5 gm). Creatinine clearance was 125 ml per minute, serum albumin level was 11 gm/L, and serum globulin level, 21 gm/L. Percutaneous renal biopsy was done and electron microscopic examination showed diffuse foot process fusion of podocytes with no electron dense deposits. Basement membrane was normal. Findings of immunofluorescence studies were negative for all immunoglobulins.

Although its occurrence may be coincidental, nephrotic syndrome due to minimal change glomerulonephritis can occur following acute decompression. The rapid change in environmental pressure probably accelerates and aggravates edema, perhaps the reverse of what occurs in up-to-the-neck immersion in water.

▶ The nephrotic syndrome may have been coincidental but more likely relates to the acute decompression sickness occurring in this young diver. It speaks again to the ubiquitous nature of long-range complications that can occur after decompression illness, which cannot be considered a short-term problem.— L.J. Krakauer, M.D.

Medical Standards for Scuba Diving
Michael B. Strauss (Harbor-UCLA Med. Ctr., Torrance, Calif.)
Sports Med. Digest 8:1–3, August 1986   1–104

The popularity of scuba diving is on the increase, resulting in the marketing of improved equipment and training programs, but medical standards for diving remain controversial.

Factors that can affect medical problems associated with diving include age, sex, pregnancy, head and neck disorders, habits and drugs, and the type of diving attempted. The respiratory, cardiovascular, gastrointestinal, and neurologic systems may be affected by diving.

Contraindications to diving are absolute and relative. Under no circumstances should a person be allowed to dive when an absolute contraindication such as epilepsy or uncorrected coronary artery disease is present. Under certain circumstances a person may be allowed to dive when a relative contraindication such as non–insulin-dependent diabetes or controlled coronary artery disease is present. A decision to allow diving when relative contraindications exist should be made by a specialist in the area of the medical problem and by a physician who is knowledgeable in diving medicine.

Although sports divers need not undergo a pretraining physical examination or submit to periodic medical examinations, virtually all recognized diving certification agencies require that a person complete a diving history questionnaire before starting scuba lessons.

There are no absolute standards for persons who should or should not dive. The general guidelines provided here will undoubtedly change as new information becomes available in this area of sports medicine.

▶ The certification programs for diving have often been casual, and after basic pool certification the degree of open water exposure is left up to the individual. This obviously leaves a large area of risk, and some of the accidents of diving clearly relate to this lack of certification and control.

I should rather see insulin-dependent diabetes consigned to a role of whether it is under excellent control or not, but other than these small points, I think the author's position is basically very sound. Periodic medical examinations after age 30 and yearly after age 40 are also something that should be done, but clearly are not done now by many divers who consider themselves in good shape. At the moment, taken at face value, this can stand as a guideline for the semicompulsive diver and may well be the absolute for the future in an increasingly regulatory society.—L.J. Krakauer, M.D.

Breath Holding in Divers and Non-Divers—A Reappraisal
J. Schneeberger, W. B. Murray, W. L. Mouton, and R. I. Stewart (Addington Hosp. Durban, and Univ. of Stellenbosch and Tygerberg Hosp., Parowvallei, South Africa)
S. Afr. Med. J. 69:822–824, June 1986   1–105

Investigators have described two phases of breath holding: an initial phase of voluntary inspiratory muscle inactivity, followed by a second phase of involuntary inspiratory efforts against a closed glottis. The duration of the quiescent phase is determined by the onset of involuntary chest wall movements resulting from the Pa_{CO_2}. Although psychological or motivational factors may be responsible for underwater blackouts, it is possible that some subjects may be at a "physiologic risk" of unexpected blackout because of an attenuated ventilatory response to hypoxia or hypercapnia, or both. It is also possible that the desire to breathe develops quickly in some individuals, thus providing little warning to the diver of an impending blackout. A study was recently undertaken to find a useful screening test for the control of breathing in novices and in divers experienced in breath holding that could identify subjects at risk of underwater blackout.

The study population consisted of seven sedentary, healthy persons familiar with breathing apparatus and eight experienced divers. The two phases of breath holding, the voluntary inactive and the involuntary active phases, were identified by noninvasive methods using the induction plethysmograph. During breath holding from normocapnia and total lung capacity it was not possible to distinguish between the two groups with respect to pattern or to duration of breath holding or alveolar gas tensions at the breakpoint. Nevertheless, the divers were able to hold their breaths much longer after hyperventilation; this was associated with a longer second phase than occurred in non-divers, and more severe nonalveolar hypoxia.

These divers exhibited a hyperventilation-dependent attenuated hypoxic ventilatory response. Some subjects had either a very short or very long second phase; these individuals were considered at risk of developing underwater hypoxia and unexpected loss of consciousness. Analysis of the phases of breath holding may be a useful screening test of both novice and experienced divers.

▶ The main basis for loss of consciousness in breath-hold divers is the sudden decrease of alveolar oxygen partial pressure which occurs when they reach the break point of a breath hold and reduce the total intrapulmonary gas pressure by a sudden ascent.

It is well recognized that prior hyperventilation contributes to such accidents by eliminating the CO_2 signal and thus further depressing alveolar oxygen pressure at the break point. In habitual divers, further factors are a depression of respiratory center sensitivity to CO_2 (Florio, J.T., et al.: *J. Appl. Physiol.* 48:1076–1080, 1979) and oxygen lack (Masuda, Y., et al.: *Jpn. J. Physiol.* 32:327–336, 1982).

The present report is interesting in distinguishing the two phases of breath holding: a first stage when there is little compulsion to breathe, and a second stage when the glottis must restrain involuntary respiratory efforts. Both phases are apparently prolonged more in the diver than in the non-diver after hyperventilation, making the regular, experienced underwater sports enthusiast at greater risk of loss of consciousness while submerged.—R.J. Shephard, M.D., Ph.D.

Marine-Acquired Infections: Hazards of the Ocean Environment
Willis J. Chang and Francis D. Pien (Univ. of Hawaii)
Postgrad. Med. 80:30–41, Sept. 15, 1986   1–106

Although the Pacific Ocean is a source of food and recreation for Hawaiian residents and visitors, many hazards are associated with the marine

---

BACTERIA ISOLATED FROM PENETRATING
MARINE INJURIES

Achromobacter xylosoxidans
Acinetobacter calcoaceticus
Bacillus species
Corynebacterium species
Enterobacter species
Escherichia coli
Propionibacterium acnes
Pseudomonas species
Staphylococcus aureus
Staphylococcus epidermidis
Streptococcus species
Vibrio species

(Courtesy of Chang, W.J., and Pien, F.D.: Postgrad. Med. 80:30–41, Sept. 15, 1986.)

---

environment since seawater contains many bacteria that are human pathogens.

Swimmer's ear (otitis externa) is a marine infection. It is characterized by itching, pain, erythema, edema, and tenderness of the ear canal and tragus. Treatment consists of débridement of the canal, application of antibiotic drops, and use of topical preparations to relieve pain.

Coral or rock cuts are frequent penetrating injuries, as are lacerations from the handling of fish or shellfish and injuries from marine equipment. Exposure to seawater may easily lead to infections of such cuts. Bacteria isolated from infected marine injuries include species found in seawater, as well as normal bacterial flora of human skin (table).

Gastrointestinal tract illnesses are associated with ingestion of contaminated seafood and swimming in contaminated waters. Enteric pathogens belonging to the genus *Vibrio* are often isolated in such cases and can cause severe, profuse, watery diarrhea and rice-water stools without tenesmus in about 1 of every 40 infected persons. Treatment consists of standard measures aimed at volume replacement and correction of electrolyte balance.

Other infections associated with marine exposure have been reported, including pneumonia, primary septicemia, conjunctivitis, and panophthalmitis. One case of endometritis has been reported in a woman who had sexual intercourse while swimming in seawater.

▶ Psychologically, we think of swimming, whether in a pool or even more so ocean, as a cleansing experience. In fact the opposite is true, and the authors' comment is noted: "Seawater has been described as a dilute suspension of bacteria, many of which are known human pathogens." The precise description of the bacteria isolated from penetrating marine injuries is excellent and is a good example of this point. The section on water-borne infection presenting as gastrointestinal tract illnesses also bears emphasis with the best-known members of the pathogenic group those of the genus *Vibrio*. Gamma globulin prophylaxis is again strongly recommended for those dividing from boats.—L.J. Krakauer, M.D.

Health Hazards Associated With Windsurfing on Polluted Water
Eric Dewailly, Claude Poirier, and Francois M. Meyer (Laval Univ. and Saint Francis of Assisi Hosp., Quebec City)
Am. J. Public Health 76:690–691, June 1986   1–107

The popularity of windsurfing is increasing. However, the sport is tolerated on waters judged to be unsafe for swimming because of water pollution. It is well known that swimming in water with fecal pollution can cause gastroenteritis, otitis, conjunctivitis, and infectious or allergic skin symptoms. The health hazards associated with windsurfing on polluted water were assessed in 79 participants in a 9-day windsurfing meet on the Saint Lawrence river in the Beauport bay area, where concentrations of fecal coliforms and enterococci are often higher than acceptable limits. Forty-one nonsurfing employees who worked at the site were also studied. All subjects were served identical meals during the meet. A questionnaire including information about exposure to polluted water and incidence of health problems was filled out by each study subject. The relative risk (RR) for each health outcome was measured as the ratio of cumulative incidence among windsurfers to that among employees.

On average, each competitor fell into the water 18 times. At least one symptom associated with exposure to polluted water was reported by 45 competitors and 8 employees. The overall RR was 2.9; the RR for gastrointestinal symptoms was 5.5. The RRs for skin infection, otitis, and conjunctivitis were also elevated. The risk increased with the number of falls into the water. All 10 competitors who fell more than 30 times reported symptoms, whereas only 44% of those who fell 10 times or less were affected. Of the 41 employees, 4 windsurfed occasionally, and they also developed symptoms during the study period.

The same water quality criteria should be applied to all recreational activities in which there is intentional, probable, or accidental direct contact with water.

▶ The risks associated with water pollution are habitually underestimated by participants in all water sports and, indeed, most people are unaware of the ubiquity of the pathogens, both bacterial and viral, in the waters used commonly for recreation. The relative risk exposure for the 9-day championship race near Quebec City appears unacceptably high. It seems that in the present world pollution must be assumed in almost all waters in any reasonable proximity to civilization, and the recreational site must be chosen accordingly. Where championship events are held with reference to pollution high environment is more of a political question. Perhaps the L.A. Olympics are an example of such decision making.—L.J. Krakauer, M.D.

Spinal Cord Injury During Windsurfing
M.K. Patel, R.J. Abbott, and W.J. Marshall (The Gen. Infirmary, Leeds, U.K.)
Paraplegia 24:191–193, 1986   1–108

Windsurfing in rough weather can impose considerable strain on the thoraco-lumbar spine, even in athletic young men. Two patients are described who sustained thoracic cord lesions while windsurfing.

The patients were aged 19 and 30 years. Both patients developed acute symptoms, including extreme pain in the chest or back and numbness on the extremities, after windsurfing on rough water. The patients adopted a position of extreme lordosis to be able to balance the craft. Both patients showed clinical evidence of thoracic cord lesions; that is, sensory and motor deficits. Plain films of the thoracic spine showed lateral wedging of the T8/9 disc in the first patient, as well as degenerative changes with calcification in the paravertebral soft tissue on the left at the T9/10 level in the second patient. Myelogram in both patients was normal. Both patients recovered rapidly.

Windsurfing in rough weather may result in injury to the spinal cord. The injury may be ischemic in origin, as there is no evidence of cord compression and as the symptoms and signs resolved spontaneously. It is possible that exaggerated movements of the spine, in the presence of previous degenerative changes at the same site, may have compromised flow in one of the radicular vessels providing arterial blood to the cord.

▶ In the inept, windsurfing has a risk of trauma to the spine from simple fall, not unlike any other sport involving motion. In addition, there is a particular risk in the competent with extreme conditions of wind and surf where particular stress is directed to the thoracic and lumbar spine. Two instances of thoracic spine pain are shown, one with a compression wedging of vertebrae. Fortunately, findings on myelographic examination were normal. It can be anticipated that there will be true spinal cord injury as the sport is associated with increased numbers and more extreme conditions. There may be a potential ischemic condition inherent in the movements of the thoracic spine in windsurfing.—L.J. Krakauer, M.D.

Terrestrial Rowing
Jay Stuller
Physician Sportsmed. 14:272–276, March 1986   1–109

Stationary rowing machines are one of the fastest-selling pieces of home exercise equipment. Strenuous rowing is as good an aerobic exercise as stationary cycling, and uses more muscle groups. Unfortunately, rowing is not the "ideal" form of exercise.

Rowing is easy on the legs and hips, but places strain on the lower back, even if the proper form is used. Not all machines are worth the money. Beginners should start with 12 strokes per minute. Aerobically fit people can start with 20 to 25 strokes per minute. It is better to work at a lower resistance level for a longer time. The target oxygen uptake zone should be maintained for 20 minutes. Proper form should always be used. A back evaluation prior to initiation of a rowing program is recommended.

The rowing machine is considered the home fitness equipment with the most benefits, but that can be debated. Rowing places a strain on the lower back, and all rowers should be aware of this.

▶ Should I buy a stationary bike? Should I buy a rowing machine? Should I walk or jog? Should I jump rope or swim? What is the best way to improve my physical fitness? *The best way is the one you will continue to do.* They all have advantages and disadvantages. You will probably continue with the one that is most enjoyable and easiest for you to perform. A great deal of money is spent on home exercise equipment that is rarely, if ever, used. We all have good intentions but just can't seem to carry through with them.

If one has a history of back problems, the rowing machine is not the best way to achieve fitness.—F. George, A.T.C., P.T.

Breakdancer's Pulmonary Embolism
Serafin Tiu, Indrani Srinivasan, Howard J. Banner, Elissa Lipcon Kramer, Nancy B. Genieser, and Joseph J. Sanger (New York Univ. Med. Ctr.-Bellevue Hosp.)
Clin. Nucl. Med. 11:402–403, June 1986   1–110

Since breakdancing became popular, a variety of musculoskeletal injuries have been described. A case of life-threatening pulmonary embolism that followed breakdancing is reported.

Boy, 16, had a 3½-week history of intermittent right upper arm swelling and a cold feeling in the fingertips, which had not responded to soaking or rest. He also described dull chest pain with exertion that had started the day before admission.

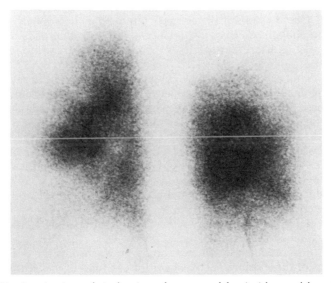

Fig 1–28.—Posterior view perfusion lung image demonstrates defects in right upper lobe and in several segments of right lower and left lower lobes. (Courtesy of Tiu, S., et al.: Clin. Nucl. Med. 11:402–403, June 1986.)

The patient was a stocker in a supermarket and had been breakdancing 1 to 2 hours daily for the previous 5 months. His right arm was grossly swollen and dusky. Findings on a sensory neurologic examination were normal, as were roentgenograms of the chest, right arm, and cervical spine. Computed tomographic examination of the right shoulder revealed thrombosis of the right axillary vein and the cephalic vein, but there was no evidence of a mass. Perfusion lung imaging revealed multiple perfusion defects that involved almost the entire right upper lobe, several subsegments of the right lower lobe, and the lateral and posterior basal segments of the left lower lobe (Fig 1–28). Pulmonary embolism was diagnosed. The patient was given intravenous heparin therapy and discharged 2 weeks later.

Besides skeletal injuries that can occur in breakdancers, life-threatening pulmonary embolism should also be considered in breakdancers with the symptoms described here.

▶ Each and every sport, and in particular those that are of relatively newer derivation, increases in intensity. The potential for trauma increases accordingly. Any break of long bone must include in the differential the risk of a life-threatening pulmonary embolism. This will be rare, but of extreme importance when it does occur.—L.J. Krakauer, M.D.

Physiology of Drugs

Do Anabolic Steroids Pose an Ethical Dilemma for US Physicians?
Marty Duda
Physician Sportsmed. 14:173–175, November 1986   1–111

Anabolic steroids will be used by athletes, with or without the help of physicians, because they are convinced that these drugs help enhance performance. One Australian physician, Tony Millar, has openly admitted prescribing anabolic steroids for athletes. Although U.S. physicians who prescribe anabolic steroids to athletes are not rare, few are willing to discuss their actions publicly.

Most U.S. physicians who are willing to talk on the matter say "no" to prescribing anabolic steroids to athletes. Robert Kerr, a well-known supplier of these agents, claims that his intentions were to steer athletes from black-market steroids of dubious quality and minimize the medical risks by prescribing safe types and dosages. However, he quit prescribing the drugs when his patients went to the black market for supplemental steroids and used far more than the dosages prescribed. McKeag believes that, "if you're true to your profession and your patient's health, there's no way you should prescribe steroids." It makes no sense to tell athletes that anabolic steroids do not work, because the athletes already know the drugs work. Football players and competitive power lifters may feel it is justifiable to use anabolic steroids, particularly when success means a lucrative livelihood in sports. These athletes should be warned of the documented side effects of these drugs, such as heart disease and liver disease. Landry says its easy flatly to condemn anabolic steroid use, but physicians should educate their patient-athletes and themselves about these agents.

Should physicians monitor athletes who use anabolic steroids? Most physicians say "maybe," but their actions do not necessarily reflect approval of use. Others believe that physicians should refuse to monitor user athletes. The ideal of fair play should be encouraged. Protecting that sense of fairness may present a potential conflict of interest for team physicians; for other physicians, there is no such conflict. Others believe that the anabolic steroid user should be suspended from the team, and any physician who abets or aids in providing a banned substance should receive the same punitive action meted to the athlete. The use of unannounced, mandatory drug testing appears to be promising as a primary deterrent of anabolic steroid use.

Anabolic Steroids: An Australian Sports Physician Goes Public
Calvin Miller
Physician Sportsmed. 14:167–170, November 1986   1–112

Tony Millar, a well-known Australian sports medicine physician and a world-renowned pioneer in sports medicine therapy and research, has openly admitted prescribing anabolic steroids for adult athletes who insist on using them. He believes that athletes who want to take anabolic steroids are best protected by receiving prescription drugs rather than resorting to black-market drugs that may be veterinary, contaminated, or of dubious composition. Only under such regimen can a physician properly monitor any adverse side effects. He advises athletes to keep their dosages at therapeutic levels, and although he knows these dosages have been supplemented, he has as yet encountered no problems. He does not prescribe anabolic steroids to adolescents, and prescribes only oxandrolone or nandrolone decanoate for all patients. He also believes that with today's sports being focused toward winning, athletes will use anabolic steroids with or without cooperation. The value system in sports needs a complete review.

Although users applaud his realistic approach, this maverick stand of Millar has caused repercussions in the medical community. The Australian Commonwealth Games Association, with its firm antidrug policy, was compelled to fire Millar as the Australian team's chief medical officer before the 1986 Commonwealth Games. Other physicians contended that Millar had done a huge disservice to sports medicine in Australia and was encouraging athletes to cheat. Further, Millar's statement encouraged athletes in doubt to use anabolic steroids.

Millar is undaunted by the negative reactions to his controversial stand on prescribing anabolic steroids to adult athletes. He believes that he is doing the right thing for his patients.

▶ It is important that these questions about anabolic steroids be aired in public and that we acknowledge that there are still some physicians who prescribe these drugs legally, and many users who obtain them illegally, some with the encouragement of coaches and trainers (see Abstracts 1–111 and 1–112). These are potentially dangerous drugs that can induce deleterious and irreversible changes in the body. Granted, strength and endurance can be improved under certain conditions. The trade-off isn't worth it. In the 1986 YEAR BOOK OF SPORTS MEDICINE, p. 145, reference was made to Haupt and Rovere's study (*Am. J. Sports Med.* 12:469–484, November–December 1984) as the landmark review of the literature. An extensive discussion was appended to that review, and I will not repeat that discussion here. John A. Lombardo updated the question in the 1986 YEAR BOOK in a special article titled "Drugs in Sports" (p. 11), and this can stand without additional comment as a fair and definitive view of the entire question of therapeutic drugs, performance aids, and recreational drugs.—L.J. Krakauer, M.D.

Cocaine and Cardiovascular Events
John D. Cantwell and Fred D. Rose (Georgia Baptist Med. Ctr., Atlanta)
Physician Sportsmed. 14:77–82, November 1986   1–113

The deaths of two well-known athletes after cocaine use have shown that cocaine alone or with other drugs can precipitate serious cardiovascular events. The authors present another case illustrating the cardiovascular effects of cocaine and discuss the likely mechanisms involved.

Man, 21, had used amphetamines orally and cocaine intranasally for several days before admission for lower substernal and left parasternal burning pain. He had no known history of heart disease, but he was a heavy smoker and had used marihuana in the past. The admission ECG showed S-T segment and T-wave abnormalities consistent with ischemia. He was admitted to the coronary care unit after severe chest pain recurred, with further S-T segment elevation. Sublingual nifedipine therapy was prescribed to relieve the chest pain, besides nitrates and calcium channel antagonists. Cardiac catheterization showed hypokinesia of the anterior wall of the left ventricle, and normal coronary arteries. Coronary spasm secondary to the abuse of cocaine and amphetamines was diagnosed. The patient has stopped abusing drugs and has remained pain free.

A cocaine-augmented catecholamine response can directly induce serious ventricular arrhythmias or sudden death or cause coronary vasospasm. The spasm can trigger coronary thrombus formation, even if the arteries are normal. Sudden total occlusion of the coronary artery, from spasm alone or spasm-induced thrombosis, can then lead to acute myocardial infarction, ventricular arrhythmias, or sudden death.

Cocaine abuse should be considered when otherwise healthy patients are seen with sudden cardiovascular events.

Acute Cardiac Events Temporally Related to Cocaine Abuse
Jeffrey M. Isner, Mark Estes III, Paul D. Thompson, Maria Rosa Costanzo-Nordin, Ramiah Subramanian, Gary Miller, George Katsas, Kristin Sweeney, and William Q. Sturner (Tufts-New England Med. Ctr., Boston, Brown Univ., Providence, R.I., Loyola Univ., Chicago, and the Medical Examiner's Offices of Suffolk Cty., Mass. and Rhode Island)
N. Engl. J. Med. 315:1438–1443, Dec. 4, 1986   1–114

Cocaine usage in the United States has reached epidemic proportions, with over 5 million persons reportedly using the drug regularly. There remains among many physicians the mistaken notion that the intranasal use of cocaine is safe. This view is challenged by the 7 cases summarized by the authors, along with 19 cases from the literature. The patients presented here all suffered a cardiac disorder that was temporally related to nonintravenous use of cocaine. Six patients used cocaine intranasally; the remaining patient was "free-basing" the drug.

Woman, 28, experienced cardiac symptoms, such as substernal chest pain, nausea, and diaphoresis 6 hours after using cocaine, when she took phenylpropanolamine and chlorpheniramine for insomnia. An ECG showed 8 mm of ST-segment depression and runs of ventricular tachycardia. A non-Q-wave infarction evolved. Cardiac catheterization several days later disclosed left ventricular anterolateral wall hypokinesis, but coronary arteriograms were normal.

In two of the other cases presented, the outcome was fatal. Six of the 7 patients in this series were male. Many patients had factors that might have predisposed them to cardiac events, such as high serum cholesterol, myocarditis, and a myocardial bridge. A fresh occlusive thrombus was found in one patient. There have been previous reports of thrombotic coronary occlusion with cocaine use. The interval between cocaine use and the cardiac event ranged from "shortly after" to the same day. Since there are no specific clinical or pathologic markers for cocaine-induced cardiotoxicity, these data indicate only a temporal, but not a causal relationship.

Cocaine can increase heart rate, blood pressure, and small vessel vasoconstriction, properties that could explain some of the cardiac events seen in these seven patients. Ischemia secondary to increased myocardial oxygen demand could precipitate arrhythmias, infarction, or aortic rupture, particularly in patients with preexisting cardiac abnormalities. Such effects might also occur even in persons with normal hearts, by means of focal constriction of the medium-sized coronary arteries. The 7 cases discussed here, along with 19 other cases from the literature, constitute compelling evidence that cocaine may precipitate life-threatening cardiac events.

While the data do not establish a pathogenetic basis for cocaine's cardiotoxicity, they do suggest several features of the presumed cardiac consequences of the drug. Such complications are not restricted to the parenteral use of the drug; most of the cases occurred after intranasal use. Seizure activity is not a prerequisite for cocaine-related disorders; it was seen in only 2 of the 26 cases. Underlying heart disease also is not a precondition for a cardiac event after cocaine usage; at least 7 of the 26 documented cases had normal coronary arteriograms. Cardiac toxicity is not limited to those who have consumed massive doses of cocaine. The presence of a contaminant in cocaine cannot be excluded as a reason for some of these cardiac events. The data document that fatal and potentially fatal cardiac consequences can be associated with cocaine usage.

▶ There is probably an increased incidence of cardiovascular events relating to cocaine (Abstracts 1–113 and 1–114) because of increasingly potent forms of the drug, combination of drugs used, and probably a broader population of use. The special article on p. 11 of the 1986 YEAR BOOK OF SPORTS MEDICINE will again stand as a reference base.—L.J. Krakauer, M.D.

Influence of Caffeine on Exercise Performance in Habitual Caffeine Users
S.M. Fisher, R.G. McMurray, M. Berry, M.H. Mar, and W.A. Forsythe (Univ. of North Carolina)
Int. J. Sports Med. 7:276–280, October 1986   1–115

The present study was undertaken to determine whether a tolerance to caffeine is acquired by habitually high caffeine consumers (600 mg per day) such that metabolic responses during exercise would not be affected. The authors also wanted to determine whether caffeine metabolic effects could be enhanced by 4 days of caffeine deprivation, followed by reintroduction before exercising.

Six women between the ages of 21 and 34 years participated. Evaluation consisted of treadmill trials in which initially 75% of the maximum oxygen uptake was determined for future trials. Within 1 week a 1-hour run was completed whereby each subject ingested a capsule of either 5 mg per kilogram of body weight of caffeine (CC) or placebo (PL). A second 1-hour run was completed within a week of the first, with each subject taking the alternate drug. The final 1-hour run was within a month of the first trial, at which time all subjects were given a caffeine capsule. Four days prior to this trial all abstained from caffeine intake.

All three exercise trials resulted in stable ventilation over the 1-hour run. Ingestion of caffeine after withdrawal (CW) yielded the greatest physiologic effects. Exercise oxygen uptake ($\dot{V}O_2$) was significantly elevated by 0.17 L per minute over the PL and CC trials. There were no significant differences in blood lactate concentration between the trials as well as over time. Preexercise free fatty acid levels were highest in the CW trial, but increased only 2.5% by the end of the exercise. Postexercise plasma norepinephrine and dopamine levels were the highest after the CW trials.

Inability to find any significant differences between the placebo and caffeine trails prior to caffeine withdrawal indicated that habitual caffeine users establish a tolerance, which reduces its effect at rest and during prolonged exercise. Furthermore, 4 days of withdrawal resensitizes one to caffeine's physiologic effects. The caffeine habits of individuals need to be controlled if precise data on the effect of caffeine are to be gathered.

Stimulants and Athletic Performance (Part 1 of 2): Amphetamines and Caffeine
John A. Lombardo (Cleveland Clinic Found.)
Physician Sportsmed. 14:128–140, November 1986   1–116

Stimulants are popular ergogenic aids, because of their ability to mask, delay, or alter the athlete's perception of fatigue. This article evaluates the roles of amphetamines and caffeine in athletic performance.

Amphetamines are indirect-acting sympathomimetic amines whose effects depend on the status of endogenous catecholamines. The role of amphetamines in enhancement of athletic performance remains controversial and reflects the variability seen with their use. They increase alertness in the fatigued person, but they can adversely affect the central nervous system (CNS) resulting in tremulousness, anxiety, insomnia, and fever. Deaths have been attributed to amphetamines.

Caffeine is a xanthine that is used mainly by athletes participating in endurance events. It does not improve performance significantly during maximal short-term exercise bouts. Caffeine increases free fatty acid utilization, masks fatigue through CNS stimulation, and increases the force of contraction of skeletal muscle. Nevertheless caffeine is harmful and can cause hyperactivity, irritability, restlessness, insomnia, and arrhythmia.

The International Olympic Committee has banned the use of amphetamines altogether, and it has banned caffeine if urine values are greater than 15 µg/ml.

▶ A clear tolerance to caffeine is shown with a return to prior work performance levels after 4 days of withdrawal. The distinction with regard to caffeine is that enhancement is limited to endurance activities and the drug does not significantly improve performance during maximal short-term exercise bouts. Caffeine has a profound impact on our culture and this may be one reason why the IOC, while considering it a harmful drug, banned it only in amounts above 15 µg/ml in the urine and not below that level. These papers (Abstracts 1–115 and 1–116) speak well for themselves.—L.J. Krakauer, M.D.

The Influence of Caffeine Ingestion on Incremental Treadmill Running
L.R. McNaughton (Tasmanian State Inst. of Technology, Australia)
Br. J. Sports Med. 20:109–112, September 1986   1–117

Caffeine has been reported to have both beneficial and neutral effects on endurance during muscular exercise. The effects of caffeine ingestion on substrate utilization during treadmill exercise were studied in 12 male athletes. Treadmill running at an initial level of 70% to 75% of maximal oxygen consumption for 45 minutes was followed by running to exhaustion. The test conditions included ingestion of a water control, a decaffeinated coffee placebo, and caffeine in dosages of 10 and 15 mg per kilogram of body weight. Treatments were given 1 hour before testing.

The average peak oxygen consumption was 57 ml/kg per minute. Subjects given large doses of caffeine performed longer before exhaustion than under the other test conditions. Respiratory exchange ratio values suggested carbohydrate sparing after large-dose caffeine ingestion. Free fatty acids increased after both doses of caffeine. Ratings of perceived exertion were lower after the large dose of caffeine than under the other test conditions.

Caffeine in large doses, given an hour before exercise, appears to increase serum free fatty acids and to lower the respiratory exchange ratio, suggesting that more energy is derived from the preferential use of fat. It is possible that caffeine ingestion has this effect only in nonelite athletes, who lack the increased lipolytic enzyme activity and mitochondrial density and size associated with endurance training.

▶ Caffeine-containing beverages have for long been popular with ultra-long distance athletes (Costill, D., et al.: *Med. Sci. Sports Exerc.* 10:155–158, 1978). Part of the benefit from such ergogenic aids is undoubtedly due to cerebral stimulation, with a lesser perception of exertion, but there is also good evidence in a number of reports, including the present one, that free fatty acid mobilization is enhanced by large doses of caffeine (15 mg/kg). Negative conclusions (Knapik, J., et al.: *Biochem. Exerc.* 13:514–519, 1983) may reflect the use of lesser concentrations of caffeine, since a somewhat smaller dose (10 mg/kg) was without effect in the present study.—R.J. Shephard, M.D., Ph.D.

Caffeine Effect on Respiratory Muscle Endurance and Sense of Effort During Loaded Breathing
Gerald A. Supinski, Saul Levin, and Steven G. Kelsen (Case Western Reserve Univ.)
J. Appl. Physiol. 60(6):2040–2047, June 1986   1–118

It is known that fatigue of the respiratory muscles may lead to hypoventilation and respiratory failure. Recently, the authors have shown that caffeine augments the contractility of the inspiratory muscles; that is, the force or pressure generated by the diaphragm at a given level of muscle excitation is increased after caffeine administration. It is possible that respiratory muscle endurance is determined in part by the balance between energy consumption and energy availability. If this is true, then the effect of caffeine on muscle tension would tend to increase muscle energy demands and might adversely affect muscle endurance. The effect of caffeine on respiratory muscle endurance was examined while subjects breathed against massive inspiratory threshold loads.

The study population consisted of 12 normal subjects, 4 female and 8 male, ranging in age from 21 to 29 years. Respiratory muscle endurance and the magnitude of sense of effort during inspiratory threshold loading was assessed following a dose of caffeine (600 mg) previously observed to increase diaphragm strength. The respiratory muscle endurance at a given level of load was determined from the time of exhaustion and from the time course of the change in the power spectrum (centroid frequency) of the diaphragm electromyogram (EMG). The intensity of the sense of effort during loaded breathing was assessed using a category (Borg) scale. At a given load, caffeine prolonged the time to exhaustion and decreased the rate of fall of the centroid frequency of the diaphragm EMG. Caffeine also decreased the sense of effort during loaded breathing in 9 of 11 subjects. However, changes in respiratory muscle endurance after caffeine administration were not explained by changes in the pressure-time index of the respiratory muscles or the pattern of thoracoabdominal movement.

Caffeine enhances inspiratory muscle endurance, while concomitantly reducing the sense of effort associated with fatiguing inspiratory muscle contractions.

▶ For a long time, it was argued that the cardiovascular system was much more significant than the respiratory system as a factor limiting endurance performance. However, in recent months, attention has been directed to respiratory muscle fatigue as an important factor limiting prolonged effort, particularly in older patients with some degree of respiratory obstruction (Cohen, C. A., et al.: *Am. J. Med.* 73:308–313, 1982; Shephard, R. J.: *Can. J. Appl. Sport Sci. In press*).

The nature of the fatigue is still discussed, but some authors have argued for a local glycogen depletion in the chest muscles. Caffeine could alter the situation in several ways—by cerebral effects, reducing the perception of effort, by increasing the availability of fatty acids, thus sparing glycogen reserves, and by increasing muscle contractility; the last of these changes could increase local energy usage and thus hasten the onset of fatigue.

The authors demonstrate a decreased perception of respiratory effort when caffeine is given in combination with loaded breathing. This could not be explained by differences in the pattern of muscle contraction. It could be that caffeine reduces the number of active respiratory neurons (Killian, K. J., et al.: *J. Appl. Physiol.* 57:686, 1984), that it has a central analgesic effect (Laska, E. M., et al.: *Clin. Pharmacol. Ther.* 33:498–509, 1982), or that there is less sense of fatigue because central stimulation increases the output to the respiratory muscles (Eldridge, F. L., et al.: *Respir. Physiol.* 53:239–261, 1983). At all events, the ergogenic benefit from caffeine extends to the respiratory as well as to the limb muscles.—R.J. Shephard, M.D., Ph.D.

Drug Testing in a University Athletic Program: Protocol and Implementation
George D. Rovere, Herbert A. Haupt, and C. Steven Yates (Wake Forest Univ.)
Physician Sportsmed. 14:69–76, April 1986   1–119

Although so-called recreational drugs are used to the same extent by intercollegiate athletes and college students who are not athletes, performance-enhancement drugs such as amphetamines and anabolic steroids are used much more often by athletes. The authors present a protocol for and describe the implementation of drug testing in an athletic drug education program in effect at their university. The advantages of contracting an off-site commercial laboratory to do the testing are also discussed.

The drug education program, for which a full-time substance abuse coordinator was hired, has three objectives: educating athletes about drug abuse, discouraging the use of drugs, and identifying and eliminating the chronic drug abuser. The program coordinator provides a drug education seminar before the start of each team's season and is available to any athlete for personal counseling. However, the team physician coordinates and is responsible for all phases of drug testing.

Because of the high projected expenses associated with setting up on-site testing, a local commercial laboratory was contracted for drug testing. This laboratory provides a screen that tests for the most commonly abused drugs at a charge of $10 per athlete. Off-site testing also eliminates the need for tight security for collected samples, since the off-site laboratory provides pickup service for which security is assured. The professional off-site laboratory also guarantees quality control, which would be difficult to maintain in an on-site facility.

When a test result is positive, corrective measures are taken, depending on whether it is the first, second, or third documented instance of drug abuse. The athlete is counseled and retested, and as long as the retest results are negative, sports participation may be continued. However, after four positive test results the athlete is automatically and permanently dismissed from the team with a recommendation for termination of the athletic scholarship.

This program has had 100% participation from athletes, cheerleaders, managers, and trainers. To date, only several first-time, but no second-time, abusers have been identified.

▶ This may be the shape of things to come in our society, but many proper questions remain. These range from whether drug testing itself is legal and ethical other than for certain specific situations, the very significant cost, and who bears this cost. There is great concern about present and future confidentiality of such programs. The long-term implications for future job employment and insurability remain.—L.J. Krakauer, M.D.

Alcohol and Its Effects on Sprint and Middle Distance Running
L. McNaughton and D. Preece (Tasmanian State Inst. of Technology. Launceston, Tasmania)
Br. J. Sportsmed. 20:56–59, June 1986   1–120

Some investigators have suggested that alcohol can be used as an ergogenic aid to improve sports performance. However, others including the American College of Sports Medicine, have concluded that alcohol has no beneficial effect on work capacity. The effects of various levels of alcohol ingestion on various running performances were examined.

The study population consisted of five sprinters and five middle-distance runners who ingested 0.01 mg/ml, 0.05 mg/ml, and 0.10 mg/ml of alcohol before running 100, 200, 400, 800, or 1,500 m. Time was used as a practical measure of performance, and blood alcohol concentration was estimated from breath alcohol concentration. Alcohol affected all but the 100-m event to varying degrees. In the 200-m run, the performance de-

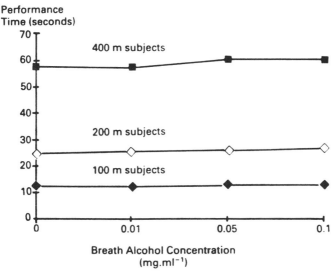

Fig 1–29.—The effects of varying amounts of alcohol on 100, 200, and 400 m performance (standard deviation was less than 0.68 second in all cases). (Courtesy of McNaughton, L., and Preece, D.: Br. J. Sportsmed. 20:56–59, June 1986.)

creased when the level of intoxication increased. Conversely, in the 400-m run, a difference was observed between the two lower levels of alcohol consumption (0.01 mg/ml vs. 0.05 mg/ml) but not between the 0.05 mg/ml and 0.10 mg/ml (Fig 1–29). The 800-m race was most adversely affected.

Alcohol is not an ergogenic aid because it was not found to improve performance. The authors recommend further research in this area.

▶ The negative effects of alcohol on race times show that any potential benefits from its energy content or a reduction in anxiety are more than offset by such factors as loss of coordination, cutaneous vasodilatation and impaired myocardial contractility.

In the present report, the authors found no adverse effect on performance over the shortest distance (100 m), and for this reason they advocated more research on alcohol in anaerobic events. However, this may be no more than a chance result from a small subject pool; M. Hebbelinck (*Arch. Int. Pharmacodyn. Ther.* 143:247–253, 1963) found a 10% decrease in speed for an 80-m dash 30 minutes after ingesting a small dose of alcohol.

Even if the rules of competition were to allow use of alcohol, it does not seem a good tactic for the runner.—R.J. Shephard, M.D., Ph.D.

Organisation of Collagen Fibrils in Tendon: Changes Induced by an Anabolic Steroid: II. A Morphometric and Stereologic Analysis
Horst Michna (Univ. of Lübeck, West Germany)
Virch. Arch. [Cell pathol.] 52:87–98, October 1987   1–121

Studies of collagen fibrils in loaded tendons following anabolic steroid treatment have shown activation of fibril organization as well as collagen dysplasia. An attempt was made to quantify the effects of anabolic steroid morphometrically in an animal study utilizing stereologic analysis.

Substantial accumulation of collagen fibrils in the extracellular matrix was observed after anabolic steroid administration. The number of dys-

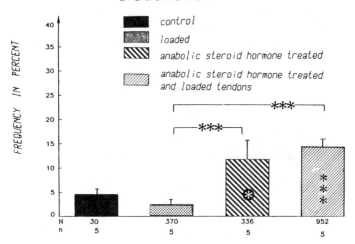

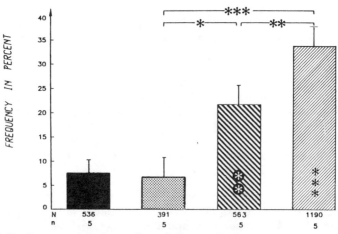

Fig 1–30.—Frequency of dysplastic collagen fibrils in tendon tissue of the different experimental groups. [Courtesy of Michna, H.: Virch. Arch. (Cell Pathol.) 52:87–98, October 1987. Berlin-Heidelberg-New York: Springer.]

plastic collagen fibrils increased with the duration of treatment. Interfibrillary and intrafibrillary dysplastic collagen fibrils had diameter distributions different from those of normal collagen fibrils in longterm studies. Mass-average diameters showed little change, but greater numbers of thinner fibrils appeared in all tendons from anabolic steroid-treated animals. The volume fraction of collagen fibrils was 20% less in study samples than in controls, while the density of fibrils increased 30%. Collagen dysplasia was especially marked in tendons from animals that were exercised and given anabolic steroid (Fig 1–30).

The changes in collagen fibrils associated with anabolic steroid therapy may be relevant to the use of these drugs in clinical medicine and in competitive sports. However, data are lacking on a correlation between the form of collagen fibrils and the biomechanical properties of tendons. Studies are needed to learn whether modification of the basic testosterone structure could reduce the degree of collagen dysplasia. This would be especially important if the drugs were used to stimulate collagen synthesis following tendon rupture.

▶ This article suggests an interesting possible complication of anabolic steroid abuse—a deterioration of tendon structure. However, two notes of caution must be sounded: first, the study was based on animals rather than humans, and second, it has to be shown categorically that the altered size distribution of the collagen fibers in tendon has an adverse impact on their mechanical function.—R.J. Shephard, M.D., Ph.D.

Altered Serum Lipoprotein Profiles in Male and Female Power Lifters Ingesting Anabolic Steroids

Jonathan C. Cohen, W. Mieke Faber, A.J. Spinnler Benade, and Timothy D. Noakes (Univ. of Cape Town Med. School and Med. Research Council of South Africa)
Physician Sportsmedicine 14:131–136, June 1986   1–122

Several studies have shown that plasma high-density lipoprotein cholesterol (HDL-C) concentration has a negative correlation with coronary artery disease. Levels of HDL-C appear to be low in male athletes who use anabolic steroids. The authors have designed a study to compare the plasma lipoprotein profiles of male and female athletes who use anabolic steroids with the profiles of those who have never used anabolic steroids.

The subjects consisted of three female and nine male amateur power lifters who had been using anabolic steroids daily for up to 24 weeks before study. The control group was composed of 40 weight-training male athletes and 9 sedentary females who had never used anabolic steroids. Nonfasting blood samples were drawn and analyzed for total serum cholesterol, HDL-C, and HDL-3-C. HDL2-C was the difference between HDL-C and HDL-3. Levels of HDL-apoprotein A-I (Apo A-I) and Apo A-II were determined by immunoprecipitation using human antibodies to Apo A-I and Apo A-II.

Compared with control male athletes, male steroid users had higher total serum cholesterol, lower HDL-C and lower Apo A-I levels. The same results were seen when female steroid users were compared with control females. The ratio of serum HDL-C to total cholesterol was 0.08 in steroid-using males and 0.28 in control males. In female steroid-users, HDL-C consisted solely of HDL3-C, indicating an absence of HDL2-C. In control females, HDL2-C made up almost 30% of HDL-C.

The fact that all steroid users had total HDL-C levels below 1.0 mmoles/L puts them in the high-risk group for coronary artery disease. Women using anabolic steroids appear to be as much at risk as men. Even when serum cholesterol and HDL-C values are compared in the steroid users and in a population considered at risk for premature atherosclerosis, the steroid users' lipid profiles were further from accepted normal values than were those of the high-risk group.

▶ There have been several recent reports drawing attention to the adverse effects of anabolic steroids upon serum lipid profiles. This report brings out both the relatively high normal HDL values which are observed in weight-trained athletes who were not using the steroids, and also the disastrous depression of HDL-cholesterol, HDL-2 cholesterol and Apo-A-I in those competitors who were taking an average of 65 mg of anabolic steroid per day (males) or 20 to 40 mg (females). The athlete who chooses to abuse anabolic steroids seems at a substantially increased risk of ischemic heart disease because of these changes in lipid profile.—R.J. Shephard, M.D., Ph.D.

Vitamins and Minerals as Ergogenic Aids
Virginia Aronson
Physician Sportsmed. 14:209–212, March 1986   1–123

Popular magazines have convinced consumers that active persons require large doses of nutritional supplements. However, nutrient supplementation requires careful consideration, particularly with regard to the potentially toxic effects of overzealous supplementation. The role of vitamins and minerals as ergogenic aids is discussed.

Overall, studies evaluating the role of vitamins in enhancing performance have failed to support their use. Furthermore, studies have shown that vitamin supplements can enhance performance only if nutrient deficiency exists. Their exercise-related functions include proper digestion, muscle contraction, and energy release from body stores for vitamin B complex, tissue maintenance and repair and resistance to infection for vitamin C, maintenance of cell integrity and muscle metabolism for vitamin E, maintenance of proper vision and resistance to infection for vitamin A, normal bone growth and development for vitamin D, and normal blood clotting for vitamin K. Excessive doses of these vitamins can result in undesirable side effects.

Certain minerals, such as sodium and potassium, chromium, selenium, zinc, and iron, are advertised as endurance enhancers. Sodium and potassium are needed during exercise to maintain normal fluid balance, regulate body systems, including heartbeat and hydration. Chromium ensures normal blood sugar metabolism, while selenium protects against oxidative damage to the tissues. Zinc maintains protein synthesis and tissue repair, and iron maintains oxygen transport to tissues for energy. However, the need for electrolyte replacement is often exaggerated, and athletes should be warned about potentially toxic side effects.

The increased energy expenditure in athletes require additional calories and fluids, which can be easily met by including generous servings of wisely selected foods. As long as an athlete's diet is balanced, there is no documented need for extra vitamins or minerals. Nutritional supplementation should be avoided unless a specific deficiency is present.

Renal Prostaglandin E_2 and $F_{2\alpha}$ Synthesis During Exercise: Effects of Indomethacin and Sulindac

Edward J. Zambraski, Robert Dodelson, Sandra M. Guidotti, and Carol A. Harnett (Rutgers Univ.)

Med. Sci. Sports Exerc. 18:678–684, December 1986   1–124

Renal tissue has a high capacity for prostaglandin biosynthesis, and prostaglandins have been implicated in inflammatory and pain responses to musculoskeletal injury. The effects of acute exercise on renal prostaglandin synthesis were studied in six physically active females with a mean age of 26.5 years, by measuring urinary PGE_2 and $PGF_{2\alpha}$ levels and by determining the effects of indomethacin, a renal prostaglandin inhibitor. Treadmill exercise testing was carried out in a double-blind design with placebo, 150 mg of indomethacin daily, and 300 mg of sulindac daily. These dosages are used clinically as anti-inflammatory treatment.

Excretion of $PGF_{2\alpha}$ decreased in the placebo condition, while PGE_2 excretion with exercise was unchanged. Baseline urinary PGE_2 was reduced by 3 days of indomethacin administration. Levels of $PGF_{2\alpha}$ were reduced by both indomethacin and sulindac. Neither drug altered the decrease in free water clearance associated with exercise. Exercise-related proteinuria was significantly increased by indomethacin but not by sulindac (Fig 1–31).

An increase in renal synthesis of vasodilatory PGE_2 may accompany acute exercise. Except for an effect on exercise proteinuria, renal prostaglandin synthesis during exercise does not seem to influence renal function. Sulindac may be less effective than indomethacin in inhibiting physiologically active renal prostaglandins.

▶ In patients with sodium depletion, heart failure, cirrhosis, and glomerulonephritis, it is well recognized that renal prostaglandins play an important role in sustaining a relatively normal pattern of renal excretion. Under the added stress of prolonged exercise, it seems that renal prostaglandins again play an important role in checking protein loss. The fact that sulindac does not interfere the renal protective action of prostaglandins, whereas indomethacin does

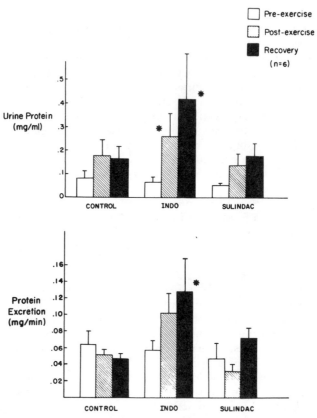

Fig 1–31.—Effects of placebo (control), indomethacin (Indo), sulindac treatments, and exercise on urine protein concentration and excretion. *denotes $P < .05$ vs. preexercise value for the same treatment. (Courtesy of Zambraski, E.J., et al.: Med. Sci. Sports Exerc. 18:678–684, December 1986. Copyright 1986, the American College of Sports Medicine. Reprinted by permission.)

seems an important argument in favor of choosing the former as an anti-inflammatory agent when treating painful musculoskeletal injuries.—R.J. Shephard, M.D., Ph.D.

Miscellaneous Topics

High Altitude Medicine

R.B. Birrer, E. Levine, R. Levine, and M. Lipski (SUNY, Downstate Med. Ctr., Brooklyn)

Ann. Sports Med. 2:155–163, 1986   1–125

An increased interest in the environment and in exercise as well as an increase in the number of people who travel to high-altitude areas has led to some serious altitude-associated problems. In the past people who visited high areas had to trek in, thus allowing time for gradual acclimatization. However, rapid ascent to high altitudes has now become common. Yet, because individual fitness and tolerance of altitude are not correlated regardless of the conditioning status, the same length of time is needed for the body to adjust to altitude. Even trained athletes need to rest every other day and to ascend about 1,000 ft per day.

Although there has been a considerable increase in the number of mountaineers who participate in high-altitude expeditions, little is known about the frequency of high-altitude–induced complaints. However, a 30-year retrospective study of 3,200 mountaineers has provided some insight. In this group there were 277 altitude-related complaints (8.7%) and 9 deaths. A total of 213 complaints were (6.7%) from mountaineers who suffered from serious systemic illness from which 3 died. In addition, there were 264 alpine accidents (8.2%) and 80 of these were fatal. Overall, approximately 24% of all mountaineers were affected by events that endangered their health or life, or both, and overall mortality was 3%.

Most of the physiologic changes encountered at high altitude are either directly or indirectly related to the low O_2 content of ambient air, which influences ventilatory and cardiovascular responses, metabolic activity of cells, renin-aldosterone-angiotensin and other hormonal systems, and the fluid and electrolyte balance of the body. It is thought that the decreased partial pressure of O_2 rather than altitude has the most direct effect on acclimatization to high altitude, which is mediated in part by hyperactivity of the sympathoadrenal system.

Life-threatening altitude-associated conditions include high-altitude pulmonary edema, encephalopathy or cerebral edema, and thrombosis and embolism. The non–life-threatening altitude-associated conditions include acute mountain sickness, systemic edema, ultraviolet keratitis, retinal hemorrhage or retinopathy, deterioration, altitude throat, chronic changes (highlanders), and cold.

With the increased accessibility and interest in high-altitude activities, physicians should be aware of the epidemiologic, physiologic, and clinical data of high-altitude medicine.

▶ In previous volumes of the YEAR BOOK OF SPORTS MEDICINE, we have dealt with high-altitude medicine and its risks in some detail. This article provides an updated review of the subject and offers statistics that are impressive in a 30-year retrospective study of over 3,000 mountaineers, with 24% risk to life in the total group from events associated with the sport. The overall mortality rate of 3%, which is cited, will vary with the risk of the activity and is appreciably higher at greater altitude and with recent patterns of rapid alpine ascent and solo climbing.

Three topics deserve particular mention because they are usually omitted in articles dealing with altitude exposure: The syndrome of high altitude systemic edema which presents after days to weeks at altitude and may occur in the absence of other signs and symptoms of altitude illness. It apparently relates to salt and water retention secondary to decreased plasma volume. Second, a good discussion is offered for the risk of ultraviolet keratitis which occurs to the unprotected eye, or partially protected eye, without warning other than occasional photophobia. Symptoms may then occur 4 to 12 hours later in the absence of any other prodrome. In the case of acute mountain sickness (AMS), these authors endorse Diamox with the alternative of parenteral steroids, clearly undesirable if possible, and note that other drugs in their review have not been effective—in particular phenytoin. This comment on phenytoin is at a variance with the paper of Wohns et al., which follows. Perhaps the side effects of Diamox have not been sufficiently stressed in the past, occurring 4 to 5 days after administration and which include paresthesias of lips, fingers, and toes, myopia, and dysgeusia. Last, in chronic mountain sickness, Birrer and colleagues speak to the use of Provera (medroxyprogesterone) as a respiratory stimulant three times daily for the chronic mountain sickness group. I am not aware of any controlled studies on this drug.—L.J. Krakauer, M.D.

Phenytoin and Acute Mountain Sickness on Mount Everest
Richard N.W. Wohns, Michael Colpitts, Thomas Clement, Anton Karuza, W. Ben Blackett, Richard Foutch, and Eric Larson (Tacoma, Wash.)
Am. J. Med. 80:32–36, January 1986   1–126

Acetazolamide and dexamethasone are effective in preventing acute mountain sickness, but both have unpleasant side effects. Since the signs and symptoms of acute mountain sickness may be related to early cerebral edema, phenytoin may prevent acute mountain sickness, provided acute mountain sickness is of neurogenic origin. To verify this hypothesis, 21 male climbers, who were members of the American Ultima Thule Everest Expedition, participated in a double-blind, randomized clinical trial of phenytoin prophylaxis for acute mountain sickness during the approach to the northeast ridge of Mount Everest. Previous expeditions to this side were associated with a high rate of acute mountain sickness, high-altitude pulmonary edema, and high-altitude cerebral edema. The study covered the ascent from Beijing to base camp, averaging 13 days.

High-altitude symptom questionnaires, filled out initially in Lhasa at 11,800 ft and in Xigatse at 12,000 feet, in Xegar at 14,000 ft, and at base camp, indicated that climbers who took phenytoin were less likely to have headaches at base camp. Analysis of variance on other indices did not show significant differences, but the power of the study was low.

Phenytoin appears to ameliorate the frequency of headaches as climbers gain altitude 16,800 ft at the Everest base camp. Phenytoin prevents acute mountain sickness presumably by altering the effect of hypoxia on the brain.

▶ The sample size was small. The drug seems to be somewhat less effective, at best, then acetazolamide, although the side effects of acetazolamide mentioned previously were avoided. The pharmacologic hypothesis is of interest in that it acts in a neurogenic fashion directly on the brain. Whether the favorable effects of this drug, such as they are, will continue to be borne out by ongoing studies in process (on Mount Rainier) remains to be seen. Whether there will be an associated beneficial effect on high-altitude retinal edema is suggested in only a small segment of the population studied and again remains to be watched in terms of the future studies.—L.J. Krakauer, M.D.

Effect of Acetazolamide on Exercise Performance and Muscle Mass at High Altitude
A.R. Bradwell, J.H. Coote, J.J. Milles, P.W. Dykes, P.J.E. Forster, I. Chesner, N.V. Richardson, and Birmingham Med. Res. Expeditionary Soc. (Birmingham Univ.)
Lancet 1:1001–1005, May 3, 1986   1–127

Exercise performance at high altitude is related to muscle loss, but the exact amount of muscle loss is difficult to assess because of concomitant fat loss and weight gain due to high-altitude edema. Acetazolamide has been used successfully to combat mountain sickness. Since it increases tissue oxygen supply, it may also decrease loss of body muscle and fat. The authors studied the effect of acetazolamide on exercise performance and muscle and other tissue loss after a slow ascent to 4,846 m at Katmandu.

The group included 21 mountain climbers (19 men), aged 22 to 56 years, of whom 12 had been on previous expeditions. None of the climbers was acclimatized to high altitude at the start of the expedition, but all were in good health. All members were given acetazolamide for 3 days before the start of the expedition. At Katmandu, subjects were randomized to receive either acetazolamide (n = 11) or placebo (n = 10).

Exercise performance at 85% maximum heart rate fell by 37% in the acetazolamide group and by 45% in the control group. The controls also experienced greater weight loss at high altitude, and the weight loss correlated with the decrease in exercise performance. During the expedition, anterior quadriceps muscle thickness fell by 8.5% in the acetazolamide group and by 12.9% in the control group, and biceps muscle thickness fell by 2.3% and 8.6%, respectively. By the end of the expedition there was loss of 5% of total body fat in the acetazolamide group and of 18% in the control group.

Acetazolamide is useful for climbers and trekkers who are acclimatized to high altitudes, not only because it effectively reduces symptoms of mountain sickness, but also because it reduces muscle and fat loss and increases exercise performance.

▶ This is a randomized study for Diamox or placebo and, inevitably, the population group is small. Perfect control studies with a significant number of subjects are hard to come by at significant altitude exposure. The data further endorse acetazolamide as the drug of choice for acute mountain sickness, as have previous studies. They go one step further and, on the assumption that this drug may increase tissue oxygen supply, they postulate a decreased loss of body muscle and fat. Their experience and data, while tentative in one sense, suggest that this did occur. This study is unique in encouraging the use of the drug in those who are acclimatized to high altitude and in suggesting it possibly is useful at extreme altitude, where prior investigators have suggested that it has a deleterious effect on maximal performance.—L.J. Krakauer, M.D.

Transient Ischemic Attacks at High Altitude
Richard N.W. Wohns (Tacoma, Wash.)
Crit. Care Med. 14:517–518, May 1986   1–128

When a patient experiences either amaurosis fugax, transient motor or sensory deficits, or a transient alteration or loss of consciousness, a workup for transient ischemic attacks (TIAs) is often begun. However, for the individual who experiences TIAs in a high-altitude environment, the diagnosis that is made and treatment that is instituted are based solely on bedside clinical criteria. Two distinct varieties of TIAs that are secondary to high-altitude exposure are described.

Man, 33, was traveling at 19,600 ft and experienced a curtain across his visual field, oculus dexter, and then blurred vision. He noticed incoordination, then visual scotomata oculus dexter. These symptoms cleared spontaneously and the patient did not have headache or any other neurologic complaint. The next night he was examined at the base campt at 17,000 ft. Examination of visual evoked potentials on both eyes revealed no change from prior examinations of 17,000 ft and at sea level. An ophthalmologic examination after dilation demonstrated a completely normal fundus in each eye without any signs of venous engorgement or hemorrhage; no emboli were observed. The subject was informed that this event was a TIA and that there was some increased risk for further TIAs and possibly a stroke with repeated exposure to high altitude. However, the subject continued his high altitude travel and did not experience a recurrence.

Man, 46, experienced a right frontal headache, blurred vision, numbness of his left hand and arm, and some mild incoordination at an altitude of 18,000 ft. The neurologic symptoms cleared and he returned to base camp where ophthalmologic examination after dilation revealed normal fundi bilaterally without signs of emboli, hemorrhage, or venous dilatation. The neurologic examination was completely normal and there were no carotid bruits. The recording of visual evoked potentials demonstrated no change from prior readings at 17,000 ft and at sea level. The subject was advised that this event increased his risk of repeated TIAs or stroke at high altitude. He elected to withdraw from mountain-climbing and has since had no difficulties.

Man, 29, had visual disturbances at high altitude on three separate occasions. These distortions lasted 15 to 30 seconds and then resolved, but sometimes they recurred at 10-minute intervals. He had no associated headache, dizziness, speech disturbance, focal numbness, weakness, or nausea. At the time of the second episode he was examined by a physician who found no neurologic abnormalities.

It is concluded that the first patient experienced an insufficiency in unilateral carotid distribution with some similarities to amaurosis fugax; the second subject most likely experienced a vertebrobasilar TIA; and the third subject suffered recurrent vascular insufficiency to the calcarine cortex. It is likely that the first subject experienced a focal ischemic event, whereas the second and third subjects apparently experienced flow-related ischemic events. The author recommends that patients who experience TIAs at high altitudes take low doses of aspirin, increase fluid intake, and be aware that repeated TIAs or stroke may occur.

▶ Transient ischemic attacks and strokes are known risks of high altitude, with Sir Edmund Hillary the classic case of a true cerebrovascular accident in a young male. The author cites three well-studied cases where the vascular etiology was different, with the patients ranging in age from 29 to 46 years. Pragmatic recommendations are made for the obligatory pragmatic treatment of such events on the mountain and are based primarily on avoiding platelet agglutination by salicylates or equivalent, and hydration.

The importance of the article to me is to raise the question of generalized salicylate prophylaxis for those visiting high altitude. Without further statistics, a definitive answer cannot be given at this time, although it certainly is an appealing recommendation with the safety record of low altitude exposure. Further, the onset of even mild symptoms in any older person at altitude is a very important prognostic indicator, and a warning sign that should not be ignored.—L.J. Krakauer, M.D.

Do Climbs to Extreme Altitude Cause Brain Damage?
John B. West (Univ. of California at San Diego)
Lancet 2:387–388, Aug. 16, 1986   1–129

The history of mountaineering is one of continual attempts to better the achievements of others. Although the primary goal used to be to conquer the world's highest peaks, since this has been accomplished, climbers now set new objectives, such as reaching the summits without oxygen. Many climbers and physicians have asked whether brain damage occurs under these extremely hypoxic conditions. Two separate issues are important. The first issue is whether there is central nervous system (CNS) impairment at great altitudes, and the second is whether exposure to the extreme hypoxia of these high altitudes causes residual impairment of CNS function. It is fairly well accepted that the extreme hypoxia of great altitudes causes functional impairment, but careful measurements on climbers are rare. Although the second issue has been hotly debated, there is evidence to suggest that exposure to extreme hypoxia at high altitudes also leads to residual impairment of CNS function. The goal of the present article was to discuss the evidence that climbs to extreme altitudes cause brain damage.

There is mounting evidence that the severe hypoxia of high altitude leads to residual impairment of neuropsychologic function. Such residual impairment was observed among 21 members of the American Medical Research Expedition to Everest after return to sea levels following about 3 months at altitudes of 5,400 to 8,848 m. Measurements made before and immediately after the expedition (Fig 1–32) revealed significant abnor-

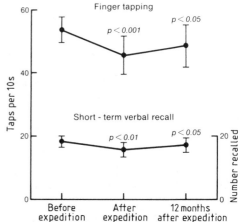

Fig 1–32.—Results of finger tapping and short-term memory tests before, immediately after, and 1 year after an expedition to Mt. Everest. (Courtesy of West, J.B.: Lancet 2:387–388, Aug. 16, 1986.)

malities in motor coordination for both hands, in shortterm and longterm verbal recall, and in the aphasia screening test. When the same tests were repeated 12 months later, persistent abnormalities were found in motor coordination for both hands, and in verbal recall. The abnormalities in motor coordination were found to continue beyond 24 months postexpedition. Others have found persistent abnormalities in a group of 12 male and 10 female Polish climbers several weeks after a Himalayan expedition. However, it is noted that not all investigators have found postexpedition abnormalities.

A significant risk exists for residual brain damage as a result of severe hypoxia at high altitude.

▶ One of my delightful colleagues at the RAF Institute of Aviation Medicine was a "Battle of Britain" fighter pilot who had frequently exceeded the ceiling of his in-flight oxygen systems in an attempt to "down" German planes. While I have no record of his personality before the second World War, it often occurred to me that he might have suffered some brain damage as a result of these escapades; certainly, his behavior patterns bore many of the hallmarks of a prefrontal leukotomy.

West here poses the same question with regard to climbers who press on toward the summit when logic tells them that the limits of their oxygen supply have been surpassed. He is in a stronger position to diagnose brain damage than I was, since careful measurements of cerebral function were made before the expedition. Persistent defects are demonstrated, even 2 years after return to sea level. West points out that the danger of impaired cerebral function is small relative to other risks of climbing (100 deaths on Everest, about 2 per expedition, due to falls, accidents in the unstable icefall, exposure, and exhaustion). However, if one should advise against boxing because of residual effects on the brain, it is logical to extend this advice to the exploration of extreme altitudes without supplementary oxygen.—R.J. Shephard, M.D., Ph.D.

High-Altitude Pulmonary Edema in Vail, Colorado, 1975–1982
Aris M. Sophocles, Jr. (Univ. of Colorado)
West. J. Med. 144:569–573, May 1986   1–130

Previous studies have suggested that there are two epidemiologically distinct forms of high-altitude pulmonary edema. Type I (nonresident-ascent) was shown to affect residents of altitudes below 2,438 m who ascend to higher altitudes for periods of 2 days or longer; the patients in whom this develops are men with a mean age in the mid-30s. Type II (resident-reascent) affects residents of high altitudes after they return from descents to elevations below 2,438 m; this disorder appears to primarily affect children and adolescents, and to affect boys and girls equally.

All cases of high-altitude pulmonary edema that were seen in Vail, Colo. (base elevation, 2,500 m) between 1975 and 1982 were analyzed. The author sought to describe the clinical and epidemiologic characteristics of the disorder found at this elevation, to look closely at unusual cases for clues to the causes of the disorder, and to examine the hypothesis that there are two distinct epidemiologic varieties of high-altitude pulmonary edema.

Between 1975 and 1982, there were 47 cases of high-altitude pulmonary edema in Vail. All of these cases occurred in visitors from lower altitudes, and the mean age of the patients was 35.6 years; 93% were men (table). The symptoms included tachycardia, tachypnea, and fever, with the mean onset of cough and shortness of breath 2.5 days after arrival. The average total ascent of the patients was 2,330 m in less than 1 day, from a mean residential elevation of 170 m. Most cases (91%) occurred between December and April, when the average daily temperature was − 4.3 C and the ambient barometric pressure was 22.37 inches of mercury.

The tendency for type I high-altitude pulmonary edema to develop is a function of the rate and the distance of the ascent, the altitude attained, and the visitor's level of activity after arrival. Men appear to be at a much greater risk than women. An etiologic role for the inappropriate secretion of antidiuretic hormone caused by hypoxia is possible.

▶ There has been increasing evidence that high-altitude edema is a problem of

THE PREVALENCE OF TYPE I HAPE AMONG MALE VISITORS TO VAIL

Year	Number of Lift Tickets Sold	Number of Males at Risk	HAPE Cases	Prevalence HAPE Cases/ 100,000
1979–1980	1,219,178	102,248	10	9.8
1980–1981	1,040,819	71,736	10	13.9
1981–1982	1,344,167	94,888	6	6.3
Totals	3,604,164	268,872	26	10.0

Hape = high-altitude pulmonary edema

*HAPE = high-altitude pulmonary edema.
(Courtesy of Sophocles, Jr., A.M.: West. J. Med. 144:569–573, May 1986. Reprinted by permission of The Western Journal of Medicine.)

weekend athletes patronizing ski resorts. This study from Vail (altitude, 2500 m) observed some seven cases per year, with symptoms appearing as anticipated (2 to 3 days after arrival at the resort).

There was no evidence that the patients could be divided into new arrivals and returning residents of high altitude; this may be because the altitude residents were in less of a hurry to rush out on the slopes than were the weekend visitors. In other cities, where the returning residents have been at risk, they have had to go to work immediately after their return (for instance, in the high-altitude mines of South America).—R.J. Shephard, M.D., Ph.D.

Control of Ventilation in Extreme-Altitude Climbers
S. Masuyama, H. Kimura, T. Sugita, T. Kuriyama, K. Tatsumi, F. Kunitomo, S. Okita, H. Tojima, Y. Yuguchi, S. Watanabe, and Y. Honda (Chiba Univ., Chiba, Japan)
J. Appl. Physiol. 61:500–506, 1986   1–131

An increased ventilatory response to very high altitude is critical in achieving high performance in mountain climbing. At more moderate altitudes, a blunted hypoxic ventilatory response (HVR) may allow native highlanders to increase their work rate more effectively than newcomers from sea level.

The value of a low HVR was assessed in ten climbers. Hypercapnic and hypoxic ventilatory responses were examined before and after the expedition and correlated with performance at extreme altitude. Five of the climbers reached an altitude higher than 8,000 m.

Responses to CO_2 were similar in the high- and low-performance groups, but hypoxic response slopes were higher in the high-performance group (table). The HVR decreased markedly after the expedition, and all subjects claimed less ventilatory drive subjectively. The Pa_{CO_2} was significantly reduced more than 1 month after the climb, indicating that the effects of acclimatization persisted. Red blood cell counts were increased, but the average level of hemoglobin did not change appreciably.

High HVR is found in extreme-altitude climbers who exhibit better performance. Depressed HVR persists more than a month after the expedition. The HVR determined at sea level may be a useful indicator of climbing performance at extreme altitude.

▶ The climber at extreme altitude uses a large part of his or her available oxygen intake in the muscles of respiration. Personal reports of some climbers give graphic accounts of the respiratory effect associated with even a single pace toward the summit of mountains such as Everest. It has thus been hypothesized that one reason why Sherpas seem to make the ascent more easily than sea-level residents is that they do not respond to hypoxia by such a large increase of ventilation; the lesser ventilatory response reduces the oxygen cost of respiration, and spares oxygen for the muscles which are used in climbing.

Not all investigators have confirmed the depressed hypoxic response of the Sherpas (Hackett, P. H., et al.: *J. Appl. Physiol.* 49:374–379, 1980). The pres-

VENTILATORY AND OCCLUSION PRESSURE RESPONSES TO CO_2 AND HYPOXIA IN CLIMBERS WITH HIGH AND LOW PERFORMANCE

High-Performance Climbers, (HPC)

CO_2 Response

Subj.	$\Delta\dot{V}i/\Delta P_{CO_2}$, $l\cdot min^{-1}\cdot Torr^{-1}$	$\Delta P_{0.2}/\Delta P_{CO_2}$, $cmH_2O/Torr$
M.Ki.	1.37	0.38
M.Y.	1.51	0.56
J.S.	1.46	0.61
J.W.	1.54	0.44
M.T.	0.89	0.13
Mean ± SD	1.35±0.24	0.42±0.17

Hypoxic Response

	Saturation Analysis		Hyperbola Analysis		
	$\Delta\dot{V}i/\Delta Sa_{O_2}$, $l\cdot min^{-1}\cdot \%Sa_{O_2}{}^{-1}$	$\Delta P_{0.2}/\Delta Sa_{O_2}$, $cmH_2O\cdot \%Sa_{O_2}{}^{-1}$	A, $l\cdot min^{-1}\cdot Torr$	C, Torr	$\dot{V}o$, l/min
M.Ki.	-0.646	-0.128	680.8	10	5.0
M.Y.	-1.672	-0.522	819.8	21	-0.5
J.S.	-0.358	-0.164	706.6	0	7.8
J.W.	-0.619	-0.356	1,025.3	5	-6.8
M.T.	-0.089	-0.056	165.6	0	9.0
Mean ± SD	-0.677 ±0.539	-0.245 ±0.170	693.9 ±292.7	7.2 ±7.8	2.9 ±5.9

Low-Performance Climbers, (LPC)

CO_2 Response

Subj.	$\Delta\dot{V}i/\Delta P_{CO_2}$, $l\cdot min^{-1}\cdot Torr^{-1}$	$\Delta P_{0.2}/\Delta P_{CO_2}$, $cmH_2O/Torr$
T.O.	1.21	0.61
K.H.	1.95	0.51
M.Ko.	1.19	0.54
Y.K.	1.18	0.81
N.O.	2.61	0.42
Mean ± SD	1.63±0.57	0.58±0.13

Hypoxic Response

	Saturation Analysis		Hyperbola Analysis		
	$\Delta\dot{V}i/\Delta Sa_{O_2}$, $l\cdot min^{-1}\cdot \%Sa_{O_2}{}^{-1}$	$\Delta P_{0.2}/\Delta Sa_{O_2}$, $cmH_2O\cdot \%Sa_{O_2}{}^{-1}$	A, $l\cdot min^{-1}\cdot Torr$	C, Torr	$\dot{V}o$, l/min
T.O.	-0.432	-0.035	277.2	11	7.2
K.H.	-0.097	-0.034	519.2	1	7.6
M.Ko.	-0.413	-0.184	225.2	26	11.7
Y.K.	-0.230	-0.033	42.2	33	7.4
N.O.	-0.421	-0.072	256.6	22	6.7
Mean ± SD	-0.319 ±0.134	-0.072* ±0.058	264.1† ±152.4	18.6 ±11.3	8.1 ±1.8

Hyperbola analysis was conducted with equation, $\dot{V}i = \dot{V}o + A/P_{ETO_2} - C$.
*Difference from high performance climbers (HPC) has borderline significance.
†Difference from HPC group is significant.
(Courtesy of Masuyama, S., et al.: J. Appl. Physiol. 61:500–506, 1986.)

ent report casts some further doubt on this hypothesis. While altitude apparently blunted the hypoxic response of all members of the expedition, when climbers were separated into good and bad performers, it was shown that those who performed well actually had a greater isocapnic response to hypoxia than those who were indifferent climbers. It would seem that at extreme altitudes (over 8,000 m), an excessive blunting of hypoxic response can be counterproductive.—R.J. Shephard, M.D., Ph.D.

Sickle Cell Trait, Exercise, and Altitude
Edward R. Eichner (Univ. of Oklahoma)
Physician Sportsmed. 14:144–157, November 1986   1–132

The impact of sickle cell trait on health is controversial. It is generally benign and does not shorten life. However, with extremes of altitude and exertion, sickle cell trait can confer some small but nonetheless real risks. There is no doubt that a small risk of splenic infarction exists at mountain altitudes in both whites and blacks. Exercise may contribute to this risk by augmenting hypoxia. The pattern of exercise-induced death in sickle cell trait consists of severe exertional rhabdomyolysis, acute renal failure, acidosis, hyperkalemia, and death in 20 to 48 hours. However, there is still no cogent evidence that sickle cell trait per se predisposes to exertional rhabdomyolysis or death.

Sickle cell trait is no barrier to outstanding athletic performance. Athletes with the trait should take the same precautions as any other athletes—no more, no less. Like any other athletes, those with the trait should avoid dehydration and overheating, should not perform vigorous exercises if they have viral infections, and should not charge into strenuous exercise if they are not used to it.

▶ This subject was discussed extensively in 1986 YEAR BOOK OF SPORTS MEDICINE, pp. 190–191, regarding the paper of Lane and Githens. It was pointed out that the trait can present in the nonblack individual and in an altitude environment higher than 7,000 ft, a splenic syndrome could develop usually indicative of splenic infarction and sequestration. Eichner emphasizes that there is still no firm evidence that the trait increases the risk of rhabdomyolysis or death. The trait should be no barrier to outstanding performance, and he does not believe that any particular precautions are indicated in those who carry the trait irrespective of color.—L.J. Krakauer, M.D.

Should Epileptics Exercise?
Virginia S. Cowart (Chicago)
Physician Sportmed. 14:183–191, September 1986   1–133

Today, many physicians have encouraged epileptic patients to lead active lives with only few restrictions on their choice of sports. The current views on exercise for epileptics are expounded.

The Epilepsy Foundation of America recommends that "persons with epilepsy can take part in sports or other vigorous activities, although a lot depends on the degree of seizure control, the type of sport, and the physician's recommendation." The risks of injury to self and others vary tremendously, according to the severity of a patient's seizures and whether or not the seizures can be controlled with appropriate medications.

Many physicians agree that sports associated with high levels of stress may not be suitable for persons with epilepsy. While common sense rules out epileptic's participation in sports in which a seizure can cause a dangerous fall—e.g., high diving and gymnastics—those with medically controlled seizures should be encouraged to participate in carefully supervised exercise programs. Swimming need not be restricted in young epileptics, provided they are well supervised. Young athletes should face virtually no school-imposed prohibitions if seizures are well controlled.

Provided seizures are well controlled, exercise and sports program will promote a healthier, more active life-style in patients with epilepsy.

▶ In most instances, the epileptic patient, child or adult, is overcontrolled in terms of activities prescribed. If seizures are under good clinical control with today's broad armamentarium of drugs, there is no reason for a sedentary lifestyle for the epileptic patient, and even vigorous activity is not precluded, provided a measure of common sense is used as to risk. Note is made of the author's comment that "60% of all children with seizure disorders who receive proper medical control early in life become seizure free and require no medication in adulthood." Thus, most exercise and sports programs are compatible with a healthy active life-style.—L.J. Krakauer, M.D.

Benefits of Aerobic Exercise for the Paraplegic: A Brief Review
L.L. Cowell, W.G. Squires and P.B. Raven (Texas Lutheran College, Seguin, and Texas College of Osteopathic Medicine, Fort Worth)
Med. Sci. Sports Med. 18:501–508, October 1986   1–134

This review summarizes literature on the effects of exercise and paraplegia. In paraplegia the loss of motor function and sensory perception as well as changes in sympathetic and parasympathetic stimulation alter cardiovascular response to exercise. Ultimately paraplegia leads to a degenerative process with decreased lean body mass (LBM), lowered aerobic capacity, an osteoporotic condition and renal dysfunction. As a result of medical advances, most complications of the paraplegic are being controlled; however, owing to reduced muscle mass these individuals have an increased risk of athrosclerosis.

After an acute spinal cord injury and during outpatient rehabilitation therapy, paraplegics are in regimented training programs. However, returning home most do not maintain their cardiovascular fitness. The energy expenditure of wheelchair locomotion appears similar or greater to that for walking, causing more cardiovascular stress due to a decreased active muscle mass. A lower fitness level is created which is the result of lack of mobility, augmented by automated wheelchair usage.

The large decrease in active muscle mass puts the paraplegic at greater risk of cardiovascular disease. The degenerative process following injury leads to noted physiological changes. The decrease in LBM decreases skeletal muscle and affects the body's energy needs. Bone demineralization and collagen catabolism constitute another aspect of the degenerative process of a sedentary lifestyle. This appears to be reversed with weight bearing and when pressure is applied across the long axis of the bone.

Because of the paraplegic's inability to ambulate, the problems associated with determining their fitness levels have led to many investigations. Paraplegics appear to respond similarly to exercise testing as able-bodied persons. As a result of using a smaller muscle mass in arm exercise, fatigue sets in sooner and only 50% to 60% of maximal work load accomplished by leg work can be attained.

Aerobic work capacity of paraplegics seems to be influenced by the injury site and activity level. Through maximal training work loads, significant improvement in aerobic capacity and muscle strength can be obtained. Wheelchair sports have resulted in large cardiac reserves, benefiting ordinary demands of mobility. As a result of possible surgical advances, the paraplegic needs to be in good cardiovascular health for easier recuperative periods.

▶ The importance of exercise is accepted by most for the general population and has been strongly encouraged. In the spinal cord injured, exercise becomes all the more important and it is emphasized that this population group can respond to an exercise regimen, to some measure, to attempt to compensate for the very marked increased risk of atherogenic disease, hypertension, and renal dysfunction. In physiologic terms, the greatest risk is the decrease in lean body mass (LBM) relating to a decreased Vo_{2max}. The autonomic nervous system is an added area of concern. This involves the sympathetic drive to the cardiovascular system as well as the lower lesions that affect bladder and bowel function.

Wheelchair sports are important and will improve cardiovascular and cardiorespiratory function in the nonsedentary paraplegic compared to the sedentary control. However, the emphasis must be on intensive discipline and rehabilitation to maintain function as long as possible—the implied hope being that neural transplantation, neural regeneration, and functional electrical stimulation via surgical implant may be available. This study offers an excellent review of the literature of this complex physiologic problem.—L.J. Krakauer, M.D.

Effect of Moderate Exercise on Esophageal Function in Asymptomatic Athletes

Lawrence J. Worobetz and David F. Gerrard (Univ. of Saskatchewan, Saskatoon, Saskatchewan, Canada, and Univ. of Otago, Dunedin, New Zealand)
Am. J. Gastroenterol. 81:1048–1051, November 1986　　　　1–135

In this study, esophageal function is examined during moderate exercise in six healthy men aged 21 to 25 years (mean age, 23 years). Each subject exercised for 2 hours on a treadmill set at a work load of 50% of their maximum oxygen uptake. Esophageal manometry was performed in the supine position immediately prior to exercise, immediately after and following a 1-hour rest in the supine position. Of the six participants, one experienced regurgitation after consuming 200 ml of water at the 1-hour interval of his run.

Lower esophageal sphincter (LES) pressure measured before exercise ranged from 18 to 27 mm (mean, 24 mm Hg). Immediately following exercise, the LES pressure increased significantly to 33% greater than the preexercise level (mean, 32 mm Hg). The mean LES pressure was reduced to 27 mm Hg (range, 22 to 30 mm Hg) after 1 hour of rest following exercise. All subjects except one showed a reduction in LES pressure after 1 hour of rest. The LES, whether pre- or postexercise, showed appropriate and complete relaxation with swallowing in all cases.

The mean amplitude and duration of esophageal peristalsis remained the same throughout the study. There were no biphasic or triphasic waves and no tertiary esophageal contractions.

Despite the small number of individuals studied, it was clearly shown that a significant increase in the LES pressure with moderate exercise occurred which appeared to gradually subside with rest. Function of the esophageal body appeared unaffected by moderate exercise.

The basis for the increase in LES pressure is unclear but may relate to the observed exercise-induced increase in serum motilin, gastrin, and catecholamine levels.

▶ In healthy asymptomatic athletes, motility of the esophagus was essentially unchanged, but the mean lower esophageal sphincter pressure demonstrated a significant increase. The emphasis is again on moderate activity and asymptomatic persons. How this relates to the common symptoms of heartburn, belching, and regurgitation in some athletes remains to be explained.—L.J. Krakauer, M.D.

Can Exercise Make Us Immune to Disease?
Heyward L. Nash
Phys. Sportsmed. 14:250–253, March 1986   1–136

It is commonly accepted that physical activity enhances psychological outlook, raises high-density lipoprotein cholesterol levels, and increases endorphin activity. However, some fitness buffs have taken this belief a step further and believe that daily exercise can ward off infection. Unfortunately, such individuals occasionally get sick because they apparently went overboard with their exercise routine. The goal of the present article is to examine what happens to the immune system during exhaustive physical activity.

Appropriate levels of exercise may enhance the immune response and may have an antistress effect. This is attributed to release of hormones into the bloodstream, including cortisone, epinephrine, opiates, endorphins, and peptides. These same hormones are usually released when a person undergoes psychological or emotional stress, and it is proposed the exercise regulates these chemicals and alleviates stress, which in turn may improve the immune response. However it is not known whether it is exercise itself or a relaxed state of mind that triggers the regulation of these chemicals. Other investigators suggest that the reverse may also be true and that acute exhaustive exercise may create too much stress and may damage the immune response. It is thought that people who exceed their optimum exercise level may in fact be courting infection. In part this may be due to changes in the ratios of helper T cells to suppressor T cells.

It is concluded that work done in the area of immunity and exercise has been flawed because "exercise physiologists don't do good work in immunology, and immunologists are not exercise oriented." The author recommends a large epidemiologic study to determine what effect exercise has on the immune system.

▶ This is one of several recent studies that suggests that overtraining or exhaustive exercise can overcome the beneficial effects of mild exercise via stress relief and endorphin production and, indeed, lead directly to infection, whether by interruption of mucociliary barriers or more importantly by basic immunologic changes in lymphocytes themselves. There seems to be little question that natural killer cell level of lymphocytes, speaking of circulatory immunity, may be abnormal for 24 hours after extreme exhaustive exercise. This has broad implications for training in many sports.—L.J. Krakauer, M.D.

Exercise Training for Special Patient Populations
Peter Hanson, Ann Ward, and Patricia Painter (Univ. of Wisconsin, Madison)
J. Cardiopulmonary Rehabil. 6:104–112, March 20, 1986   1–137

Exercise training is considered to be beneficial in the treatment of patients with coronary heart disease and is widely used in cardiovascular rehabilitation. Prescribed exercise training may also be useful in the management of other chronic cardiovascular and metabolic disorders. The authors reviewed the literature to assess the effect of exercise training in patients with insulin-dependent (type 1) and non–insulin-dependent (type 2) diabetes mellitus, hypertension, and chronic renal failure.

Initial studies of training in diabetics showed increased peripheral insulin sensitivity and attenuation of hyperglycemia during exercise and after exercise training. Later training studies in patients with uncomplicated type 1 diabetes showed that significant increases in maximum oxygen consumption can be achieved. Most studies in type 2 diabetics showed increased peripheral insulin sensitivity and improved glycemic control, but the degree of improvement appeared to vary with the intensity of exercise training, diet, and simultaneous weight loss.

In patients with mild to moderate hypertension, blood pressure is partially normalized by aerobic exercise training. Patients with end stage renal disease also benefit from improved exercise tolerance and reduction in hypertension.

Exercise training in these patient groups requires careful evaluation of clinical and exercise-testing data. Consideration should be given to potential side effects of prescribed pharmacologic agents. Possible risks or contraindications to exercise training should be assessed before a patient is enrolled in an exercise training program.

▶ We tend to concentrate on the healthy athlete in our comments on the pros and cons of exercise training. It is appropriate to note that exercise training has a role, not only in cardiovascular rehabilitation, a common practice, but in various chronic cardiovascular and metabolic disorders as reviewed by these authors. The psychological aspects of some of these diseases, such as end stage renal disease and advanced diabetes, can be discouraging both for the therapist and patient. That there are objective figures of improvement in Vo_{2max}, however, stands as a measure of physiologic improvement and the importance of individualization and a very graduated low level program is stressed. An important point: exercise testing or training is contraindicated in patients with potassium levels greater than 5.5 mEq/L.—L.J. Krakauer, M.D.

Objective Measurements of Customary Physical Activity in Elderly Men and Women Before and After Retirement
J.M. Patrick, E.J. Bassey, J.M. Irving, A. Blecher, and P.H. Fentem (Univ. Med. School, Queen's Med. Ctr., Nottingham, England)
Q.J. Exp. Physiol. 71:47–58, 1986   1–138

There is a need for effective methods to assess customary physical activity in elderly persons in order to determine the level of customary physical activity necessary to maintain physical capacities for an independent lifestyle. Subjective methods for assessing physical activity involving questionnaires and diaries may be reliable in groups which partake of regular vigorous recreational activity, but have been shown to be unreliable in groups such as the elderly with moderate to low activity levels. The advent of miniature magnetic tape systems has permitted the authors to develop methods in which biosignals related to the intensity of physical activities can be recorded in parallel with a time signal over long periods using body-borne equipment. This method was used to establish physical activity levels of workers just before retirement, to determine whether or not there were changes at retirement, and whether these changes would affect their physical condition as measured by the heart rate response to submaximal exercise.

The authors used computer analyses to obtain indices of the intensity and duration of periods of physical activity using biosignals based on heart rate and footfall signals. Threshold values were set for each subject at a heart rate related to a standard walking speed of 4.8 km per hour (3 miles per hour). Four activity indices were established in terms of time spent

THE STANDARDIZED HEART RATE (ADJUSTED TO A WALKING SPEED OF 4.8 km · h⁻¹) AND THE FOUR INDICES OF CUSTOMARY PHYSICAL ACTIVITY IN THREE GROUPS OF SUBJECTS BEFORE AND AFTER RETIREMENT FROM WORK (MEAN ± S.E.M.)

| | | Steel-workers | | Factory-workers | | |
| | | Men | | Men | | Women |
		Pre-retirement	Post-retirement	Pre-retirement	Post-retirement	Pre-retirement	Post-retirement
	$n =$	16	25	17	17	22	16
H.R.$_{4·8}$ (beats min⁻¹)		$92·1 \pm 3·3$	$91·4 \pm 2·1$	$91·5 \pm 3·0$	$93·5 \pm 2·4$	$96·2 \pm 2·0$	$98·1 \pm 2·5$
Time sustained (min)		87 ± 18	136 ± 22	91 ± 26	109 ± 23	89 ± 19	61 ± 22
Intensity sustained (beats)		1390 ± 384	2134 ± 396	1336 ± 381	1750 ± 434	1207 ± 282	868 ± 345
Walking time (min)		68 ± 14	51 ± 7	46 ± 9	41 ± 5	50 ± 6	34 ± 7
Walking intensity (beats)		913 ± 169	718 ± 105	624 ± 121	578 ± 89	651 ± 96	426 ± 114

(Courtesy of Patrick, J.M., et al.: Q.J. Exp. Physiol. 71:47–58, 1986.)

above this threshold and the intensity of the heart rate elevation above it, applying criteria relating to the duration of periods of activity or the concurrent activation of the walking signal. The study population consisted of three groups of subjects, aged older than 60 years, who were studied before and after retirement: 25 were steelworkers and 39 were factory workers. These individuals exhibited rather low levels of activity. After 1 year of retirement, the female factory workers showed a substantial decrease in activity; however, in men this was observed only after several years of retirement had elapsed (table).

The body-borne tape recorders used for these measurements of physical activity are unobtrusive and well tolerated even by elderly subjects, and they have been shown not to influence the activity being measured. The recordings of heart rate and footfall during the day provide a large amount of objective information which preserves the duration and sequence of separate periods of activity. This information can be used flexibly to provide appropriate numerical indices of physical activity. Regarding the physical activity levels of the elderly subjects, it is concluded that they were too low for optimum maintenance of physical condition and body composition.

▶ One of the key, unanswered questions of sports medicine at present is just how much activity does the general public take? Recent estimates of the proportion of the general North American population who take enough exercise to sustain physical condition have ranged very widely from 9% to 78% (Shephard, R. J.: *Fitness of a Nation.* Basel, Switzerland, S. Karger, 1986). Most of the rather dubious information available to date has been obtained by the fallible approach of retrospective questionnaires.

J. M. Patrick and associates have here adopted the alternative tactic of using simple instrumentation to actually record activity patterns. While in theory such instrumentation can be applied to large samples of the population, in practice their report is limited to 80 subjects. The footfall instrument presupposes that the main activity of the day is walking—more true for some people such as retirees than for others who are working at various industrial tasks. The heart-rate recorder presupposes that the heart rate is not substantially increased by factors other than exercise—for example, the effect of anxiety or high environmental temperatures must be minimal if activity patterns are to be indicated faithfully.

The heart-rate data obtained in Nottingham mirror those previously reported for the retirement age (Sidney, K. H., and Shephard, R. J.: *J. Gerontol.* 32:25–32, 1977). The average heart rate of the elderly is in the low 90s, with most subjects showing little evidence of significant physical activity.—R.J. Shephard, M.D., Ph.D.

Hot Weather, Exercise, Old Age, and the Kidneys
Patricia A. Eisenman (Univ. of Utah)
Geriatrics 41:108–114, May 1986   1–139

It is generally acknowledged that walking and other exercise programs offer benefits to many older persons. However, on hot days any benefits of exercise to the person older than age 50 years may be paralleled by an increased risk of dehydration and hyperthermia. The author discusses the effects of aging on the heat-regulating responses of the body and offers strategies for minimizing risks of dehydration and heat injury during exercise in warm weather.

Hyperthermia is a serious problem encountered during foot races in hot weather in persons of all ages. Earlier studies have shown that thermoregulatory responses in older exercising persons are blunted as a result of diminished sweat production capabilities in response to prolonged heat

---

COMPARISON OF SYMPTOMS OF CLASSIC AND EXERTIONAL HEAT STROKE

Characteristic	Classic	Exertional
Age	Older	Young
Occurrence	Epidemic form	Isolated cases
Body temperature	Very high	High
Presdisposing illness	Frequent	Rare
Sweating	Often absent	May be present
Acid–base disturbance	Respiratory alkalosis	Lactic acidosis
Rhabdomyolysis	Rare	Common
DIC*	Rare	Common
Acute renal failure	Rare	Common
Hyperuricemia	Mild	Marked
Elevated muscle enzymes	Mild	Marked

*Disseminated intravascular coagulation.

[Courtesy of Eisenman, P.A.: Geriatrics 41:108–114, May 1986. Reprinted with permission from Medicine (Baltimore) 61:196, 1982. © by Williams & Wilkins, 1982.]

stress. Thermoregulatory mechanisms can become impaired if a person exercises on successive days without adequate rehydration. Since thirst is not an accurate measure of water need, exercisers often do not balance fluid intake with fluid loss. Fluid replacement may lag 2 or 3 days behind actual needs if thirst alone is relied on, and symptoms of dehydration or heat injury may then occur.

Symptoms of dehydration and heat injury after exertion differ from symptoms of classic heat stroke. Whereas exertion-induced heat stroke is seen most often in young, healthy athletes who train in hot, humid weather, classic heat stroke has been associated most often with the elderly who are unable to cope with environmental heat waves (table). However, with more elderly persons participating in physical activity, the likelihood of older persons manifesting symptoms of exertional heat stroke is on the increase.

Preventive strategies in hot weather include reducing the intensity of activities, exercising for shorter periods, exercising only in the morning or evening, wearing loose clothing, and replacing fluids lost through sweating about every 15 minutes. Such precautions should minimize the likelihood of dehydration and heat injury for older exercisers.

▶ The table is of good value in this article: concise and descriptive. Classic heat stroke is the more common problem in our elderly and is perhaps more serious. With increased exercise participation the point is made that some of the milder variants may present in this population group. Thirst is a poor guide in the elderly. Dehydration can almost be assumed ubiquitous with activity or with the extremes of temperature elevation. Those in this age group who do exercise should be trained in preventive hydration.—L.J. Krakauer, M.D.

Does Ketanserin Relieve Frostbite?

Michael Vayssairat, Pascal Priollet, Albert Hagege, Edward Housset, and Jacques Foray (Hôp. Broussais, Paris, and Hôp. de Chamonix Mont-Blanc, Chamonix, France)
Practitioner 230:406–408, May 1986   1–140

Treatments of deep frostbite have been many and have yielded conflicting results. The successful use of ketanserin, a selective antagonist of serotonin 2 receptors, in a patient with severe frostbite is described.

Man, 19, had severe frostbite of both hands. Examination revealed severe bilateral finger edema with blister formation and large areas of skin necrosis with hypesthesia. Conventional management was instituted, but healing was slow. On the ninth day, large areas of skin necrosis were still present. Ketanserin, 20 mg orally three times daily, was added. Healing progressed considerably, and the patient was discharged on day 20 with completely healed hands.

Ketanserin is useful as a complementary treatment in frostbite.

▶ This drug is a selective antagonist of the serotonin 2 (5-HT$_2$) receptors. This is used as a complementary oral measure to standard therapy and it was so used in this single case. It may have a role in the future care of frostbite, but will warrant much more extensive study for certainty.—L.J. Krakauer, M.D.

Aerobic Capacity After Contracting Infectious Mononucleosis
Michael J. Welch and Leigh Wheeler (U.S. Military Academy, West Point, N.Y.)
J. Orthop. Sports Phys. Ther. 8:199–202, October 1986   1–141

Infectious mononucleosis can be disabling to athletes of all ages. Traditional treatment includes bed rest, fluids, and fever control during the acute phase of the disease, followed by extended periods of limited physical activity. If an athlete remains inactive too long, a significant amount of detraining occurs, whereas premature return to full activity might precipitate side effects or relapses. The authors used an objective method to assess the optimum period of limited physical activity after the acute phase of infectious mononucleosis.

Of 16 cadets in whom infectious mononucleosis had been diagnosed, 9 were randomly assigned to a rehabilitation exercise group and 7 to a control group after hospital discharge. All participants were given an aerobic capacity test on a motor-driven treadmill. The exercise group began light training on a bicycle ergometer and increased training intensity over the initial 2-week period. The control group did not participate in any physical activity during the same period. After a second period of self-paced activity for both groups, the cadets were again evaluated for aerobic capacity on a treadmill. There were no significant differences between the groups in aerobic capacity, metabolic cost, or run time to exhaustion on the two aerobic tests.

Prolonged bed rest does not appear to be indicated for patients recovering from infectious mononucleosis. Noncontact activities may be resumed as soon as a patient becomes afebrile.

▶ Note that the study group consisted of 16 healthy young West Point cadets. Taken at face value, prolonged bed rest did not seem to enhance the recovery from this potentially disabling illness. Caution must be raised about extrapolating from this to older age groups or to those with coexisting disease or impaired immune capacities. In this instance of infectious mononucleosis, rest and the recovery phase reminds one of the Chalmers study of infectious hepatitis.—L.J. Krakauer, M.D.

Isolation of *Legionella pneumophilia* From Canadian Hot Springs
B.J. Dutka and P. Evans (National Water Research Inst., Canada Ctr. for Inland Waters, Burlington, Ontario, and Bureau of Microbiology, Health Protection Branch, Health & Welfare Canada, Ottawa)
Can. J. Public Health 77:136–138, March/April 1986   1–142

The incidence of *Legionella* was determined at three Canadian hot and warm spring sites, Fairmont, Radium, and Banff, using culture and direct fluorescent antibody (DFA) techniques. *Legionella pneumophilia* was either recoverable from or detected by DFA studies in samples from all of the three hot springs examined. Chlorination of the water in the upper pool of the radium hot springs probably reduced the bacterial count at least to a level under that detectable by culture and serologic procedures.

Legionella detection by DFA is not as accurate as that recovered by culture since *L. pneumophilia* antiserum has been known to react with non-*Legionella* organisms. However, in this study as culture technique yielded positive results at two of the sites, DFA detection alone at the third site carried more weight than it otherwise would.

While four different media were used to support *Legionella* growth from at least one water sample, no one medium alone would have recovered the organism from all positive culture sites. This emphasized the importance of using more than one medium type in performing surveys as such.

Inhibitors of other organisms in the growth media are known to lower *Legionella* recovery. Therefore, present quantitative results represented a low estimate of the population present.

Recognition of *Legionella* presence in hot spring water could be helpful in epidemiologic studies of those illnesses where the more usual sources have been eliminated, although it should be noted that no obvious aerosol or other means of disseminating the organisms is present in these waters.

▶ In simple objective terms, this potentially dangerous organism has been found at three diverse hot springs in Canada. It must be reasonably assumed that this is present at other hot springs. Why there has not been clinical infection associated with this sort of exposure is unknown. Chlorination will reduce the bacterial count without question. It is also of incidental interest to know that chlorine protection itself is not innocuous, especially in its gaseous form or in its acidic form with penalties on the teeth of those exposed repetitively as well as acting as a respiratory allergen and direct URI irritant. Aerosols have usually been necessary, or at least implicated, in the dissemination of the disease previously. None were present at these sites. The world was easier when we knew less.—L.J. Krakauer, M.D.

Stress and the Athlete: Coping With Exercise
Patrick Murphy
Physician Sportsmed. 14:141–146, April 1986   1–143

Stress and sports often seem to go hand in hand. To succeed many athletes have to endure overwhelming pressure, and failure can lead to despair. However, stress and pressure can also have a positive effect, because some athletes appear to thrive on pressure. Whether stress is positive or negative, it is clear that athletes who must train several hours per week in pursuing athletic excellence push their body and mind to the limit and must cope with stress daily.

Stress can be defined as a process that consists of the stressor, which is based on many factors such as personality, race, and gender, and a response in the form of eustress (euphoria) or distress. Any given stimulus or dose can be perceived differently by different people and can be perceived differently by the same person at different points in time. Clearly, athletes inflict upon themselves varying degrees of stress and how they handle that stress often determines whether they will perform successfully or whether they will continue with their exercise programs.

Signs that a person is under too much stress include difficulty in falling asleep, loss of appetite, difficulty in enjoying sex, and difficulty in concentration. The most common response to stress is worry, but stress among athletes can often manifest itself in the form of perceived pain or injuries. The greatest cause of stress in child athletes appears to be their parents and the major cause of stress in professional athetes appears to be their coaches.

One of the primary consequences of stress has been shown to be staleness, which is both a physiologic and a psychological phenomenon. Although it is difficult to identify the distressed athlete, it is crucial to do so, and it is likely that the best person to make this identification is the coach.

Unlike a disease, stress cannot be cured; therefore, it is important for the athlete to identify the source of stress. Once that source is identified it is essential to determine why it is causing stress. The authors points out that the definitive answer for helping athletes cope with stress lies in more research in both the fields of psychology and physiology.

▶ This subject and article are included because I think it is necessary to deal with the concept of stress when one is dealing with competitive athletics. Stress can be positive or negative and is multifactorial with the sport, the nature of the goal involved, and most important, the inherent makeup of the individual involved. I don't believe there are answers at the moment as to why and how individuals handle stress. Very much depends on parents and coaches. Sophisticated counseling for some individual athletes may be critical.—L.J. Krakauer, M.D.

Increase of Circulating Beta-Endorphin-Like Immunoreactivity Correlates With the Change in Feeling of Pleasantness After Running
Johannes Wildmann, Arnd Krüger, Mathias Schmole, Jürgen Niemann, and Heinrich Matthaei (Göttingen, West Germany)
Life Sci. 38:997–1003, March 17, 1986   1–144

It is known that activities such as running and exercise are followed by a variety of physiologic responses; these responses are thought to be partially mediated by the secretion of catecholamines and several peptide hormones. Plasma levels of ACTH and β-endorphin are elevated concomitantly, and these agents might be responsible for increases in plasma cortisol, growth hormone, and prolactin concentrations. In addition to physiologic responses, there are also well-documented mood changes associated with running and exercise including an increased feeling of pleasantness. The endorphins may play a role in eliciting these mood effects. The goal of the study was to determine whether mood change and increase of plasma β-endorphin after long distance running are correlated.

The study population consisted of 21 male long-distance runners. Each subject participated in two 10-km runs 1 week apart and their β-endorphin-like immunoreactivity (β-EIR) was assayed in plasma before and immediately after running. Mood was assessed by an adjective check list prerun and postrun. Self-reliance and good mood scored higher after running. Although both mood elevation and plasma β-EIR increase were found to exhibit considerable individual variability, there was a significant correlation in the mean values of the two runs betwen individual β-EIR increases and the changes of rating in feeling of pleasantness. High β-EIR increases corresponded to positive mood change postrun.

Although no simple conclusion can be drawn as to the relationship between endorphinergic alterations and emotional elation, the study did provide the first clear demonstration of a correlation between circulating β-EIR increase and feeling of pleasantness.

▶ To date, much of the work on β-endorphin release has relied on the suppression of endorphin effects by administration of naloxone. The immunoassay of β-endorphin activity is a useful alternative.

The present sample participated in two 10-km runs. The subjects reported that a feeling of "pleasantness" was an important reason for running (22 points), although interestingly, fitness (29 points) and performance (26 points) were more significant motivators in this group.—R.J. Shephard, M.D., Ph.D.

Use of UV-A Sunbeds for Cosmetic Tanning
B.L. Diffey (Dryburn Hosp., Durham, England)
Br. J. Dermatol. 115:67–76, July 1986   1–145

As a result of the social desirability of obtaining a tan, suntan salons have thrived during the past decade. Long-term risks of exposure to sunbeds emitting ultraviolet A (UV-A) radiation are not yet known. The results of a national survey of sunbed users, which was made in 1985 in England, are reported.

A total of 1,013 clients of commercial suntan salone, 168 males and 845 females, including 514 females aged 16 to 30 years, completed questionnaires. Eighty-seven clients were taking the suntan treatments because they had acne or psoriasis. Most subjects (61%) used a sunbed for half-hour sessions, but exposure times ranged from 10 to 60 minutes. Most clients (98%) reported a slight or deep tan after using a sunbed (table). A high proportion (83%) reported feeling better psychologically since they started the sunbed treatments. However, the psychological benefits appeared to be closely related to the degree of tan obtained.

The incidence of reported acute side effects was 28%. Eight percent of subjects developed a skin rash or felt nauseated during or immediately

Ability to tan in sunlight	Degree of tan with sunbed		
	Deep	Slight	None
Easily	295	317	4
Slightly	84	265	12
Never	3	13	6

TAN ACHIEVED WITH SUNBED RELATED TO TANNING IN SUNLIGHT*

*χ^2: $P < .001$.
(Courtesy of Diffey, B.L.: Br. J. Dermatol. 115:67–76, July 1986.)

after exposure. The incidence of itching, nausea, and skin rash in females aged 16 to 45 years who were taking oral contraceptives was higher than that in those who were not using any medications.

The results of this study are probably biased, since only satisfied customers could be counted on to come in for repeated treatments, whereas those that were either unhappy with the results obtained or who experienced adverse reactions would be unlikely to return.

▶ The statistics for increased risk of skin cancer, and melanoma in particular, are real. Against this background the use of the artificial ultraviolet environments is hardly to be recommended and is a commercial exploitation of many health clubs and individual businesses of the society as a whole. Such warnings are unlikely to deter people who derive a psychological benefit from ultraviolet exposure whether it be in a box or on a beach.—L.J. Krakauer, M.D.

2 Biomechanics

Biomechanical Study of Full-Contact Karate Contrasted With Boxing
Michael L. Schwartz, Alan R. Hudson, Geoffrey R. Fernie, Ken Hayashi, and
Allan A. Coleclough (Univ. of Toronto)
J. Neurosurg. 64:248–252, February 1986   2–1

In boxers, cumulative brain injury results from repeated blows to the head and correlates with the number of bouts fought. Much less is known about full-contact karate (kickboxing), wherein punches and kicks are actually landed, rather than being focused, to culminate just short of an opponent as practiced in traditional karate. A combatant can win on points, but the surest means of victory is a knockout. Consequently, fighters strive to land blows to the head.

Since violent angular acceleration of the head may occur with punches or kicks, a biomechanical study was conducted to investigate the relative forces of kicks and punches in full-contact karate. A dummy head was mounted 175 cm above the floor (to simulate a 50th-percentile man standing erect) and 125 cm above the floor (to simulate the man in a crouched position) on a universal joint allowing motion about three axes. The mechanism was designed to provide constant rotational stiffness, while springs provided constant restorative movements about the three axes. The dummy was fitted with a mask of visco-elastic foamed material to simulate the texture of soft tissue. Fourteen karate experts delivered punches, using bare hands, "safety-chop" hand protectors, and 10-oz boxing gloves, and kicks with bare feet or safety-kicks to the dummy.

Accelerations ranging from 90 G to 120 G were recorded. On the average, punches to the side of the "head" produced greater peak accelerations than did kicks to the front and side, which in turn produced greater acceleration than punches to the front of the "head." The use of safety chops and safety-kicks did not reduce acceleration of the dummy, but the use of boxing gloves significantly reduced the peak acceleration of punches.

In boxing and full-contact karate, blows are frequently directed toward the head, resulting in violent acceleration of the head. If full-contact karate is practiced widely, cases of kickboxer's encephalopathy will soon be reported.

Biomechanical Consequences of Sport Shoe Design
E.C. Frederick
Exerc. Sports Sci. Rev. 14:375–400, 1986   2–2

The methodologies used to characterize the mechanical properties of sport shoes, the effects of these properties on performance, and the etiology of sports injury are examined in detail in this comprehensive review.

The biomechanical consequences of sport shoe design are affected by interaction of the shoe, the surface it contacts, and the body. The biomechanical tools used to study sport shoes consist both of physical measurements which mechanically characterize the shoe or its component materials, or human subject tests, in which people subjectively gauge the body's response to shoes possessing various properties.

It was found that most of the effects of sports shoes on human biomechanics are a consequence of the body's response to the shoe and not the result of the shoes' mechanical properties in isolation. Given the many possible shoe designs and the body's tendency to adjust predictably to particular characteristics of shoes, we now have a convenient model for the study of biomechanical adaptation, as well as a new way to manipulate human kinetics and kinematics.

▶ With the "running craze" came the design and redesign of the running shoe, then the design and redesign of every other type of athletic shoe. It is not necessary to have special shoes for every athletic event in which one participates. The author of this review explains how we got to where we are and how the shoe is not a powerful tool for manipulating human movement.—Col. J.L. Anderson, PE.D.

The Practical Biomechanics of Running
Robert S. Adelaar (Virginia Commonwealth Univ.)
Am. J. Sports Med. 14:497–500, November–December 1986   2–3

An understanding of the biomechanics of the foot in static and dynamic conditions is essential for the proper evaluation of gait and clinical problems associated with running. The author discusses the physiology, kinematics, and muscle interaction of walking, jogging, and running cycles and reviews the current biomechanical literature.

The variation in speed between running, jogging, and walking causes different gait patterns (Fig 2–1). The walking cycle consists of a stance phase (65%) and a swing phase (35%). Heel strike, midstance, forefoot off, swing phase, and opposite heel strike are the components of the walking cycle. Running is equivalent to about 60% of the walking cycle time, and jogging is equivalent to about 70% of the walking cycle time. As velocity increases, the stance phase decreases, and a double unsupported phase, called a float phase, occurs. The double support limb phase disappears. It is essential to understand the phases of gait in walking in order to understand the running cycle.

During the first phase, heel strike is equivalent to about 15% of the stance phase. The tibia is rotated internally from an externally rotated position at heel strike, and the ankle moves passively toward plantar flexion. During the second phase, the relationships between hindfoot eversion and inversion are important in midfoot pronation, distribution of forces, and positioning of the plantar grade forefoot surface. During the third phase, the arch is stabilized by the hindfoot position and plantar fascia

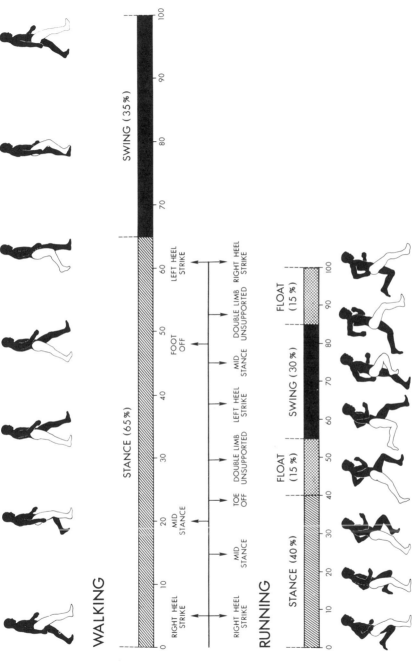

Fig 2–1.—Comparison of the phases of the walking and running cycle. The running gait cycle is different from walking because of the increase in the double limb unsupported time or float phase, decrease in stance phase, and increase in swing phase. (Courtesy of Adelaar, R.S.: Am. J. Sports Med. 14:497–500, Nov–Dec 1986.)

186 / Sports Medicine

windlass mechanism. Long and short flexors and intrinsics are also very active in initiating footoff. During this phase, the foot supinates and raises the arch in preparation for the swing phase.

▶ Understanding the phases of gait is certainly important; so is understanding the biomechanical interaction of foot placement in running and walking and the linkage from the ankle to the knee and the hip. Many athletes, after they reach the age of 30, begin to develop pain in the Achilles or the knee. Often they are told they have to give up their favorite sport such as running, tennis, or handball. We have had great success at West Point by prescribing the Roberts rear foot controls in shoes used for exercise or even in dress shoes. Almost everyone, including this author, has found the pain the Achilles and the pain behind the patella gone within a couple of days. If I remove the rear foot controls, which are designed to correct excessive pronation, the pain returns in both areas. Expensive orthotics made by a podiatrist did not give the same relief of pain.—Col. J.L. Anderson, PE.D.

Kinematic Accommodation of Novice Treadmill Runners
David A. Schieb (Univ. of Northern Colorado)
Res. Q. Exerc. Sport 57:1–7, March 1986   2–4

Subjects who are used for treadmill studies are given various amounts of exposure prior to acquisition of data. First-time treadmill performers frequently make kinematic adjustments until a stable, consistent gait pattern with minimal stride-to-stride variability is achieved. However, the actual time required before the individual feels comfortable with the treadmill seems to depend on such factors as the length of time into the run, the amount of prior overground running experience, and various psychological factors.

To determine the effects of treadmill training on the kinematic accommodation and habituation process of novice treadmill runners, the author observed six experienced male college distance runners who were novice treadmill runners. These subjects trained on a treadmill that was operating at 4.0 m per second for 15 minutes a day for 10 days. The subjects were filmed each day in the frontal and sagittal planes at 1, 8, and 14 minutes into the run. Stride length, temporal data, and vertical and lateral horizontal displacements of the center of gravity were assessed with a computer digitizer system.

Significant alterations occurred in the kinematics of treadmill running between days 1 and 2 of the 10-day training period. On days 1 through 3 significant changes in stride occurred between minutes 1 and 8 but not between minutes 8 and 14.

Minimal amounts of treadmill training are necessary for a subject to accommodate fully to the treadmill.

▶ For experienced college distance runners, one would not expect that it would take long for them to adapt to running on a treadmill. It would be interesting to replicate this study using inexperienced runners to see how long it would take them to adapt.—Col. J.L. Anderson, PE.D.

Effects of Stride Length Alteration on Racewalking Economy
D.W. Morgan and P.E. Martin (Arizona State Univ.)
Can. J. Appl. Sports. Sci. 11:211–217, December 1986   2–5

This study was undertaken to investigate the effects of stride length (SL) alteration on racewalking economy in a group of competitive racewalkers. Four male and three female competitive racewalkers participated. The average age, weight, and height were 32.4 ± 14.4 (SD) years, 59.9 ± 10.5 kg, and 169.1 ± 10.8 cm, respectively. Mean training duration was 27.0 ± 9.7 months, and weekly mileage was 34.4 ± 15.9 miles.

Following two test sessions in which $\dot{V}O_{2max}$ and freely chosen stride length (FCSL) were determined, each subject completed 6-minute racewalking bouts at five randomly ordered SL conditions (FCSL and −10%, −5%, +5%, and +10% of leg length from the FCSL). This was done while walking at a velocity approximately equal to their 10-km training pace.

For the five SL conditions, actual and predicted group mean $\dot{V}O_2$ values implied that the subjects were most economical walking at the FCSL, with progressively higher energy costs manifested at the +5% and −5% and the +10% and −10% leg length conditions, respectively. Between subjects' FCSL and optimal SL (OSL), a mean absolute difference in $\dot{V}O_2$ of 0.6 ml.kg^{-1}.min^{-1} was observed. A mean absolute SL difference of 3.2 cm (3.6% of mean leg length) was linked with this deviation in $\dot{V}O_2$.

For most subjects, walking at stride lengths longer and shorter than the FCSL was less economical than walking at the FCSL. However, individual differences in $\dot{V}O_2$ responses at the various stride length conditions were manifested. The minor differences in $\dot{V}O_2$ and stride length seen between the FCSL and OSL conditions supports the hypothesis that trained subjects adopt locomotion patterns which are nearly optimal in terms of the aerobic demands. Data suggested that from a performance standpoint, modification of the FCSL is not needed for most racewalkers. However, lengthening or shortening the FCSL toward more optimal conditions may be beneficial to the elite performer who exhibits a substantial deviation in $\Delta\dot{V}O_2$.

▶ Maybe this study shows the value of trial and error training. If we assume that the freely chosen stride length (FCSL) is developed over time as the race walkers practice and develop their techniques and they freely choose stride length that is very close to the optimal stride length (OSL) then what more needs to be done. Will race walkers of the same physical builds, height, weight, length of limbs, develop the same FCSL over time? Is there a proven method to compute the OSL and program the new race walker to adopt the OSL in a shorter period than it would take to develop the FCSL by trial and error?—Col. J.L. Anderson, PE.D.

The Biomechanics of the Long Jump
James G. Hay
Exerc. Sports Sci. Rev. 14:401–446, 1986   2–6

The United States Olympic Committee is involved in a project designed to provide useful scientific information to coaches and athletes who are preparing to participate in the Olympic games. The author reviews the available scientific literature on the biomechanics of the long jump.

The long jump consists of four consecutive parts: the approach, the takeoff, the flight, and the landing. The optimum approach length for a given athlete is determined by the athlete's sprinting ability and the method used to begin the approach. The takeoff is determined by an athlete's execution in each of three phases: an initial phase during which the angle of the knee joint remains mostly unchanged; a middle phase in which the included knee joint angle decreases; and a final phase in which the knee-joint angle increases. The flight path of an athlete is fixed by the speed, angle, and height of takeoff. Air resistance has only a small modifying influence on flight performance. Landing efficiency is affected by the optimum position of the body at landing, but there is still much speculation about what constitutes an optimum body position.

Some studies have been done on how the magnitude and direction of the wind affect performance in the long jump. Findings suggest that, in general, the magnitude and direction of the wind have relatively little influence on the distances recorded. However, it is possible that for a given athlete on a given day, the wind may affect performance profoundly.

The 8.90-m leap of Bob Beamon in the 1968 Olympic Games in Mexico City still stands as a world record to date. Since no scientific films were taken of the men's long jump event, the parameters of this jump have been analyzed with the aid of available news film and photographic sequences. It appears that Beamon achieved such a great distance as a result of a fast approach run and an almost perfect takeoff.

The author concludes with the observation that the overall quality of the papers reviewed was poor, while many of the data presented in tables and graphs were outright wrong. He states that future progress in the area of sports biomechanics is likely to be very slow if the level of scholarship does not improve considerably in the future.

▶ This author, Hay, has spent many years studying and teaching the development of athletic skills through biomechanical analysis. When he speaks we should all listen. His comments concerning the overall quality of the papers he received from a number of countries (Czech, English, French, German, Japanese, Polish, and Russian) left no doubt that they left much to be desired. He found the data-gathering unimaginative, with little or no technological innovation in most of the studies. He found variables not defined, crucial measurements techniques not described, and major results not presented or discussed. Data in the tables were in error. Accepting what he says as fact, is there any wonder that it is difficult to build on the research of other investiga-

tors? We must do a better job or we will just continue spinning our wheels.—
Col. J.L. Anderson, PE.D.

The Tennis Stroke: an EMG Analysis of Selected Muscles With Rackets of Increasing Grip Size
Stanley Adelsberg (Hosp. for Joint Diseases Orthopaedic Inst., New York)
Am. J. Sports Med. 14:139–142, March–April 1986   2–7

Despite the large volume of research on tennis, little is known about the electromyographic (EMG) analysis of the tennis stroke. The tennis stroke involves changes in motor unit activity and changes in the positions of body segments that are organized in a particular time and space sequence in accordance with the stroke that is being executed. Many tennis injuries, such as tennis elbow, have been attributed to a variety of causes, including technique, racket characteristics, warm-up, age, sex, and experience.

It is hypothesized that there are certain patterns of EMG activity of the muscles of the forearm and shoulder during the forehand and backhand strokes when different racket grips are used and that this pattern of activity may be associated with tennis elbow or other complaints.

The author evaluated the EMG activity of the muscles involved in the

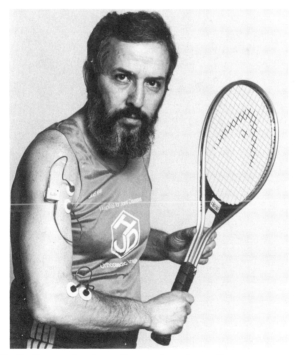

Fig 2–2.—Tennis player with racket and EMG electrodes in place. (Courtesy of Adelsberg, S.: Am. J. Sports Med. 14:139–142, March–April 1986.)

tennis forehand and backhand strokes in a group of four tennis players who were instructed to hit a ball that was thrown at a constant speed and angle from a ball-throwing machine. The EMG activity of the anterior deltoid muscle and the forearm extensor groups was recorded with the subjects using racket grip sizes of 4 1/4, 4 1/2, and 4 3/4. (Fig 2–2).

There was a specific pattern of sequence phasing in all subjects, and the amplitude ratio between the muscles was constant. Changes in grip size revealed a decrease in amplitude of both the anterior deltoid and the forearm extensor group.

It is concluded that the force changes which occur at the shoulder and the forearm are not significant enough to suggest changes in grip size when there are complaints of tennis elbow.

▶ We should not be too surprised that changing the tennis racquet grip by 1/2 in did not produce force changes significant enough to help in the prevention or treatment of tennis elbow. It is much more likely that such factors as experience, skills, and muscular conditioning are variables more important in explaining the causes of tennis elbow. Probably most of us have had problems with tennis elbow when we have tried to play much more than we are conditioned to play. We have also seen the person who hits the backhand stroke with the elbow bent and leading the racquet and then noticed the band worn just below the elbow. That person also wants to know how to treat tennis elbow.—Col. J.L. Anderson, PE.D.

Mechanical Efficiency in Rowing
Tetsuo Fukunaga, Akifumi Matsuo, Keizo Yamamoto, and Toshio Asami (Univ. of Tokyo)
Eur. J. Appl. Physiol. 55:471–475, September 1986   2–8

The purpose of this study was to estimate gross, net, work, and delta efficiencies during rowing and investigate the similarities and differences in the efficiency of rowing previously reported. Five varsity oarsmen participated who were aged 20.8 ± 1.5 years, 173.6 ± 4.0 cm tall, and weighed 67.1 ± 4.0 kg.

Measurement was performed using a rowing tank in which water was circulated at 3 $m \cdot s^{-1}$ by a motor driven pump. The subjects rowed with the stepwise incremental loading in which the intensity increased by 10% of the maximum force of rowing (max F_c) every 2 minutes. Power (W_o) was calculated from the force applied to the oarlock pin (F_c) and its angular displacement (Θ_H). Oxgen uptake ($\dot{V}O_2$) and heart rate were measured every 30 seconds during rowing. Anaerobic threshold was determined from expired gas variables with the Wasserman method.

The Θ_H indicated about 45 degrees at the moment when the oar blade went into the water, and it was about 30 degrees at the moment the blade came out of the water. The peak value of F_c in a stroke was about 1,500 N. The times when the oar went in and out of the water were 0.76 second and 1.16 second on average, respectively.

Anaerobic threshold of the oarsmen was 74.6 $\pm$ 6.01% $\dot{V}O_{2max}$. Linear increases of F_c were observed with increasing $\dot{W}o$, whereas displacement of the oar handgrip (D_o) was independent of $\dot{W}_o$. A small increment in stroke frequency occurred with low rowing intensities.

With unladen rowing ($\dot{W}_o = 0$), $\dot{V}O_2$ was 1.12 $\pm$ 0.11 1.min^{-1} (mean $\pm$ S.D.). With low intensities below about 100 W of $\dot{W}_o$, $\dot{V}O_2$ increased curvilinearly with increase in $\dot{W}_o$. At higher intensities, a rectilinear relation was seen between $\dot{V}_o$ and $\dot{W}_o$, and gross efficiency ranged from 15% to 20%. Efficiencies were independent of intensity within a range of 45% to 75% $\dot{V}O_{2max}$. Mean mechanical efficiencies obtained in the region of 124 to 182 W of $\dot{W}_o$ indicated the highest value for work efficiency (27.5%) and the lowest for gross efficiency (17.5%).

The increment in $\dot{W}_o$ was caused mainly by increase in F_c, while being independent of D_0. In tank rowing, compared to regular boat rowing, the pin and foot braces are rigidly fastened to the floor. Thus, the force of inertia stored in the shell is not present, and additional muscle strength is needed to accelerate the body forwards. This may increase energy expenditure at a given rowing frequency in the tank and yield a lower efficiency in tank rowing than when rowing in a moving boat.

▶ This study is a good example of using biomechanical analysis to investigate mechanical efficiency of athletic performance. It would have been valuable to use three-dimensional cinematography to record the rowing patterns and analyze what happens to the pattern as fatigue sets in. This would help in deciding what parts of the body need strengthening or where additional training is needed.—Col. J.L. Anderson, PE.D.

Effect of Seat Position on Maximal Linear Velocity in Wheelchair Sprinting
C.M. Walsh, G.E. Marchiori, and R.D. Steadward (Univ. of Alberta, Canada)
Can. J. Appl. Sports Sci. 11:186–190, December 1986   2–9

One of the most prevalent problems facing the wheelchair athlete is where to position the seat in order to achieve maximum efficiency and speed. The relationship between seat position and linear velocity in wheelchair sprinting was investigated. The study was also concerned with the identification of anthropometric measures that might act as predictors in selecting the ideal seat position.

Nine male subjects, aged 19 to 33 years, with varying physical disabilities were included. Linear velocity was determined for nine different seat positions by analyzing the filmed performance of subjects wheeling at maximum speed on a wheelchair ergometer. Prior to performing at each seat position, the following measurements were taken; the vertical distance from the axilla to the top of the wheel and from the fingertip to the bottom of the handrim, and the vertical and horizontal distances from the greater trochanter to the axle of the rear wheel.

No significant differences between the maximal linear velocities at each of the nine seat positions were found. This suggested that within the range of seat positions chosen, maximal linear velocity was minimally affected. Observed variability in the shoulder-hub angle during each test position may have affected these findings; despite the fact that subjects were instructed to maintain a stable trunk position deviation occurred. The negative effects of poor seat positions could be lessened by altering the degree of upper body lean. The lack of significant correlations between anthropometric measurements and linear velocity could also be accounted for by the variability in shoulder-hub angle.

Significant negative correlations were revealed between time on the handrim and linear velocity and time on the handrim and pushing frequency. The stepwise regression results indicate the importance of time on and off the handrim in the prediction of velocity in wheelchair sprinting. These findings are in opposition to other reports. The high negative correlation observed supports the notion that an increase in pushing frequency may be more critical than time on the handrim in producing maximum linear velocity.

Maximal velocity in wheelchair sprinting appears to be increased by shortening the time on the handrim and increasing the pushing frequency. With improved trunk stabilization, the shoulder-hub angle and anthropometric variables could contribute to the linear velocity.

▶ It is good to see this study because these investigators are treating the disabled wheelchair racers as the athletes they are. We need people to learn more about training disabled athletes. Competition is just as important for the disabled as for the able-bodied athletes. We need to develop training techniques for disabled athletes so they have the opportunity to improve their performances and become the best athletes they are capable of being.—Col. J.L. Anderson, PE.D.

Sit-To-Stand Movement Pattern: A Kinematic Study
Sharon Nuzik, Robert Lamb, Ann VanSant, and Susanne Hirt (Virginia Commonwealth Univ.)
Phys. Ther. 66:1708–1713, November 1986   2–10

Although standing from a seated position is performed often during a given day, no adequate studies have been done on the most efficient pattern of movement. The authors developed a clinically relevant visual model of the body rising from a seated position from film data obtained from healthy volunteers.

The study was done with healthy volunteers, 38 women and 17 men, ranging in age between 20 and 48 years, who were filmed in the sagittal plane while rising from a seated position on an armless wooden chair with a seat height of 46 cm. Each procedure was recorded on film in three consecutive trials, but only one trial from each subject was selected for analysis.

Data points were established at various points of the body. These body points defined the angles of interest. The data points were analyzed at 5-

degree increments with a computer program and movement patterns were reconstructed on a computer screen by connecting the data points of each phase into a total of 21 stick figures. The moving stick figures formed a schematic diagram of the entire movement cycle.

It is hoped that after this model has been further refined, a physical therapist will be able to assess abnormal movement patterns in a patient by either observing or filming that patient's movement sequence and comparing it with the norms set by this model.

▶ The sit-to-stand movement pattern may not seem like an important thing to young, healthy people, but it becomes more important as people get older. This study is limited because it uses only a hard armless chair and healthy subjects. It is much more difficult to move from sit-to-stand from a low, soft chair. The pattern also changes when arms are available for the subject to use. This study is a beginning. It is the type of study that beginning students studying the techniques of biomechanical analysis would start with. It is also the type of study that can be expanded and built on to provide information on something that will be more and more important as our population gets older.—Col. J.L. Anderson, PE.D.

Activity in Torso Muscles During Relaxed Standing
A.P. Woodhull-McNeal (Hampshire College, Amherst, Mass.)
Eur. J. Appl. Physiol. 55:419–424, August 1986   2–11

The present study aims to determine the minimum necessary and sufficient activity of torso muscles during relaxed standing compared to lying. The muscles studied consisted of the major superficial muscles of posture: erector spinae, external obliques, and rectus abdominis. Activity in the forearm extensors and forearm flexors was also evaluated. Surface electrodes were used for examining electromyographic activity in six women, aged 19 to 24 years, with no history of major back problems. Six additional similar subjects were studied as a pilot group.

While subjects were relaxed and lying down, each of the torso muscles exhibited 0.2 μV of activity and the forearm muscles 0.1 μV. For a minimum of ten 10-second samples per subject, the erector spinae, external oblique, and rectus abdominis muscles showed a median activity of 1.0 μV, 2.5 μV, and 0.7 μV respectively, during quiet standing. Comparison of medians for each of the torso muscles showed a significant increase during standing. Activity in the forearm flexors and extensors was not significantly greater during standing than lying. A positive correlation was observed between activity in the erector spinae and the external obliques during standing.

Slight but constant activity in the superficial dorsal and ventral muscles of the torso appeared necessary for quiet standing. No consistent increases appeared in the nonpostural forearm muscles. Evidence of consistency was found between the right and left erector spinae muscles.

Data supported the biochemical model in which opposing sets of muscles act as "guy wires" for the torso. There was no support for hypotheses of passive support for the torso, nor do torso muscles act in either/or fashion as both, anterior and posterior muscles are active together. Appropriate opposing sets of muscles are activated at a low level around joints in unstable equilibrium by unknown mechanisms.

▶ Few researchers pay much attention to the upright posture of humans. I appreciate this study because it examined the minimum necessary activity of torso muscle during relaxed standing. However, I would also liked to have gained some information concerning the energy costs of standing while holding the body in an upright posture that is associated with "good posture." How much more muscular activity would it take to stand using good posture compared to relaxed standing? Is it possible for older people to maintain good upright posture as they age? What effect would exercise to strengthen the erector spinae, the external obliques, and the rectus abdominis muscles have on helping older people maintain good upright posture?—Col. J.L. Anderson, PE.D.

Objective Anterior Cruciate Ligament Testing
Raymond J. Boniface, Freddie H. Fu, and Kaveh Ilkhanipour (Univ. of Pittsburgh)
Orthopedics 9:391–393, March 1986   2–12

It is frequently difficult to perform a clinical assessment of the anterior cruciate ligament (ACL) of the knee. The Lachman test, i.e., the anterior drawer test, which is performed in 20 degrees of knee flexion, is thought to be the best single indicator of a deficiency of the ACL. Other tests such as the pivot shift test may also provide useful information. However, these tests may be difficult to carry out and to interpret when the patient is muscular, or after an acute injury, when discomfort and guarding limit manipulation of the knee and hemarthrosis may mask a subtle finding. Several devices are commercially available which claim to provide an objective assessment of laxity.

The authors tested the Stryker knee laxity tester (Fig 2–3) to determine its usefulness in evaluating the ACL. The study population consisted of 123 athletes with no history of knee injury, 30 patients with arthroscopy-proved injury to the ACL, and 11 injured patients with an intact ACL at arthroscopy. The anterior and posterior tibial displacement was recorded at 20 degrees of knee flexion and 20 lbs of force in each direction.

Anterior laxity and side-to-side difference correlated with injury to the ACL; posterior and total anteroposterior laxity did not. In normal subjects mean anterior laxity was observed to be 2.5 mm, and only 8% of normal knees had anterior laxity of 5 mm or more. However, 10% of normal subjects had a side-to-side difference of 2 mm or more. In the group with tears of the ACL mean laxity was found to be 8.1 mm, with 94% measuring 5 mm or more. Eighty-nine percent of subjects with unilateral injury to the ACL had an increase of 2 mm or more on the injured side. Ten of ten acute tears of the ACL were detected by using these criteria, and there

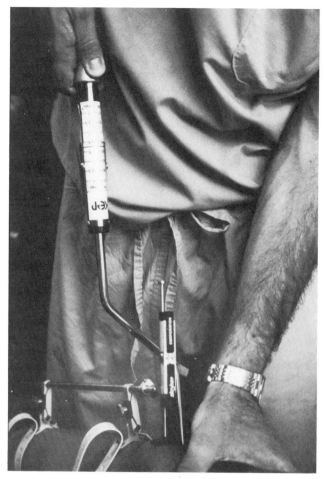

Fig 2–3.—Anterior drawer at 20 degrees of knee flexion. The force applied is measured at the calibrated handle and the extent (mm) of laxity is read at the gauge over the patella. (Courtesy of Boniface, R.J., et al.: Orthopedics 9:391–393, March 1986.)

were no false positive results. In the injured knees with intact ACL measurements were not significantly different from normal.

Objective measurement of knee laxity is a useful complement to clinical knee examination.

▶ This study demonstrates the positive application of a commercially available knee laxity tester to objectively measure anterior knee laxity and to improve knee injury assessment. The authors found they could diagnose anterior cruciate ligament deficiency more accurately; they could quantify any increase in laxity to grade the severity of the injury; and they can use the device to objectively reassess patients after ACL reconstruction. The Stryker knee laxity tester was inexpensive, easy to use in the clinic or emergency room, and well tolerated by the patient when 20 lbs or 89 newtons of force was used. There are other knee laxity testers commercially available which may also meet the above criteria.—Col. J.L. Anderson, PE.D.

Knee Menisci: Correlation Between Microstructure and Biomechanics
A. Beaupré, R. Choukroun, R. Guidouin, R. Garneau, H. Gérardin, and A. Cardou (Laval Univ., Quebec)
Clin. Orthop. 208:72–75, July 1986   2–13

Menisci are fibrocartilaginous structures which contain a varied architecture of collagen bundles. However, little is known about structural organization in relation to the potential role in biomechanics. On the basis of clinical and experimental observations it is thought that menisci may play a direct role in the mechanics of knee function. Menisci appear to be essential in the transmission of load, stability, and lubrication of the joint.

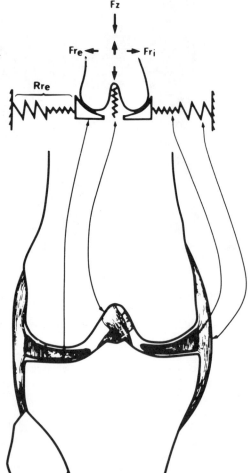

Fig 2–4.—Illustration of mechanical model suggested by ultrastructure of meniscus. (Courtesy of Beaupré, A., et al.: Clin. Orthop. 208:72–75, July 1986.)

To define the microstructural organization of collagen bundles and analyze the biomechanical functions, the authors examined 60 menisci of human knees by conventional histologic studies and scanning electron microscopy (SME).

Sections made in the frontal plane in the middle portion of both lateral and medial menisci revealed an essentially similar structure. Vertical sections that were made in the midportions of the Menisci demonstrated two structurally different regions: a mesial part that included the inner two thirds and a peripheral part that was formed by the outer one third. The organization of collagen bundles in the mesial part showed a radial pattern, and those of the peripheral part were larger and circumferential. The articular surfaces of the mesial part were lined by thinner bundles that were parallel to the surface; the outer portion was covered by synovium.

This structural organization suggested specific biomechanical functions (Fig 2–4), mainly compression mesially with tension peripherally and a direct translation of forces from the inner wedge-shaped part to the outermost region. The covering layer is thought to be well suited for surface-to-surface motion. Outward displacement of the menisci by the femoral condyles is probably resisted by solid anchorage of the peripheral circumferential fibers to the intercondylar bone. The resistance to such displacement is likely to force the femoral condyles inward.

Such an organization of menisci has implications for stability of the knee joint and the pathology of meniscal injuries.

▶ This explanation of the structural organization of the menisci should be of interest to us all. The understanding of the mechanics of knee function is going to be important as we continue our work in preventing, treating, and rehabilitating knee injuries.—Col. J.L. Anderson, PE.D.

Isokinetic Torque Levels for Knee Extensors and Knee Flexors in Soccer Players
B. Öberg, M. Möller, J. Gillquist, and J. Ekstrand (Univ. Hosp., Linkoping, Sweden)
Int. J. Sports Med. 7:50–53, February 1986   2–14

It has been shown clinically that abnormal torque differences between antagonists and/or contralateral muscle groups increase the probability of muscle or joint injury, or both. However, to discuss functional imbalance or muscle weakness, it is important to know the normal torque values of athletes in various sports. Although such data have been published on several sports, no data have been published on players from different levels of soccer.

The present study was designed to establish isokinetic torque values for knee extensors and knee flexors in male soccer players and a reference group of non-soccer players. A second goal was to investigate the hamstring-quadriceps ratio and the fast-speed–slow-speed ratio in soccer players.

The study population consisted of a national team (13 players; mean

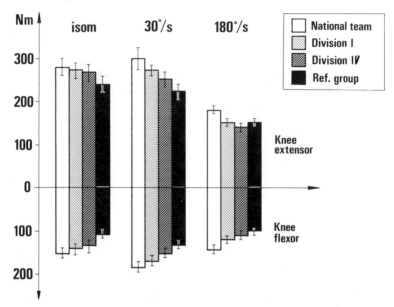

Fig 2–5.—Torque levels (Nm) for knee extensors and flexors. Mean torque values and SD are given for each group. (Courtesy of Öberg, B., et al .: Int. J. Sports Med. 7:50–53, February 1986.)

age, 26 years), 1 team from division I (15 players; mean age, 24 years), 12 teams from division IV (180 players; mean age, 25 years) and 32 non-soccer players (mean age, 21 years).

It was found there were differences in strength between divisions (Fig 2–5). Correction for body surface area did not change the outcome. The knee flexor-knee extensor ratio was markedly higher for soccer players than for non-soccer players. In addition, the fast-speed–slow-speed ratio for knee extensors was found to be higher for non-soccer players and for national team players than for players from divisions I and IV.

Torque levels in knee extensors and flexors are higher in soccer players than in nonplayers. The differences in torque levels among players from different divisions suggest that soccer training at higher grades gives greater strength or that the stronger player also is the more skilled player, or both. The finding that the knee flexor-knee extensor ratio was lower for most of the soccer players suggests that soccer training improves the strength of the knee flexors. The finding that the fast-speed–slow-speed ratio for knee extensors was lower for most of the soccer players than for the nonplayers argues that soccer training has more effect on slow than on fast movements. The authors suggest further research to determine whether this ratio plays any role in prevention of injuries.

▶ If we could get an agreement on the protocol for conducting this kind of research for various athletic skills we could greatly improve our training methods. For instance, player profiles could be developed and we could determine what physiological performance variables are important for players at different positions and different levels. Why is this so difficult?—Col. J.L. Anderson, PE.D.

Shoulder Joint Load and Muscular Activity During Lifting

Ulf P. Arborelius, Jan Ekholm, Gunnar Németh, Ola Svensson, and Ralph Nisell (Karolinska Inst., Stockholm)
Scand. J. Rehabil. Med. 18:71–82, 1986   2–15

Repetitive lifting is responsible for numerous neck-shoulder disorders. Mechanical factors have been suggested as possible agents for various disorders of the locomotor system in the shoulder-neck area. In this study, load on the shoulder joint and muscles was investigated in 15 healthy volunteers who were instructed to lift a moderate burden (12.8 kg) from the floor to table level. Lifting was performed in four different ways: with straight knees, with flexed knees and burden lifted in front of the knees, with flexed knees and burden between knees, and with flexed knees but subject allowed to step toward the table before completion of the lift. Electromyographic (EMG) recordings of shoulder and arm muscular activity were received from electrodes placed over the muscles. Calculations of loading moments of force were performed using a static biomechanical model. The loading moments were compared using ANOVA and a specialized statistical computer program.

The initial loading moment was lowest in the straight knee lift; the peak load moment occurred late in all the lifts. Upon completion of the lifts, both load and activation were lower in subjects allowed to step before depositing the burden. In contrast to the loading moments, muscular activity was quite varied; the most active shoulder muscles were the anterior and the lateral parts of the deltoid and the serratus anterior. The subjects in this study had to exert approximately 75% of their maximum shoulder flexor strength to lift the moderate weight used in the experiment.

▶ It is interesting to note the number of studies being done involving the shoulders and the concern for injuries to the shoulders. Here at West Point, we see more shoulder injuries among our student population now than ever before. I feel this is because of the change in the way our society viewed the importance of exercise over the past 10 or more years, when running was seen as all that was needed to maintain health and performance. We are now trying to pull back from that—not by stopping running, but by also doing exercise to strengthen the skeletal muscles.—Col. J.L. Anderson, PE.D.

Fine Wire Electromyography Analysis of Muscles of the Shoulder During Swimming

Gordon W. Nuber, Frank W. Jobe, Jacquelin Perry, Diane R. Moynes, and Daniel Antonelli (Centinela Hosp., Inglewood, Calif.)
Am. J. Sports Med. 14:7–11, January–February 1986   2–16

Shoulder pain is a common orthopedic problem among athletes. Competitive swimmers are frequently disabled by shoulder pain. This fine wire electromyogram (EMG) analysis of the shoulder was performed on 11 swimmers to provide a baseline against which pathologic conditions could be compared. Five studies were performed under dry conditions and seven under aquatic conditions.

The EMG data were synchronized with a film analysis to determine what muscles were used at different phases of the swim stroke. The muscles studied were the biceps, subscapularis, latissimus dorsi, pectoralis major, supraspinatus, infraspinatus, serratus anterior, and deltoid.

The supraspinatus, infraspinatus, middle deltoid, and serratus anterior were predominantly used during recovery phase. The latissimus dorsi and pectoralis major predominantly functioned as pullthrough phase muscles. The biceps were active in both phases. The serratus anterior functions near maximal muscle test during each stroke and could fatigue with repetition.

A training program that strengthens the scapular rotators may help alleviate impingement syndrome in swimmers. This article also presents a reproducible method to evaluate the shoulder musculature during swimming.

▶ The authors took on a major task in attempting to use fine wire electromyography with swimmers in the pool. Although they were unable to gather and analyze all of the data they were after, this is of value to other researchers because of the methodology used and the information they were able to collect. Their finding that particular attention should be paid to strengthening the muscles concerned with scopular rotation during the recovery phase is valid if impingement in the shoulders occurs primarily in the recovery phase. The work on this research needs to continue to see whether the problems with EMG signals can be solved to give more complete data collection.—Col. J.L. Anderson, PE.D.

Muscle Activity and Fatigue in the Shoulder Muscles During Repetitive Work: An Electromyographic Study
H. Christensen (Univ. of Copenhagen)
Eur. J. Appl. Physiol. 54:596–601, February 1986   2–17

The increasing mechanization of industrial work processes has simplified the movements that are involved but has increased the number of movements per unit time. Although these simple movements require less energy, the velocity and monotony represent a local stress on the skeletal muscles. One of the side effects of this mechanization seems to be an increased incidence of pain in the locomotor system, especially for employees who do light industrial work, workers at assembly lines, and others for whom the working processes are characterized by light repetitive movements. Most of the symptoms are located in the back, neck, shoulders, and upper arms.

To evaluate the degree of activity and fatigue in shoulder muscles during

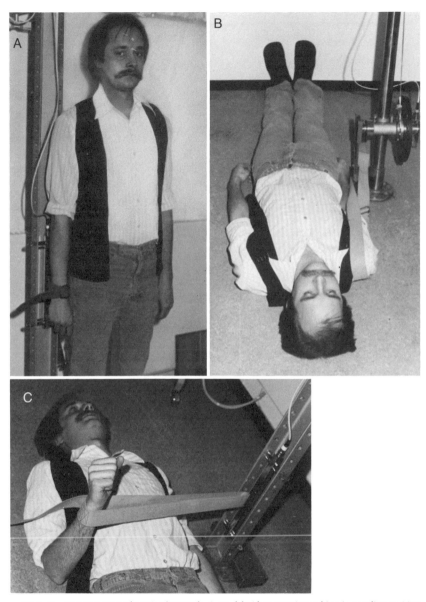

Fig 2–6.—Measurements of maximal strength. **A,** m. deltoideus anterior: subject in standing position with strain gauge at wrist while forward flexion of arm was made. **B,** m. trapezius pars descendens: with subject in supine position and feet flat against wall strain gauge is placed around shoulder via a nonelastic strap (patient has to lift both shoulders). **C,** m. infraspinatus: with subject in supine position with arm flexed at 90 degrees and strain gauge placed around wrist outward movement of lower arm was performed. (Courtesy of Christensen, H.: Eur. J. Appl. Physiol. 54:596–601, February 1986.)

an entire working day when monotonous and repetitive work was being performed, the author measured the amplitude distribution probability function (ADPF) and the power spectrum of the surface electromyogram (EMG) from the m. deltoideus anterior, m. infraspinatus, and m. trapezius par descendens in seven persons who were working at a pillar drill.The recordings were made six times during a working day, and the ADPF was analyzed from two or three work cycles from each recording.

Static levels of contraction were 11.0% of maximal voluntary contraction (MVC) (Fig 2–6) in m. deltoideus anterior, 8.5% of MVC in m. infraspinatus, and 20.5% of MCV in m. trapezius, without any change throughout the day.

Both the static and medium levels of contraction were too high in the performance of this particular task when these values were compared to previous suggested upper limits of levels of ADPF. When the power spectrum of the EMG was analyzed during isometric contractions of the shoulder muscles, it was found that the mean power frequency decreased during the day in m. trapezius only, indicating muscular fatigue in this area.

▶ Although this is an industrial engineering research study, it involves the same type of activity and fatiguing of muscles we seen in training for sports competition. The industrial engineers could learn something from the sportsmen and develop regular training sessions for their workers to help them delay the onset of fatigue. The workers would become more productive. This is being done in Japanese factories.—Col. J.L. Anderson, PE.D.

Rotator Cuff Function During a Golf Swing
Frank W. Jobe, Diane R. Moynes, and Daniel J. Antonelli (Centinela Hosp. Med. Ctr., Inglewood, Calif.)
Am. J. Sports Med. 14:388–392, September–October 1986   2–18

Although golf is not often considered a strenuous sport, golf-related injuries are beginning to receive attention. In a recent review of patients with injuries attributable to golf, a high number of injuries of the rotator cuff at the shoulder were identified. The authors studied shoulder muscle activity bilaterally in golfers in an effort to gain insight into this type of injury and to design prevention and rehabilitation programs for golfers.

The study included seven adults male right-handed professional golfers who had no shoulder problems. Their average age was 36 years. Indwelling electrodes were inserted on the right side into the major shoulder muscles. Resting and maximal muscle test recordings were made for each muscle, and the data were transmitted to a recording console. Each golfer was then filmed in the course of executing his normal golf swing. The entire testing procedure was repeated on the left side. Each filmed swing was divided into four segments: takeaway, forward swing, acceleration, and follow-through (Fig 2–7), and data from each segment were then analyzed.

All portions of the deltoid were inactive on the right side throughout the swing, and likewise inactive on the left side, except for a brief spurt

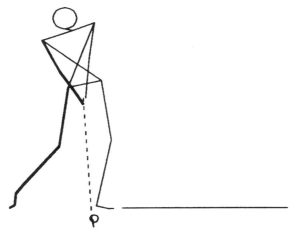

Fig 2–7.—Ball contact initiates follow-through. (Courtesy of Jobe, F.W., et al.: Am. J. Sports Med. 14:388–392, September–October 1986.)

from the anterior portion during the moments preceding ball contact. Rotator cuff injuries appear to be associated with a lack of conditioning, proper warm-up, and flexibility exercises which precede play in other sports, but are usually absent in preplay regimens of golfers. Moreover, the golfing population tends to be older than in other sports, and thus at higher risk for rotator cuff tears.

The authors suggest that golfers add exercises which strengthen the shoulder muscles to their warm-up regimen.

▶ Weekend golfers should also take note of this paper. They, more than the professional golfers, need to add conditioning, warm-up, and flexibility exercises to their precompetition preparations. They can also improve their performance—meaning distance off the tee—by using muscle-strengthening exercises for the latissimus dorsi, pectoralis major, and rotator cuff during their days when not on the golf course. These exercises will also lessen the risk of injuries to the shoulders.—Col. J.L. Anderson, PE.D.

Mechanical Efficiency of Pure Positive and Pure Negative Work With Special Reference to Work Intensity
O. Aura and P.V. Komi (Univ. of Jyväskylä, Finland)
Int. J. Sports Med. 7:44–49, February 1986   2–19

Mechanical efficiency is frequently used as a means of describing the efficiency of human beings in motion. The efficiency of positive work of an isolated muscle has been shown to have values ranging from 0.20 to 0.25. The values that have been reported for mechanical (net) efficiency in positive work situations range from 19% to 27%, although some authors have calculated the work of the delta efficiencies, which have baseline definitions different from the mechanical (net) efficiency. In most of these

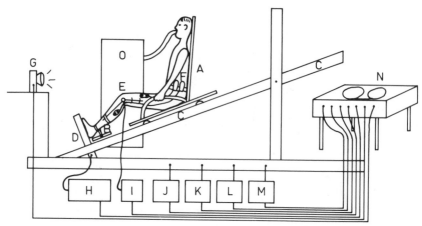

Fig 2–8.—Experimental procedure used in study. (Courtesy of Aura, D., and Komi, P.V.: Int. J. Sports Med. 7:44–49, February 1986.)

studies less attention was paid to the effects of work intensity on the mechanical efficiency of the pure positive work. Available information on the mechanical efficiency of the pure negative work is also slightly obscure, particularly when negative work is related to the work intensity.

To investigate the mechanical efficiencies of the pure positive and pure negative work with a special effort to examine the influence of the work intensity on the efficiency, the authors studied 36 male subjects who performed separate concentric (CONC) and eccentric (ECC) exercises on a "sledge" apparatus (Fig 2–8).

Work intensities in positive work varied between 40% and 90% and in negative work between 30% and 120% of the maximum CONC exercise (Fig 2–9). In 54 exercises of positive work (CONC), mean mechanical efficiency was 17.1% and its value correlated negatively with work intensity, and with the average angular velocity of the knee. In 103 exercises of negative work (ECC) the mechanical efficiency was on average 80.2%, and its value correlated positively with work intensity. Both intersubject and intrasubject variations were large (32% to 163%). The integrated electric activity (EMG) of the leg extensor muscles increased with an increase of work intensity in both the positive and negative work situations.

Less efficient recruitment of muscle units in higher positive work rates may be the reason for the decrease in mechanical efficiency, whereas better regulation of stiffness via increased preactivation may cause high values of mechanical efficiency in higher work intensities in negative work situations.

▶ Coaches, athletic trainers, and teachers need to understand the differences between concentric (positive) and eccentric (negative) work. Both can be used to help athletes develop muscular strength and endurance more effectively. By understanding and taking advantage of the differences in the mechanical efficiencies of positive and negative work, it is possible to continue exercising the

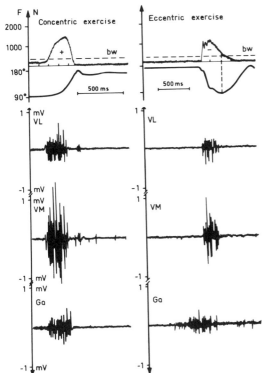

Fig 2–9.—Data recorded during experiments; pure positive work (*left*) and pure negative work (*right*). Curves from top to bottom: force, knee angle, EMG vastus lateralis, EMG vastus medialis, and EMG gastrocnemius. (Courtesy of Aura, D., and Komi, P.V.: Int. J. Sports Med. 7:44–49, February 1986.)

same muscles using negative work after positive work can no longer be performed. At West Point, we have found this to be valuable in helping the cadets improve their muscular strength and endurance to higher levels and faster than if they use only positive work.—Col. J.L. Anderson, PE.D.

Force, Speed and Power Output of the Human Upper Limb During Horizontal Pulls

D.W. Grieve and J. van der Linden (Royal Free Hosp., London)
Eur. J. Appl. Physiol. 55:425–430, August 1986   2–20

It is known that isometric pulling strength of an arm changes rapidly with hand position when both the elbow and shoulder are involved in pulls at shoulder height, but very slightly if only the elbow is used. Speed of movement and limb posture affect the horizontal manual force at shoulder level. The authors studied a group of volunteers to assess how force, speed, and power output of horizontal pulling with the upper arm is affected by the height of pull.

The study was done with 14 right-handed male volunteers who performed horizontal pulls with maximal effort at eye, shoulder, and elbow level from their positions of full reach after their trunk and shoulder girdle had been rigidly constrained in a chair by two tight straps. The pulls were done against a water-filled viscous dynamometer with a variable resistance proportional to the square of the velocity. Isometric strengths of each individual were measured in outer, middle, and inner ranges of reach at each of the three heights of pull.

The height of pull does not affect static or dynamic performance significantly. Even though pulling at eye, shoulder, and elbow height differs significantly in biomedical mechanical parameters, performance at each of these three levels was similar. The total work performed in a complete pull increases with resistance.

▶ The authors' hypothesis that performance would be affected by the height of the pull seems reasonable. Maybe the reason the performance was unaffected by the height of the pull was because the grip strength of the subjects became the weakest link in the chain and additional force could not be exerted at any height because the subjects were afraid the grip would fail. I have seen evidence of this when administering the flexed-arm hang to young women. Often it is the grip strength that the subject is afraid will fail and she lowers her body even though the upper arm and shoulder girdle muscular still is not fatigued.—Col. J.L. Anderson, PE.D.

Skeletal Muscle Profiles Among Elite Long, Middle, and Short Distance Swimmers

Elizabeth S. Gerard, Vincent J. Caiozzo, Benjamin D. Rubin, Carlos A. Prietto, and Dennis M. Davidson (Univ. of California, Irvine and La Jolla)
Am. J. Sports Med. 14:77–82, January–February 1986   2–21

This investigation compared skeletal muscle fiber composition and strength in 30 national caliber swimmers, 20 male and 10 female, who were classified according to the distance of their competitive event. It was hypothesized that the long-distance swimmers would have the highest amount and percentages of type I fiber. The short-distance swimmers would have the highest leg strength and power values.

The long-distance group had the highest values of percent type I muscle fiber composition. They had the lowest values of leg power and strength. Subjects with 50% or more type I fibers had significantly lower values for leg power and strength parameters.

The hypothesized relationship between type I muscle fibers and leg power and strength values was seen in this study. The composition of the muscle fibers was consistent with the different demands of the event lengths in which the swimmers specialized.

▶ I remember taking a class taught by Dr. Jim Cousilman at Indiana University in 1964, and he explained how he could identify long-distance, middle-distance, or short-distance swimmers by administering one simple test. That test was the vertical jump. He then proceeded to show us the data he had collected on the university men's swimming team. That was 23 years ago, and we do not seem to have anything better to use today.—Col. J.L. Anderson, PE.D.

3 Sports Injuries

Epidemiology

Activity in the Spinal Cord-Injured Patient: An Epidemiologic Analysis of Metabolic Parameters
Stephen R. Dearwater, Ronald E. Laporte, Robert J. Robertson, Gilbert Brenes, Lucile L. Adams, and Dorothy Becker (Univ. of Pittsburgh)
Med. Sci. Sports Exerc. 18:541–544, October 1986   3–1

Owing to medical advances which have increased life expectancy, cardiovascular disease has become a major cause of death in spinal cord injury (SCI) patients. In this study the metabolic differences between extremely inactive disabled SCI patients, active disabled persons, and able-bodied persons were analyzed. A total of 73 sedentary male SCI patients in a rehabilitation center, 17 male SCI athletes, and 126 able-bodied male controls, with a mean age of 29 years, were included. High-density lipoprotein cholesterol (HDL-C), the subfractions HDL_2 and HDL_3, serum glucose and serum insulin levels were evaluated from fasting morning blood samples.

Male SCI athletes had significantly higher (P<.001) total HDL-C (42.7 mg•dl^{-1}) than the SCI sedentary group (34.7 mg•dl^{-1}) with concomitant lower (P<.05) total cholesterol levels. The HDL-C levels for the SCI athlete were slightly below the mean for male sedentary controls (46.1 mg•dl^{-1}), in spite of the athletes relatively aggressive behavior.

Physical inactivity appeared to influence both subfractions ($HDL_{2\&3}$) of total HDL-C as both components were significantly lower (P<.05) in the SCI sedentary than in the SCI athlete. A significantly higher concentration of the HDL_3 levels was seen in controls.

While all three groups were within the normal range for glucose concentrations, in both SCI groups these levels were significantly lower than in the control group. All the insulin values were within normal limits, with no significant difference between groups.

The low concentrations of total HDL-C and HDL_2 observed in the sedentary SCI group could be at least partially explained by inactivity. While the HDL_3 of the able-bodied controls was responsible for a more elevated HDL-C compared to the SCI athletes, this subfraction has been shown in the past to have less association to coronary heart disease. In spite of their physical activity differences, blood glucose levels in both SCI groups were similar, suggesting neuronal control of glucose metabolism. The lower glucose and similar insulin values suggest possible increased insulin sensitivity in the SCI groups which does not appear to be a function of physical activity. While the effects of chronic inactivity on lipid and glucose metabolism in the SCI groups have been shown, response to an exercise regimen is less clear.

▶ This article follows the previous one in looking at this study group in greater biochemical detail with particular attention to cholesterol fractions, glucose and insulin. The important observations were that total levels of HDL-C in both subfractions were significantly lower in the male SCI sedentary population than in SCI athletes or the able-bodied, but that the HDL_2 level was significantly elevated in the SCI athlete and similar to the control. Surprisingly to me, glucose levels were similar in the two SCI groups and lower in both SCI groups than in the able-bodied controls. The similarity of glucose and insulin levels in both SCI groups despite marked difference in activity suggests that these parameters are not associated with activity. A neuronal control of glucose metabolism is postulated in these disabled groups.—L.J. Krakauer, M.D.

The Epidemiology of Aerobic Dance Injuries

James G. Garrick, Donna M. Gillien, and Patrice Whiteside (St. Francis Mem. Hosp., San Francisco)
Am. J. Sports Med. 14:67–72, January–February 1986   3–2

Within the past 15 years, aerobic dance has grown to be the largest organized fitness program in the United States directed primarily at women. There have been few reports of injuries, but there exists growing concern among physicians about the safety of this activity. Among 11,414 individuals treated for athletic injuries over the past 5 years in a facility dealing specifically with injuries of athletes, it has been reported that 5.4% have been due to aerobic dance, the fourth highest causative activity. The type, frequency, severity, and possible causes of injuries associated with aerobic dance activities were identified.

The study population consisted of 351 students and 60 instructors from six facilities, who were followed for 16 weeks with weekly telephone calls. There were 29,924 hours of documented activity and 327 reported medical complaints. Only 84 of these complaints (0.28 per hundred hours) resulted in any disability and only 2.1% required medical care. Nearly two thirds of the injuries were associated with the shin/leg, foot, and ankle, and instructors were twice as likely to be injured as students. Higher injury rates were reported for participants with a history of prior orthopedic problems and a lack of involvement in other fitness activities. The injury rates were found to be influenced by the design and conduct of the aerobic program, but not by the brand of shoe or type of flooring.

Aerobic dance offers students the potential for fitness enhancement with a minimal risk of injury.

▶ It is certainly gratifying to read the survey of a physical activity in which knees are not mangled, bones are not broken, and spinal cords are not severed.—J.S. Torg, M.D.

The Effectiveness of Knee Bracing for the Prevention of Sports Injuries

George D. Rovere and G. Scott Bowen (Wake Forest Univ.)
Sports Med. 3:309–311, 1986   3–3

The use of knee bracing for the prevention of sports injuries remains controversial. According to the American Academy of Orthopedic Surgeons, the ideal prophylactic knee brace should (1) supplement stiffness of the knee to injury-producing loads from both contact and noncontact stresses, (2) be anatomically adaptable to the wearer's knee, (3) be cost effective and durable, (4) have documented efficacy in preventing injuries, and (5) not interfere with normal function, increase risk factors elsewhere in the lower extremity, or be harmful to other players. The effectiveness of knee bracing in preventing injuries was evaluated in several athletic teams wearing prophylactic braces.

There has been one report documenting 4-years with and 4-years without prophylactic knee braces worn by a collegiate football team during practice sessions and games. There were no significant differences in the number, kind, and severity of anterior cruciate, medial collateral ligament, or meniscal injuries in braced and nonbraced athletes. However, another study demonstrated a 70% decrease in surgical repairs of medial collateral ligament injuries during the study period. Another report of a 2-year study without bracing and a 2-year study with bracing indicated that knee injuries and surgeries did not differ significantly between groups. A controlled laboratory study on the mechanical effects of lateral knee bracing suggested potential problems in such bracing, including preloading of the medial collateral ligament, shifting of the center axis, which preloads the cruciate ligaments, slippage of the braces, which causes forced concentration, and bending of the brace, which creates a fulcrum effect. Player response to bracing was mixed, cost of bracing was $400 per player per season, and complaints of triceps surae muscle cramping were more common during the braced period.

Until their efficacy can be documented more thoroughly, the routine use of prophylactic braces is not recommended.

Evaluation of the Use of Braces to Prevent Injury to the Knee in Collegiate Football Players
Carol C. Teitz, Bonnie K. Hermanson, Richard A. Kronmal, and Paula H. Diehr (Univ. of Washington)
J. Bone Joint Surg. [Am.] 69-A:2–8, January 1987   3–4

Preventive or prophylactic braces have been used by numerous collegiate football players in an attempt to prevent injury to the knee, even if the knee had never been injured before. The results of studies on the effectiveness of such devices have been contradictory, with some studies reporting less knee injuries and other studies reporting an increase in knee injuries with knee braces. The authors conducted a study to compare the incidence and severity of injuries to the knee in collegiate football players who wore preventive knee braces and those who did not.

Data were collected in 1984 from 71 schools with a total of 6,307 players and in 1985 from 61 schools with a total of 5,445 players. All schools belonged to the National College Athletic Association. In 1984, preventive knee braces were worn by all players of 2 schools, by some players of 62 schools, and by none of the players of 7 schools. In 1985, braces were worn by all players of 4 schools, by some players of 55 schools, and by none of the players of 2 schools.

In both 1984 and 1985, injury rates were significantly higher in players who wore braces than in those who did not, regardless of the type of brace used.

Based on these findings, the use of so-called preventive knee braces may actually be harmful and their use cannot be recommended.

▶ The widespread use of prophylactic knee braces in football (Abstracts 3–3 and 3–4) may well have been a successful commercial venture. However, from the standpoint of an effective preventative endeavor, it has been a failure. As demonstrated by Teitz et al. (Abstract 3–4) ". . . it appears that the so-called preventative braces for the knee did not lead to a decrease in the number of severity of injuries to the knee; there actually was an increase in the rate of injury. The increased rate in players who wore braces may have been the result of decreased agility caused by the braces, carelessness of players who believed that they were protected, or preloading of the medial collateral ligament in players who had genu varum." The use of these devices despite a lack of objective biomechanical and clinical information to substantiate the manufacturers' claims of effectiveness is regrettable.

See also the introduction to chapter 6.—J.S. Torg, M.D.

Patterns of Knee Injuries in Wrestling: A Six Year Study
R.R. Wroble, M.C. Mysnyk, D.T. Foster, and J.P. Albright (Univ. of Iowa)
Am. J. Sports Med. 14:55–66, January–February 1986   3–5

Collegiate wrestling has a high injury rate, often second only to that of football. Knee injuries incurred by members of the University of Iowa wrestling team in a 6-year period were reviewed. Fifty-one of 136 wrestlers evaluated sustained injuries to 64 knees. Twenty-eight wrestlers had more than one knee injury. An average of 19 days was lost with each knee injury. The most frequent diagnoses were prepatellar bursitis and lateral sprains. Twenty-six meniscal injuries were observed. A majority of evaluable injuries occurred during practice. Takedowns were involved in a majority of instances. About half the injuries were primary.

Thirty of the 136 injuries were managed operatively in 21 athletes.Meniscectomy was the most frequent procedure, followed by prepatellar bursectomy. Other management included immobilization, aspiration/injection, physical therapy, drugs, and rest. About half the wrestlers were considered to be compliant, while seven were frankly noncompliant. Recurrent injuries were substantially more frequent in noncompliant subjects. The same wrestlers who tend to do well in a rehabilitation program are those who are prone to reinjury.

Knee injuries are an important cause of serious time-loss injury in collegiate wrestlers. The knee is in danger during takedowns, especially when on the defense. Noncompliance is endemic among wrestlers. The exposure time is very high, and "contact" time accounts for a very high proportion of total exposure in wrestling. Further studies may help prevent knee injuries and make collegiate wrestling a safer activity.

▶ This is an interesting study that reports an incidence of 30 knee injuries per 100 wrestlers per year, with 11.5 knee injuries per 100 wrestlers per year requiring a week or more time loss. However, most of the injuries are due to patellar bursitis, and medial and lateral collateral ligament sprains. It is interesting to note that there are only 4 anterior cruciate ligament tears in this group of 136 injuries.

On the basis of exposure data which revealed injury rates in competitive matches to be 40 times those of practice, the authors "feel strongly that all wrestling meets should have physicians in attendance." It would appear that most of the injuries described could certainly be managed initially by an experienced certified athletic trainer. Although a physician experienced in management of athletic injuries should certainly be available at all times, I personally question the need for on-site physician coverage of every game, match, and meet.—J.S. Torg, M.D.

Mouth Protectors and Oral Trauma: A Study of Adolescent Football Players
Mark W. Garon, Arthur Merkle, and J. Timothy Wright (Univ. of Alabama, Birmingham)
J. Am. Dent. Assoc. 112:663–665, May 1986   3–6

The incidence of oral trauma in organized football has decreased dramatically with the use of oral protectors. The use of mouth protectors and its relation to oral trauma in other sports is unknown. A total of 754 junior high school and high school football players from Birmingham, Ala., were evaluated to determine the extent of sports-related oral trauma among players. Many of these players had participate in and reported injuries in other organized and unorganized sports. The players underwent physical and oral evaluation and were asked a series of questions regarding the use of mouth protectors and any history of sports-related oral trauma.

There were 93 oral injuries and 29 concussions sustained while participating in various sports. More than half (52%) of the oral injuries and more than one third (38%) of the concussions were sustained in sports other than organized football. Baseball, basketball, and unorganized football showed a high prevalence of hard tissue oral trauma with virtually none of the players wearing mouth protectors. In contrast, most of the oral injuries sustained by football players who typically wore mouthguards involved soft tissues.

Mouth protectors are beneficial for participants in virtually all sports, but particularly baseball and basketball. The current mouthguard protector designs are helpful in preventing hard tissue trauma, but additional soft tissue protection is needed in football mouth protectors.

▶ Common sense supports the value of mouth protectors in any activity where the oral structures can sustain a direct blow. However, the authors' conclusion that "... it is apparent that mouth protector wear would be beneficial for participants in other sports, especially baseball and basketball" is not supported by the data. Specifically, the study is retrospective, not randomized, and did not employ statistical analysis.

It would appear, on the basis of these observations, that a prospective and randomized study be performed in groups of baseball and basketball players that when subjected to statistical analysis will substantiate the thesis that mouth guards in these groups will protect against dental injuries.—J.S. Torg, M.D.

Maxillofacial Fractures Sustained in Bicycle Accidents
Christian Lindqvist, Sirkka Sorsa, Tapio Hyrkäs, and Seppo Santavirta (Helsinki Univ. Central Hosp.)
Int. J. Oral Maxillofac. Surg. 15:12–18, February 1986   3–7

The increasing popularity of cycling and the use of seat belts in automobiles have increased the proportion of maxillofacial fractures caused by bicycle accidents. Ninety-three patients seen from 1981 to 1983 with facial bone fractures sustained in bicycle accidents were reviewed. There were 52 males with a mean age of 31 years and 41 females with a mean age of 29.5 years. One fifth of patients were younger than 15 years of age. The patients represented 7% of all those seen during the review period with facial bone fractures. A majority of cyclists were injured in accidents involving only 1 vehicle.

Two thirds of patients had mandibular fractures, while one third had midface fractures. More than 40% of patients had multiple fractures. Condylar and subcondylar fractures were the most common mandibular injuries. A majority of midface injuries were lateral. Twenty-nine patients underwent surgery, including 12% of patients with mandibular fractures. All dislocated zygomatic fractures were managed by open reduction. Osteotaxis was used for some maxillary fractures. Forty-seven working patients had an average sick leave of 2 weeks.

Bicycle accidents are an increasingly prominent cause of maxillofacial fractures, including many condylar fractures of the mandible. Injuries may be severe and often are associated with dental injuries and multiple trauma to other organs. Protective helmets should be strongly recommended for use by bicyclists, but most available helmets fail to protect the facial area properly, especially the chin.

Bicycle Accidents and Injuries Among Adult Cyclists
Douglas Kiburz, Rae Jacobs, Fred Reckling, and Judy Mason (Univ. of Kansas)
Am. J. Sports Med. 14:416–419, September–October 1986   3–8

Bicycling accidents comprised the greatest recreational source of emergency room visits last year, numbering over 500,000. To evaluate cycle morbidity, 492 active adult bicyclists, with a mean age of 34.3 years (range, 6 to 86 years), responded to a survey to determine cycle use and accident patterns. Average cycling experience was 10.7 years.

Nearly all cyclists (95.3%) used cycling for recreational purposes. Nearly half (46.3%) had been involved in an accident (mean, 1.4 accidents; range, 0 to 27), with 34.8% involving moderate or severe injuries. Lone cyclists accounted for nearly half (46%) of accidents. The majority of the accidents occurred in May through August. Cyclists were at fault 58.7% of the time. Significant factors contributing to bicycle accidents included rider reck-lessness (58.7%), cycle malfunction (14.9%), environmental factors such as debris, corners, rough roads, curbs (36.9%), turns (22.9%), hills (13.4%), and companion riders (15%). Soft tissue injuries to the extremities were very common. Head injuries were involved in 16.7% of accidents, but only 8.8% were due to concussion. Of those injured, 9.3% required hospitalization, averaging 7 days, and 22.5% missed days from work or school. The use of gloves significantly reduced hand injury, and the use of helmets reduced hospitalization time and the severity of injury.

Bicycling is associated with considerable morbidity. The majority of bicycle accidents involve lone cyclists and are associated with environmental factors. The use of helmets and gloves may not prevent accidents but can significantly reduce the number and severity of injuries.

▶ It is interesting to compare the observations of the authors with those of two other reports of bicycle accidents and injuries recently published. Kruse and McBeath (*Am. J. Sports Med.* 8:342–344, September–October 1980) using a questionnaire sent to 1,200 randomly selected college students determined that 29% have been involved in an accident during the previous 3 years, and 13% within the immediate year. Roadway conditions were reported as a major contributing factor by 52% of the respondents. The automobile was a major contributor to the accident in 26% of the incidents. Bohlmann (*Phys. Sportsmed* 9:117–124, May 1981) collected data on 3,700 competitive cyclists. It was determined that in this group the most frequent causes of injuries were flat tires and collisions.—J.S. Torg, M.D.

All-Terrain Vehicle Accidents: The Experience of One Hospital Located Near a Major Recreational Area
George W. Trager, Glen Grayman, and Sidney Harr (Desert Hosp., Palm Springs, Calif.)
Ann. Emerg. Med. 15:1293–1296, November 1986   3–9

The all-terrain vehicle (ATV), which is small and has three or four wheels, is designed to be ridden by one operator over sand, snow, or on rocky, rough terrain. Its instability and use for recreation, often in conjunction with alcohol, have led to concerns about its safety. A joint retrospective and prospective study was carried out to characterize those most at risk for becoming victims of ATV accidents and the types of accidents they suffer.

The emergency room records of patients treated following ATV accidents were reviewed for the retrospective part of the study. The prospective part was conducted by giving questionnaires to the next 25 people treated at the emergency room after ATV accidents. Both groups of patients, totaling 169, were classified by age, sex, type of injury, stay in hospital, type of surgery undergone, if any, and history of the accident.

Women comprised 24% of the cases. Hospitalization was required for 30%, and two patients died. Age ranged from 3 to 76 years. Approximately 31% had been drinking. The most common injuries were burns, contusions, abrasions, and lacerations. The prevalent type of bone injury was to the clavicle, ribs, or sternum. The accident rate was 10 accidents per 1,000 ATV rider days. Most of the accidents involved the three-wheeled type of ATV.

The rate of injury with ATVs is comparable to that of snow skiing. Moreover, many of the injuries are minor and can be minimized by the use of protective clothing. Nevertheless, the three-wheeled ATV is inherently unstable and tends to be ridden by people under the influence of alcohol or too young to control the vehicle. Design modifications to reduce the incidence of the driver's leg being caught under the rear wheel should reduce the accident rate.

The Three Wheeler (Adult Tricycle): An Unstable, Dangerous Machine
C. Doyle Haynes, S.D. Stroud and C.E. Thompson (Emory Univ., Auburn Univ., Opelika, Ala., and Univ. of Texas, Houston)
J. Trauma 26:643–648, July 1986   3–10

In 1982 to 1985, 125 patients in the east Alabama area sustained injuries secondary to all-terrain vehicle (ATV) accidents. Of this total, 21 (17%) were hospitalized and 104 (83%) were treated and released. The majority (85%) were less than 25 years of age, with 53% less than 15 years. Patient ages ranged from 2 to 48 years; the mean age was 18 years.

The mode of injury was determined in 79 patients; 39 (49%) of the accidents were caused by rollover of the ATV. The most commonly injured area was an extremity, specifically, the foot. Lower extremity injury was also the most common injury in the 21 hospitalized patients. It is the authors' opinion that few of the injured wore any protective clothing.

The ATV of today weighs from 300 to 500 lbs, has a recommended occupancy of one, and travels on three oversized tires up to 50 mph. The area required to make a safe turn at a given velocity is much greater compared with that of the four-wheeler. This factor contributes to accident frequency. Warning messages provided by manufacturers are very small and located in hard-to-find places. Recreational aspects of the ATV are generally publicized without similar publication of proper precautionary measures. ATVs are not automatically covered by any federal safety regulations concerning age and helmet use, yet more accidents with this vehicle have been recorded than with the recalled Ford Pinto.

It is concluded from this review that the ATV is unstable and difficult to control. Children under 16 years of age are at greatest risk of injury. Most deaths recorded occurred from head injuries.

Reduction in morbidity and mortality is believed to be possible through greater public awareness of the serious dangers posed by ATV use. Instructional courses are advised for teaching riding skills; mandatory protective clothing should be worn. It is further recommended that young children not be allowed to ride ATVs except under strict supervision. With such precautions the massive onslaught of injury and death should be decreased.

▶ Haag has documented in a United States Consumer Product Commission memorandum of Feb. 20, 1986, the continuous increase in the occurrence of all-terrain vehicle related injuries. Specifically, in 1982, 8,585 such injuries were reported as treated in hospital emergency rooms. This number increased to 27,554 in 1983 and 66,756 in 1984. Trager et al. (Abstract 3–9) emphasized that 31% of those involved in accidents had been drinking. They further calculated the accident rate as 10 accidents per 1,000 ATV rider days. Most sobering is that the Consumer Product Safety Commission estimates that from 1982 to 1984 there were, in this country, 104 deaths associated with the use of these vehicles.—J.S. Torg, M.D.

Injury Patterns in Nordic Ski Jumpers: A Retrospective Analysis of Injuries Occurring at the Intervale Ski Jump Complex From 1980 to 1985
James R. Wright, Jr., Edward G. Hixson, and Jay J. Rand (Olympic Regional Development Authority and US Olympic Training Ctr., Lake Placid, N.Y., Washington Univ., St. Louis, and Gen. Hosp. of Saranac Lake, N.Y.)
Am. J. Sports Med. 14:393–397, September–October 1986   3–11

Nordic ski jumping is widely believed to be a dangerous sport, although athletes and officials contend that strict regulations keep ski jumping a relatively safe sport. The medical literature has no studies of the types and frequency of injuries associated with the sport. This retrospective study aims to assess injuries among nordic ski jumpers.

The accident report from injuries occurring at Intervale Ski Jump Complex for 5 years formed the basis of the study. The total number of jumps that were made during training was not recorded, so only jumps made during competitions could be included in this study. The total number of falls was estimated from the score that the jumper was given by the judges. This method of analysis tended toward underestimation of the total number of falls.

Forty-seven jumpers with confirmed injuries received a total of 72 injuries. The most common complaints were contusions. Eleven jumpers suffered fractures, most of which were nondisplaced and occurred in the upper extremities. Eight jumpers required hospitalization, and none of the injuries resulted in permanent disabilities. Injury rates for the World Cup and all other competitions were 1.2 and 4.3 injuries per 1,000 skier-days respectively.

This study suggests that the injury rates for ski jumping and recreational alpine skiing are similar. Most ski jumping injuries are contusions, abrasions, and mild concussions. The rate of fractures and sprains is lower among jumpers than alpine skiers. Visceral injuries made up only 10% of all injuries. None of the injuries led to permanent disability. Thus, the dangers of nordic skiing appear to be overestimated.

▶ The authors recognize that this study has all the inherent problems of a retrospective review. They also acknowledge that there are no data available to estimate injury rates for practice jumping, which was the setting in which majority of the injuries occurred. Thus, the reported injury rates for competitive jumping was based on a relatively small number of injuries. Noteworthy is the fact that none of the injuries resulting in permanent disability. However, at best the conclusion should read: "this study suggests that the dangers of nordic ski jumping have been overestimated" at the Intervale Ski Jump in Lake Placid from 1980 to 1985.—J.S. Torg, M.D.

Necropsy Study of Mountaineering Accidents in Scotland
W.A. Reid, D. Doyle, H.G. Richmond, and S.L. Galbraith (Univ. of Leeds, Southern Gen. Hosp., Glasgow, and Raigmore Hosp., Inverness, Scotland)
J. Clin. Pathol. 39:1217–1220, November 1986   3–12

Mountaineering accidents account for 20 to 30 deaths per year in Scotland. Although each death is investigated by an official, the cause of death is often ascribed to "multiple injuries," and few necropsies are done. Necropsies with neuropathologic examinations were conducted on victims of mountaineering accidents in order to determine true cause of death.

Over a 5.5 year period, 121 fatal mountaineering accidents occurred. Necropsies were performed on 42 of these cases; the brain was formalin fixed for neuropathologic study, and a history of the accident was taken. The victims' ages ranged from 14 to 54 years, and 37 were male. All but two of the accidents involved falls.

Head injury was the major factor in 21 cases, hypothermia in 4 cases. Brain damage was more commonly focal (hematomas, contusions, or lacerations) than diffuse. Spinal injuries often occurred with other major injuries. Serious chest injuries occurred in 18 cases, but abdominal injuries were uncommon.

More than half of the victims with severe head injuries had few other injuries, and they likely would have survived had the head injury been prevented. Of the five victims wearing crash helmets, only one suffered a head injury. The other injuries occurring among climbers who suffered a fall or crushing were spinal fractures, chest injuries, abdominal injuries, and fractures located in the pelvis, face, and legs.

▶ An interesting article that essentially raises more questions than it answers. It would be nice to know the approximate size of the population at risk as well as the frequency of exposure. In 21 of the 42 persons autopsied, head injury was identified as the cause of death. The authors note that only one in eight of the climbers in this study was wearing a crash helmet and state that because of the variety of circumstances no general conclusion about the value of helmets can be made. Certainly, head protection in this activity is an aspect deserving consideration. Other factors such as supervision, experience, trail marking, and weather protective clothing should be evaluated. This study could serve as the first step to preventing mountaineering accidents.—J.S. Torg, M.D.

Head, Neck, and Spine Injuries

Retinal Injury and Detachment in Boxers
Joseph I. Maguire and William E. Benson (Thomas Jefferson Univ., Philadelphia)
JAMA 255:2451–2453, May 9, 1986   3–13

Wills Eye Hospital has recently treated a large number of boxers with retinal injuries. Nine boxers with ten injured eyes were evaluated and treated at this hospital from April 1983 to October 1985. Eight of these patients had retinal detachment, while the ninth patient had a traumatic tear without detachment.

Eight eyes had rhegmatogenous retinal detachments, and two eyes had retinal tears without subretinal fluid. Six detachments were secondary to a retinal dialysis; three of these were giant tears. All tears were clearly caused by blunt trauma to the eye. Six were located superonasally, three were inferonasally, and one was superotemporally located. All affected eyes underwent surgery. The retinal detachments were treated with a scleral buckling procedure and cryotherapy. Simultaneous vitrectomy was used in the cases with giant tears. Cryotherapy was used for retinal tears without subretinal fluid. Four of these patients required reoperation.

This evidence suggests that the retinal tears in boxers are caused by direct blows to the eye by a fist. This is extremely relevant in view of the current American Medical Association stance in favor of the abolition of this sport.

▶ It is important to note that most of the subjects studied were totally asymptomatic until they noticed decreased visual acuity. Although the authors could not relate the occurrence of these injuries in boxers on an exposure basis, they did note that in a 2-year period 5% of their patients in the third decade of life treated for rhegmatogenous retinal detachments were boxers.—J.S. Torg, M.D.

Concussion Injury in College Football: An Eight-Year Overview
W.E. Buckley (Pennsylvania State Univ.)
Athletic Training 21:207–211, Fall 1986   3–14

The fatality rate in organized football is approximately 3 per 100,000 participants per year. Most of these fatalities were due to head and neck injuries. Cerebral concussions account for a high percentage of nonfatal injuries to the central nervous system. However, since concussions are considered benign, with transient pathologic findings, no accurate analysis of this type of injury has been performed. The author reports the results of his investigation of the nature and extent of concussion injuries in college football.

Data collected by the National Athletic Injury/Illness Reporting System were analyzed according to standard statistical methods. The investigation covered an 8-year period between 1975 and 1982. An average of 49 college teams contributed injury information relative to concussion injury, representing 36,749 athlete seasons and 395 team seasons. Severity of injury was based on a time-loss criterion: an injury resulting in less than 7 days' time-loss was classified as minor, whereas an injury resulting in more than 7 days' time-loss was classified as a significant injury.

The incidence of concussion injury during the 8-year study period was relatively low, but fairly consistent, with a slightly decreasing rate per 100 athletes during the 1979, 1980, and 1981 playing seasons. Of the 2,124 athlete injury incidents identified as concussion injury, 208 were classified as significant. A comparison of injury rates showed the risk of concussion during games to be nine times as high as during practice sessions. Other parameters evaluated in this study include the influence of which team position was played by the athlete, what type of activity caused the injury, and what was the situation when the injury occurred.

▶ Articles such as this allow me to get on a soap box again and preach against the use of the helmet or face mask in blocking and tackling. The helmet or face mask should never be the initial point of contact when blocking or tackling. Coaches who teach this technique are wrong and may be causing irreparable damage to their athletes. Shoulders, arms, and chests are for blocking and tackling. Many head and neck injuries could be prevented if coaches would teach safe and proper methods of blocking and tackling.—F. George, A.T.C., P.T.

Sports and Recreation Are a Rising Cause of Spinal Cord Injury
Charles H. Tator and Virginia E. Edmonds (Toronto Western Hosp. and Univ. of Toronto, Ontario)
Physician Sportsmed. 14:157–167, May 1986   3–15

Spinal cord injuries related to sports and recreation appear to be increasing in Canada, both absolutely and relative to other causes of spinal injuries. Between 1948 and 1983, 141 cases of spinal cord injury resulting from sports and recreation were studied to identify specific activities, risk factors, and target groups necessary to provide an epidemiologic base for designing effective programs for preventing sports-related spinal injuries. The results of separate surveys of diving and hockey injuries are also reported.

The incidence of spinal cord injuries related to sports and recreation increased from 15.4% in 1948–1973 to 28.3% in 1980–1983. The majority of the injuries were sustained by males (85.5%) and patients in the 11–20 and 20–30 age groups (75%). Shallow-water diving accounted for more than half (58.9%) of all spinal cord injuries, followed by motor sports (9.2%) and hockey (5%). Most of the injuries were in the cervical region (80.1%), and most caused complete paralysis below the level of injury (54.6%).

The aquatic survey, made in cooperation with the Royal Life Saving Society, revealed 33-water related spinal cord injuries, most due to diving. Except for one, all injuries were cervical. Shallow-water diving with the head striking the pool or lake bottom was the leading mechanism, with fracture-dislocation the most frequent type of spinal injury. Drinking or drugs were associated factors in almost 30% of the cases and suspected in another 26%. Spinal cord injury was sustained by 28 of 42 injuries among hockey players; 12 showed complete paralysis below the level of injury. Most of the injuries were in the middle to lower cervical region. Fracture-dislocation was the most common type of injury. A push or check into the boards with the helmeted head striking the boards with the neck slightly flexed accounted for most of the injuries.

Sports and recreation are causing a growing number of spinal injuries, most of which are major. The public should be made aware of the risks of such activities as shallow-water diving and of the importance of neck muscle conditioning in hockey and other contact sports.

▶ Perhaps most important, the authors note that "prevention has been stressed insufficiently" with regard to these injuries. Also of note is that the mechanism of injury for both aquatic and hockey cervical spine injuries is one in which the head strikes an object and the cervical spine is subjected to an axial load. Such a mechanism has been well established as being responsible for cervical spine injuries resulting from tackle football in the United States. Just as football-induced quadriplegia has been reduced by appropriate rules changes (Torg, J. S.: *JAMA* 254; 3439–3443, Dec. 27, 1985) education, rule and equipment changes, or both could possibly reduce cervical spine injuries in diving activities and ice hockey.—J.S. Torg, M.D.

Neurapraxia of the Cervical Spinal Cord With Transient Quadriplegia
Joseph S. Torg, Helene Pavlov, Susan E. Genuario, Brian Sennett, Ronald J. Wisneski, Bruce H. Robie, and Caren Jahre (Univ. of Pennsylvania and New York Hosp.-Cornell Univ.)
J. Bone Joint Surg. [Am.] 68-A:1354–1370, December 1986   3–16

A syndrome of neurapraxia of the cervical spinal cord with transient quadriplegia was delineated in 32 athletes, males with a mean age of 20 years. Twenty-nine subjects were injured while playing football. Spinal stenosis was determined by the ratio method (Fig 3–1). Seventeen patients had evidence of developmental stenosis of the spinal canal. Four patients

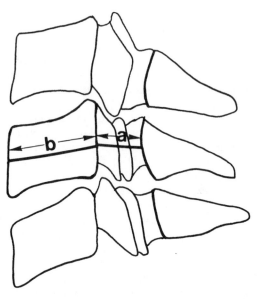

Fig 3–1.—The ratio of the spinal canal to the vertebral body is the distance from the midpoint of the posterior aspect of the vertebral body to the nearest point on the corresponding spinolaminar line (a) divided by the anteroposterior width of the vertebral body (b). [Courtesy of Torg, J.S., et al.: J. Bone Joint Surg. (Am.) 68-A:1354–1370, December 1986.]

had evident ligamentous instability, while 6 had intervertebral disc disease. Congenital cervical anomalies were seen in five patients.

The sensory changes included burning pain, numbness, tingling, and loss of sensation. Motor changes ranged from weakness to complete paralysis. Patients usually recovered completely within 10 to 15 minutes, but full recovery sometimes was delayed for as long as 48 hours. Cervical spine roentgenograms failed to demonstrate fracture or dislocation in any case. Significant spinal stenosis was demonstrated in 24 evaluable patients.

A history suggesting neurapraxia of the cervical cord was found in 1.3 per 10,000 in a survey of athletes at 503 colleges. A reduced anteroposterior diameter of the spinal canal between the third and sixth cervical vertebrae (Fig 3–2) appears to be the key finding.

Patients with associated cervical spinal instability or acute or chronic degenerative changes should avoid further contact sports activities. Subjects having developmental spinal stenosis—or spinal stenosis associated with congenital abnormality—should be managed individually.

Congenital Cervical Stenosis Presenting as Transient Quadriplegia in Athletes: Report of Two Cases
Amy L. Ladd and Pierce E. Scranton (Seattle)
J. Bone Joint Surg. [Am.] 68-A:1371–1374, December 1986   3–17

When an athlete who appears to be quadriplegic immediately after an injury rapidly recovers all neurologic function and has normal routine roentgenograms and computed tomographic scans of the cervical spine, it is important to recognize stenosis of the cervical spine as a possible di-

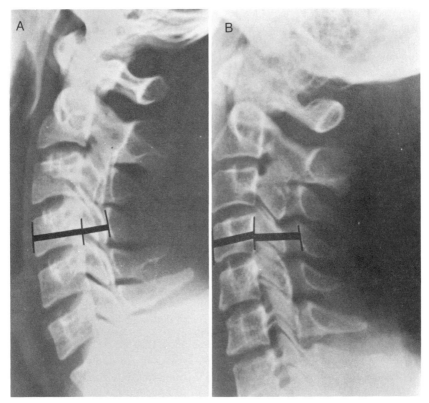

Fig 3–2.—A comparison between the ratio of the spinal canal to the vertebral body of a stenotic patient versus that of a control subject is demonstrated on lateral roentgenograms of the cervical spine. The ratio is approximately 1:2 (0.50) in the stenotic patient (**A**) compared with 1:1 (1.00) in the control (**B**). [Courtesy of Torg, Joseph S., et al.: J. Bone Joint Surg. (Am.) 68-A:1354–1370, December 1986.]

agnosis before deciding that the athlete can resume full-scale activities. The authors present two case reports of athletes who were found to have congenital cervical stenosis after they experienced transient quadriplegia.

Case 1.—Man, 23, who was black and a professional running-back, sustained an injury to the neck which rendered him quadriplegic immediately. However, motor and sensory function returned within 2 minutes after the injury, and a subsequent neurologic examination was normal. Two weeks after having returned to full activity, he was injured again and had another episode of transient quadriplegia. A neurologic examination was again normal, but a metrizamide-enhanced myelogram showed anterior and posterior narrowing and a filling defect at the level of the disk between the third and fourth cervical vertebrae. The patient retired from professional football and was neurologically normal at follow-up 6 years later.

Case 2.—Man, 25, who was black and a professional wide-receiver experienced flaccid quadriplegia for about 2 minutes after sustaining a head injury. Although he had normal neurologic findings, a metrizamide-enhanced myelogram was recommended in light of the experience gained with the previous case. A filling defect was found anteriorly and posteriorly between the third and fourth vertebrae and a bulging of the disk between these vertebrae. The patient retired from professional football and was neurologically normal at follow-up 3 years later.

▶ The diverse conclusons of these two articles regarding the management of athletes with diagnosed congenital developmental cervical stenosis requires explanation. Ladd and Scranton (Abstract 3–17), on the basis of two case reports from an unpublished and undocumented personal communication, state that in instances of a decrease in the sagittal diameter of the cervical canal " . . . a potentially dangerous situation may arise if a physician permits such an individual to continue to participate in contact sports when there is certain or even equivocal radiographic evidence that stenosis is present." On the other hand, Torg et al. (Abstract 3–16), reporting on 32 instances of neurapraxia of the cervical cord as well as a review of nearly 1000 cervical spine injuries resulting from football which included 223 players who were known to have sustained injuries with associated quadriplegia, derive different conclusions. Specifically, although youngsters with developmental stenosis and associated instability or degenerative changes should be precluded from further competition, the vast majority of youngsters with developmental stenosis with or without congenital malformations can be treated on an individual basis. Essentially what we have in the first instance are ill-founded conclusions based on two case reports and unsubstantiated "antidotalism."—J.S. Torg, M.D.

Injuries of the Spine Sustained During Gymnastic Activities
J.R. Silver, D.D. Silver, and J.J. Godfrey (Stoke Mandeville Hosp., Aylesbury, and Childwell, Liverpool, England)
Br. Med. J. 293:861–863, Oct. 4, 1986   3–18

Spinal injuries can occur during gymnastic activities. During a 30-year period, 38 patients, aged 12 to 54 (mean age, 20) were seen for gymnastic accidents. There were 33 men and 5 women. The causes of spinal injury in these patients are presented and prevention techniques are suggested.

There were 31 spinal injuries, resulting in complete paralysis in 24 cases, incomplete paralysis in 7, and no deficit in 2; information was incomplete in 5 patients. Most of those injured were club standard, county standard, or national standard, and one was professional. The cord injuries were predominantly at the fourth to the seventh cervical segments, most of which were flexion injuries. The accidents occurred largely because gymnasts landed on their heads, the force being transmitted to the cervical spine. Most of the injuries were sustained in a gymnasium and were caused by inadequate supervision. The falls resulted largely from static exercises and falls from ladders, ropes, and wall bars.

Serious cervical injuries can occur during gymnastic activities and can cause severe paralysis. Supervision must be adequate at all times, with regard to the use of the gymnasium and its equipment and performance of gymnastic programs. The public, as well, should be made aware of the dangers of doing somersaults in the road. Greater skill of the athlete does not afford protection from injury, as an advanced gymnast remains a beginner with every new exercise he tries.

▶ It is interesting to note that in the United States catastrophic cervical spine injuries resulting from gymnastic activities are synonymous with trampoline and minitrampoline (*Pediatrics* 74:804–812, November 1984). In England the trampette has been implicated consistently. It is described as follows: "The trampette is a little understood, much abused piece of equipment. It is a muscle replacement, its angle aids rotation, it preserves energy, and it allows people, especially children, to achieve height and carry out exercises of spatial orientation. It enables people to do exercises, such as somersaults, that they do not have the muscles to achieve spontaneously. . . . The trampette's greatest danger is that it enables the gymnast to gain uncontrolled height, which can be corrected by neither gymnast nor catcher."

Also to be noted is that in instances where the mechanism was observed, the injured gymnast are described as "landing on his head. . . ." This certainly suggests the axial load mechanism, which has been documented as being responsible for cervical spine injuries in football, ice hockey, and diving. (*Med. Sci. Sports Exerc.* 17:295–303, 1985).—J.S. Torg, M.D.

Lumbar Spondylolysis and Spondylolisthesis in College Football Players: A Prospective Study
John R. McCarroll, John M. Miller, and Merrill A. Ritter (Methodist Hosp. of Indiana, Methodist Ctr. for Sports Medicine, and Indiana Univ., Indianapolis)
Am. J. Sports Med. 14:404–406, September–October 1986   3–19

A high rate of lumbar spondylolysis has been reported in college football players. A prospective study was made of films of the lumbar spine of 145 incoming freshman football players from 1978 to 1983, and the athletes were followed closely for lower back problems.

Nineteen (13%) of the 145 had initial findings of spondylolysis or spondylolisthesis. Ten of the 31 players with low back pain had previous radiographic findings of spondylolysis. Three (2.4%) of 126 others developed such findings. Overall incidence of spondylolysis was 15%. There were 15 cases at the L5-S1 level and 1 case at L4–5. All cases of spondylolisthesis involved L5-S1; none had progressed beyond grade 1.

Five other subjects had spina bifida occulta that was not associated with low back pain. Eight subjects had transitional vertebrae; only 2 of them had low back pain. Two of three subjects with degenerative lumbar disk changes presented with low back pain.

None of the athletes with spondylolysis or spondylolisthesis failed to complete their college football career. One athlete had disk surgery and later became a professional player.

Spondylolysis is more frequent in college football players than in the general population. The problem appears to arise in adolescence during athletic activity or other stress. Players other than linemen are susceptible.

Emphasis should be placed on proper blocking and tackling techniques, weight training, and other methods of conditioning.

▶ It is interesting to note that the data presented in this paper compare with those reported by Ferguson et al. (*Am. J. Sports Med.* 2; 63–69, March–April 1974) where the incidence of spondylolysis and spondylolisthesis amongst a group of twenty-five interior intercollegiate linemen were 24% and 8%, respectively. Also, Semon and Spengler (*Spine* 6:172, 1981) reported an apparent incidence of lumbar spondylolysis of 21% in a group of intercollegiate football players.—J.S. Torg, M.D.

Sacroiliac Dysfunction in Runners

Terry J. Whieldon and Thomas W. Winiewicz (State Univ. of New York at Buffalo and St. Jerome's Hosp., Batavia, N.Y.)
Athletic Training 21:15–19, Spring 1986   3–20

Many runners have nonspecific low back and/or buttock pain on one side and a history of multiple treatments. Only refraining from running

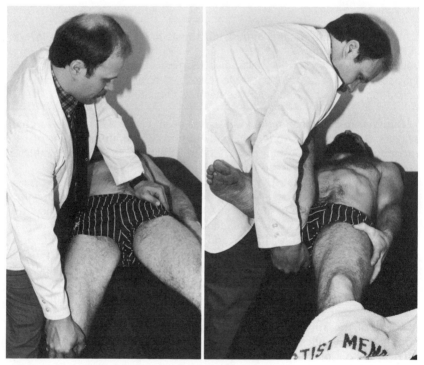

Fig 3–3 (left).—Posterior ilium correction technique.
Fig 3–4 (right).—Anterior ilium correction technique. (Courtesy of Whieldon, T.J., and Winiewicz, T.W.: Athletic Training 21:15–19, Spring 1986.)

has controlled the pain. Sacroiliac joint trauma may result from various athletic activities or a change in terrain for runners. A forceful heel strike also may be a factor. Abnormal running mechanics may lead to improper sequencing of heel strike, stance phase, and pelvic rotation, resulting in abnormal anterior pelvic rotation on the sacrum, and ultimately iliac wedging and locking.

Often a specific incident is described, or there may be a history of increasing pain as the running mileage increased. Walking frequently aggravates sacroiliac dysfunction, as does lateral trunk flexion toward the involved side. Pain on descending stairs implicates the sacroiliac joint. Standing postural screening begins the objective examination. The standing flexion, sitting flexion, and long sitting tests may be used to evaluate sacroiliac joint function. The sitting flexion test is specific for motion of the sacrum within the ilia.

Muscular correction methods are used to unlock the ilium from the sacrum and restore normal sacroiliac joint motion. These techniques (Figs 3–3 and 3–4) have effectively reduced or relieved symptoms of unilateral hip and low back pain in athletes. The technique used is based on demonstrating an abnormally rotated ilium with associated sacroiliac dysfunction.

▶ Treatment of sacroiliac joint dysfunction has become very popular the past few years. Treatment techniques are varied but all stress the importance of a thorough evaluation before treatment begins. The skill of the evaluator is most important as many of the tests are subjective and may be misinterpreted. Very often evaluators in the same clinic will disagree on the findings. The treatment rationale must be based on the clinical evaluation. Muscle energizing techniques are probably the most conservative and safest techniques to use. Joint mobilization techniques should be attempted only by those with a good knowledge and experience with these techniques.

A word of caution. Every time I attend a workshop or clinic, regardless of the subject, seven of the next ten injured athletes I see has a form of that particular ailment, and I must put all my new found skills into practice. Be cautious with newly learned techniques.—F. George, A.T.C., P.T.

Upper Extremity Injuries

Hook of the Hamate Fractures in Athletes

Richard D. Parker, Mark S. Berkowitz, Malcolm A. Brahams, and William R. Bohl (Mt. Sinai Med. Ctr., and Lutheran Med. Ctr., Cleveland)
Am. J. Sports Med. 14:517–523, November–December 1986   3–21

Hook of hamate fractures are more frequent than previously thought, and are found in baseball, golf, tennis, and racquetball players. Five athletes with six such fractures were seen in the past 8 years. Four were professional baseball players, and were injured when batting. Two injuries were caused by a fall on the outstretched hands. The patients were males, 22 to 29 years of age. Pain was the initial symptom, and a dull ache persisted at

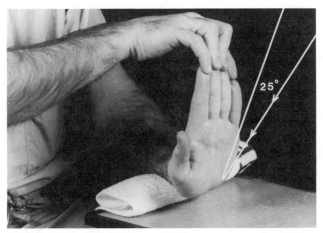

Fig 3–5.—Technique of obtaining a carpal tunnel view of the wrist. (Courtesy of Parker, R.D., et al.: Am. J. Sports Med. 14:517–523, November–December 1986.)

the ulnar aspect of the wrist. Grip strength was decreased. The hook was primarily excised in four cases, and two patients had secondary surgery. All were able to resume physical activity within 1 month of surgery, and returned to the previous level of activity within 6 weeks.

Carpal tunnel views (Fig 3–5) are helpful when a hook fracture is suspected. Several views may have to be obtained with small degrees of cassette rotation to obtain a clear view of the entire hook (Fig 3–6). Oblique views (Figs 3–7 and 3–8) with the forearm in midsupination and the wrist dorsiflexed also are helpful. Tomography and CT will provide a more detailed evaluation of the margins of the hook fracture.

Nonoperative management in a short arm case often fails, while surgical excision of the hook consistently relieves pain and permits full wrist motion with normal grip strength. Patients return to previous activity within 6 to 8 weeks. The chief complication of surgery is the risk of anesthesia. No functional loss results from excision of the hook. Nonoperative management may be followed by nonunion, tendinitis, or rupture of the finger flexor digitorum profundus or sublimis tendons.

▶ An excellent article dealing with the problems presented by hook of the hamate fractures. The interested reader is referred to the original article.—J.S. Torg, M.D.

Intra-Articular Fractures of the Distal End of the Radius in Young Adults
Jerry L. Knirk and Jesse B. Jupiter (Harvard Univ.)
J. Bone Joint Surg. [Am] 68-A:647–659, June 1986   3–22

Intra-articular fractures of the distal part of the radius are difficult to manage in young adults and are associated with a high frequency of ar-

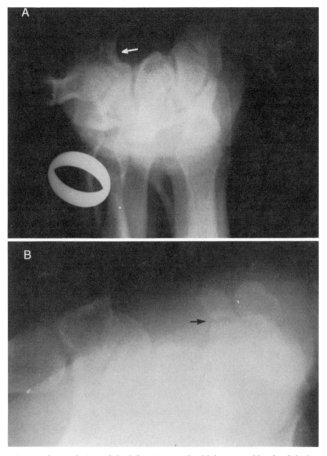

Fig 3–6.—A, carpal tunnel view of the left wrist reveals old fracture of hook of the hamate (*arrow*) with sclerotic border. **B,** carpal tunnel view of right wrist reveals fracture through the base of the hamate (*arrow*). (Courtesy of Parker, R.D., et al.: Am. J. Sports Med. 14:517–523, November–December 1986.)

thritis. This retrospective study of 43 fractures in 40 young adults was initiated to determine the issues important in treatment. The mean follow-up time was 6.7 years.

At follow-up, 26% of the fractures were rated excellent, 35% good, 33% fair, and 6% poor. There was evidence of arthritis in 28% of the fractures. Twenty-four fractures healed with incongruity of the radiocarpal joint and 91% of these had evidence of arthritis. However, of 19 fractures healed with a congruous joint, only 11% developed arthritis. A depressed articular surface was responsible for incongruity in 75% of the incongruous joints. It was anatomically reduced by closed methods in only 49% of all cases.

Accurate articular restoration was the most critical factor of successful

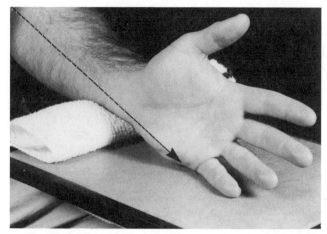

Fig 3–7.—Technique of obtaining oblique view of wrist. (Courtesy of Parker, R.D., et al.: Am. J. Sports Med. 14:517–523, November–December 1986.)

treatment. Nonunion of the ulnar styloid process decreased treatment success. However, restoration of the dorsal tilt and radial length was not usually critical.

▶ This is an excellent study that confirms the premise that an intra-articular-

Fig 3–8.—Oblique view of right wrist reveals subtle hook of hamate fracture (*arrow*). (Courtesy of Parker, R.D., et al.: Am. J. Sports Med. 14:517–523, November–December 1986.)

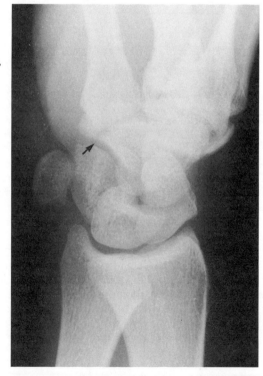

fracture of the distal radius in a young adult is a complex injury with considerable associated morbidity. Also to be noted, in addition to the fact that 65% had roentgenographic evidence of post-traumatic arthritis, there was associated medial nerve compression in 23% of the patients.

The authors suggest that initial attempt at closed reduction be made using longitudinal traction and manipulation. If an anatomical reduction is achieved an external fixation device with frame is applied. If there is impaction with incongruity of the joint measuring more than 2 mm after closed reduction, they suggest consideration of open reduction and internal fixation with cancellous bone graft to support the articular surface of the distal part of the radius.—J.S. Torg, M.D.

A Mechanical and Electromyographical Analysis of the Effects of Various Joint Counterforce Braces on the Tennis Player
Jack L. Groppel and Robert P. Nirschl (Univ. of Illinois at Urbana-Champaign)
Am. J. Sports Med. 14:195–200, May–June 1986   3–23

In 1973, the authors introduced the term and use of counterforce bracing. This concept was based on the theory that this bracing technique acted as a diffusing counterforce, thereby decreasing either the quantity of internally generated muscle contractile tension or altering and directing potentially abusive forces overloads to less sensitive tissues and possibly to the brace itself. This concept in bracing differs substantially from those concepts of protection from impact or extrinsic overload and is designed to decrease those forces which occur from intrinsic muscle contraction or excessive movements of tendon and certain joint parts.

Although counterforce braces now have been used clinically by thousands of patients for the purposes of injury prevention, protection during rehabilitation and protection during return to normal activity, it is not known which physical changes accomplish the positive effect. A biomechanical analysis was conducted of braced and unbraced tennis players (serve and backhand strokes).

The study population consisted of nine tennis players; three were skilled competitors, three were intermediate recreational players, and three were inexperienced novice players. The authors used three-dimensional cinematography and electromyographic techniques to analyze the serve and backhand strokes of the subjects. They compared three commonly used counterforce braces (lateral elbow, medial elbow, and radial-ulnar wrist) with the unbraced condition. The braces led to positive biomechanical alterations in forearm muscle activity and angular joint acceleration which were dependent upon the brace and joint area analyzed.

It is concluded that there is a positive effect for the tennis player when using the counterforce brace.

▶ We have used counterforce braces in our treatment of lateral epicondylitis with a high incidence of success. Our treatment usually consists of some type of cryokinetics (usually cold whirlpool at 55 degrees for 20 minutes) anti-inflammatory medication, flexibility exercises, and a counterforce brace. When the pain subsides strengthening exercises are begun. We have also used hydracortisone injections, ultrasound and phonophoresis in problems which do not respond to more conservative treatment. We recommend that the brace be worn 24 hours a day when the injury is acute or painful.—F. George, A.T.C., P.T.

Reconstruction of the Ulnar Collateral Ligament in Athletes
Frank W. Jobe, Herbert Stark, and Stephen J. Lombardo (Univ. of Southern California and Kerlan-Jobe Orthopaedic Clinic, Inglewood, Calif.)
J. Bone Joint Surg. [Am.] 68-A:1158–1163, October 1986   3–24

The anterior part of the ulnar collateral ligament is a major stabilizer at the elbow, and elongation or tearing of the structure leads to an unstable, painful elbow, particularly in athletes who throw a baseball or javelin. The ligament was reconstructed in 16 throwing athletes, most of them professional baseball pitchers, between 1974 and 1982. The patients, all men, were aged 20 to 31 years at the time of surgery. In eight cases the rupture occurred as a sudden catastrophic event, but nearly all patients had been symptomatic on throwing for months or years. Five patients had had previous elbow surgery. Valgus instability was a consistent finding. Holes were placed in the medial epicondyle and ulna for placement of a donor tendon, usually the palmaris longus, in a figure eight fashion (Fig 3–9).

Ten patients returned to participation at the same level of competition, and one at a lower level. Most patients returned to full activity within 1 year after reconstructive surgery. Five patients retired from professional athletics, but not because of the operation. Two of the athletes who resumed activity required secondary surgery for ulnar palsy and recovered completely. Another patient was reoperated on for medial epicondylitis and removal of scar tissue from the ulnar nerve.

Several professional throwing athletes in this study were able to return to competition after reconstruction of the damaged ulnar collateral ligament. Slow revascularization of the graft by means of the sheath of granulation tissue growing from adjacent tissue presumably occurs. Presently athletes of any caliber who are unable to play at all with an unstable elbow

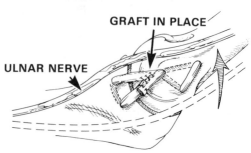

Fig 3–9.—The graft forms a figure of eight and the ulnar nerve is transferred anteriorly (*shaded arrow*). [Courtesy of Jobe, F.W., et al.: J. Bone Joint Surg. (Am.) 68-A:1158–1163, October 1986.]

are operated on. The lengthy period of rehabilitation requires a highly motivated patient.

► An interesting and well-documented study. However, certain questions have gone unanswered. First, what were the indications for surgical intervention—acute onset of valgus instability? In that only 10 of the 16 patients returned to participation in their former activity level, one must ask if similar or better results could not have been obtained with conservative management. Also, it is noted that the ulnar nerve was transposed anteriorly in all instances. What role did this part of the procedure have in success or failure of the operation? To be noted: "there was a high incidence of complications related to the ulnar nerve. Two patients have postoperative ulnar neuropathy that required a second operation . . . Three others reported some transient postoperative hypoesthesia along the ulnar aspect of the forearm that resolved after a few weeks or months." Also to be noted was relatively prolonged recuperative period. "In the patients in our study, the shortest interval from operation to effective pitching was 11 months, and the longest interval was 19 months."— J.S. Torg, M.D.

Ulnar Collateral Ligament Tears of the Elbow Joint
Shigehito Kuroda and Koh Sakamaki (Kashima Rosai Hosp., Ibaragi, and Chiba Kawatethu Hosp., Chiba, Japan)
Clin. Orthop. 208:266–271, July 1986   3–25

Sixteen cases of ulnar collateral ligament (UCL) tear without intra-articular complications were treated in an 11-year period. Nineteen other cases were associated with intra-articular complications. Thirteen patients with isolated UCL tear were followed up for 2 years or longer after injury. The mean age was 22 years. Eight injuries occurred when subjects fell or stumbled. Ten cases of valgus stress in the elbow-extended position were documented. Arthrograms showed hemarthrosis and extracapsular leakage of contrast; stress roentgenography confirmed joint instability and valgus instability, the latter averaging 15 degrees.

Ten patients underwent repair of torn ligaments under general or intravenous regional block anesthesia. End-to-end suturing was done at the midportion of the UCL, and side-to-side suturing was employed when longitudinal tears were present (Fig 3–10). If a small avulsing fracture of the ligamentous attachment was noted, sutures were passed through drill holes. After an average follow-up of 39 months, 2 conservatively treated patients had elbow pain when working or playing sports. One patient who underwent surgery reported numbness in the fifth finger. Three patients lacked 5 to 10 degrees of extension, and one lacked 5 degrees of flexion. Valgus instability averaged 5 degrees in patients undergoing surgery and 8 degrees in conservatively managed patients. The only roentgenographic abnormalities were minimal bone spur formation in two cases and late closure of the medial epicondylar epiphysis in one case.

Women not involved in sports activities do not require operative repair of UCL tears, and arthrography therefore is not necessary. Active women

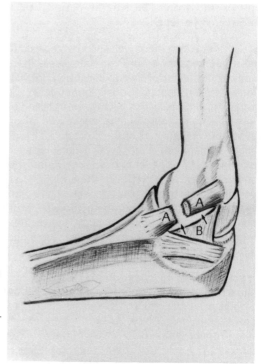

Fig 3–10.—Schematic drawing of complete cordlike part tear of the U.C.L. Additional longitudinal tear (*arrows*) between the cordlike part (*A*) and the fanlike part (*B*) was recognized in all cases of complete tears. (Courtesy of Kuroda, S., and Sakamaki, K.: Clin. Orthop. 208:266–271, July 1986.)

and men should, however, undergo operative repair following arthrographic examination.

▶ Of 13 cases of acute ulnar collateral ligament instability, 10 were surgically repaired and 3 were treated conservatively. Of those treated surgically, preoperative stress roentgenographic examination revealed valgus instability of an average of 14.9 degrees (range, 5 to 27 degrees). At follow-up, the operatively treated patients had an average 5.1 degrees laxity while conservatively treated patients had an average of 8.0 degrees. We must assume, then, that the surgical procedure resulted in only a difference of 3 degrees laxity between the surgically and conservatively treated patients. There was no functional assessment of the patients. This study does not support the conclusion that "valgus instability is necessarily disabling in patients performing heavy labor or vigorous sports and should be treated surgically."—J.S. Torg, M.D.

Stress Fractures of the Olecranon in Javelin Throwers
A. Hulkko, S. Orava, and P. Nikula (Univ. Hosp., Oulu, Keski-Pohjanmaa Central Hosp. and Sports Injury Clinic Medirex, Kokkola, Finland)
Int. J. Sports Med. 7:210–213, 1986   3–26

Valgus and extension overload of the elbow in pitching or throwing can produce various types of trauma, including stress fracture of the olecranon.

Four javelin throwers were treated for this injury between 1977 and 1984. The three males and one female had a mean age of 23 years. All had good throwing technique but had had elbow pain for weeks or months before diagnosis. One patient had acute painful dislocation of the fracture during a throw.

One patient was managed conservatively and had healing in 18 months, followed by return to full athletic activity. Two other patients were operated on using a tension band and two Kirschner wires, and in the third case, the tip of the olecranon was excised. The former injuries healed in 4 months, but one of these patients had a refracture that was treated with bone pegs and a compression screw. The other patient had ulner nerve release performed 10 months after primary operation. The injury treated by excision of the olecranon tip healed in 2 months, and the patient then was able to throw normally.

Stress fracture of the olecranon tip in throwing athletes results from the tip repeatedly making violent contact with the olecranon fossa in maximal extension. The distal stress fracture in a javelin thrower calls for operative treatment, using a tension band and two parallel Kirschner wires if a transverse fracture line is present. Established nonunion or stress fracture across the epiphyseal plate is managed by bone grafting. Comprehensive training efforts are needed to rehabilitate these athletes.

▶ The particular lesions described in this article must be differentiated from stress fractures involving the olecranon epiphyseal plate (Torg, J. S., et al.: *J. Bone Surg.* 59A:264–265, March 1977; and Kovach, et al.: *Am. J. Sports Med.* 13:105–111, March–April, 1985). It does not appear that the particular stress fracture presented in this article involves the growth plate, and I would agree that excision of the involved olecranon tip is perhaps the most efficacious way of managing this particular problem.—J.S. Torg, M.D.

Open Reduction and Internal Fixation of Comminuted Radial Head Fractures
Richard A. Sanders and H. Graeme French (Hughston Orthopaedic Clinic, Columbus, Ga., and Tulane Univ.)
Am. J. Sports Med. 14:130–135, March–April 1986   3–27

Currently, comminuted radial head fractures of the elbow are treated either by excision of the radial head or early motion without surgery. Although both methods give satisfactory results in most patients, some patients have had poor results after radial head excision. On the other hand, early motion without surgery has also been associated with undesirable results which cannot be corrected by late radial head resection. The authors report the results of open reduction with internal fixation as a treatment of radial head fractures and assessed the results of this treatment on distal radioulnar joint and elbow joint function, and on elbow joint stability.

A total of eight patients, ranging in age between 20 and 40 years, who had sustained comminuted radial head fractures was treated with open reduction and internal fixation. Four male and two female patients were available for follow-up study beyond fracture healing. All patients were operated on between the second and seventh day after injury.

At follow-up, four patients reported mild, intermittent elbow pain associated with weather changes or very heavy exertion, but the other two patients had no elbow pain. Two patients had developed a loss of 45 degrees of supination, but the other four patients showed no functional deficit. One patient experienced proximal migration of the radial head, but this may have been due to an intercarpal injury at the time of elbow dislocation.

Open reduction and internal fixation of comminuted radial head fractures is technically feasible and produces satisfactory results.

Late Results of Excision of the Radial Head for an Isolated Closed Fracture
I. Goldberg, J. Peylan, and Z. Yosipovitch (Tel Aviv Univ.)
J. Bone Joint Surg. [Am.] 68-A:675–679, June 1986   3–28

Fractures of the radial head are most often treated nonoperatively if they are undisplaced type I fractures, whereas severely comminuted type III fractures are most often treated by excision of the radial head. However, there is no consensus on the best treatment for type II fractures with displacement of segments of the radial head. The authors conducted a retrospective study to evaluate the long-term results of radial head excision performed in patients with isolated closed type II or type III fractures. Three case reports are also presented.

The study comprised 21 female and 15 male patients, who were available for follow-up, ranging in age between 18 and 75 years, including 20 patients with type II fractures and 16 patients with type III fractures. All patients were operated on by radial head excision shortly after sustaining their injury. The dominant arm was injured in 21 patients (58%) and the nondominant arm in 15 patients (42%). Follow-up ranged from 3 to 27 years, or an average of 16.4 years.

At follow-up, 31 (86%) of 36 patients stated that they were satisfied with the results, and 34 patients (94%) reported that they had returned to their preoperative occupations. Three patients had lost 30 degrees or more of flexion of the elbow or of pronation or supination of the forearm. In eight patients (22%), a measurable proximal migration of the radius was found of more than 1 mm, but this movement had not resulted in any harmful effects. Although osteoarthritic changes were found on roentgenograms of the operated arm in all the patients, functional scoring was not affected by these changes.

Satisfactory results can be obtained with surgical treatment of type II fractures of the radial head. However, since results of nonoperative treatment as reported in the literature have been equally favorable, the authors have adopted the nonoperative approach to the treatment of all type II fractures.

Results of Delayed Excision of the Radial Head After Fracture

Mark A. Broberg and Bernard F. Morrey (Mayo Clinic and Found.)
J. Bone Joint Surg. [Am.] 68-A:669–674, June 1986   3–29

There is controversy over the best method of treatment for Mason type II and type III fractures of the radial head. Most authors favor early radial head excision in order to decrease the incidence of late pain and loss of motion. Others are of the opinion that patients with this type of fracture will do equally well with nonsurgical treatment and that, in case of failure, radial head excision can still be performed. However, unfavorable results have been reported with such delayed procedures. The authors evaluated the results of delayed radial head excision in patients whose closed management of the fracture had failed.

The study comprised 11 male and 10 female patients, ranging in age between 10 and 60 years, who underwent delayed excision of the radial head between 1 month and more than 20 years after they sustained their original injury because initial nonsurgical treatment had failed. All patients were followed postoperatively for at least 3 years, with follow-up ranging from 3 to 32 years. Four (19%) of 21 patients had a Mason type II fracture, and the other 17 patients (81%) had a Mason type III fracture.

Although 90% of the patients reported that they were satisfied with the final functional outcome of the surgery, objective evaluation showed that only 2 patients (10%) had excellent results, 14 (67%) had good results, 4 (19%) had fair results, and 1 patient (4%) had poor results. Preoperatively, 1 patient had no pain, 8 had mild pain, and 12 had moderate pain, but none of the patients complained of severe pain.

In conclusion, the overall objective clinical result was good or excellent in 77% of the patients, suggesting that delayed excision is a viable option for patients with a fracture of the radial head in whom nonoperative treatment has failed or late symptoms have developed.

▶ These three articles (3–27, 3–28 and 3–29) present distinctly different approaches to the problem of dealing with comminuted fractures of the radial head. Sanders et al. (Abstract 3–27) advocate open reduction and internal fixation; Goldberg et al. (Abstract 3–28) recommend early radial head excision, whereas Broberg and Morrey (Abstract 3–29) advocate initial nonsurgical management with delayed excision of the radial head as indicated.

The dilemma created by essentially similar results from the three treatment methods is a manifestation of the retrospective, nonrandomized approach of the authors. What is needed is a prospective, randomized, multi-institutional study with treatment and follow-up protocols and data subjected to statistical analysis.—J.S. Torg, M.D.

Brachial Plexus Stretch Injuries: The Need for Accurate Evaluation and Management Techniques

Anthony Glodava
Athletic Training 21:357–359, Winter 1986   3–30

Serious spinal injuries, including fractures and dislocations, sustained by athletes during contact sports such as football, hockey, or wrestling have been well documented. However, brachial plexus or cervical nerve root stretch injuries do not always receive proper attention since the signs and symptoms of such injuries are often transient. As a consequence, underlying deficits of strength and endurance that predispose an athlete to more serious injuries are often not investigated further. The author discusses the proper diagnostic procedures that should be followed when brachial plexus or cervical nerve root stretch injuries are encountered by the athletic trainer or the team physician.

When an injury occurs after a collision during contact sports, the athlete often experiences immediate and complete paralysis, a sensation of burning and stinging that radiates down the entire arm, hand, and fingers of the involved side, and a persistent heaviness and generalized weakness of the upper arm. Symptoms usually subside after a few minutes. After serious cervical injury has been ruled out, the brachial plexus should be evaluated on the sidelines by neurologic testing and a differential diagnosis should be made between nerve root lesions and brachial plexus stretch injuries based on the history of pain. Local pain of one dermatone that does not travel down the arm indicates a nerve root injury rather than a brachial plexus stretch injury. When a loss of sensory, reflex, muscle strength, or endurance is noted, a player should be removed from further competition for the day in order to prevent a more serious injury.

Treatment includes ice application, immobilization with a sling, anti-inflammatory medication, and range-of-motion and resistance exercises where indicated. When repeated brachial plexus stretch injuries occur, permanent removal from competition should be considered since such repetitive injuries will result in chronic weakness of the upper arm musculature.

▶ How serious are these injuries? Should the athlete rush back onto the field as soon as the severe pain subsides? What tests can be performed on the sideline to ensure that the athlete is safe to return to the game? Brachial plexus injuries are encountered frequently and must be treated properly.

The athlete should not return to the game until he has regained normal strength and motion of the neck and involved upper extremity. The burning and stinging should have subsided completely, and protective measures should be taken. This is another controversial subject. Do neck collars help? How about cervical straps? Is there a way to prevent this injury from recurring? It is one injury that has a very high reoccurrence rate.—F. George, A.T.C., P.T.

Examination of the Shoulder Complex
Richard W. Bowling, Paul A. Rockar, Jr., and Richard Erhard (Univ. of Pittsburgh)
Phys. Ther. 66:1866–1877, December 1986   3–31

A detailed evaluation of the shoulder complex with an emphasis on functional objective examination will allow optimal management of shoulder problems. Resisted tests are done after available range of motion has

TABLE 1.—Correlation of Events in Inflammatory Process With Clinical Examination Findings and Treatment of Synovial Joints

Stage of Inflammation	Pain	Range of Motion	Motion Barrier	Treatment
Early	constant felt at rest predominant feature distal reference zone before motion barrier	capsular pattern	muscular (fast guarding) empty	pain control modalities immobilization
Intermediate	intermittent felt during movement synchronous with motion barrier may become more intense and more distal with repeated forceful movement	capsular pattern	muscular (fast-slow guarding)	pain control gentle movement
Late	pain not severe only felt with forceful movement after motion barrier proximal extent of reference zone	capsular pattern	capsular	vigorous mobilization exercise (automobilization)

(Courtesy of Bowling, R.W., et al.: Phys. Ther. 66:1866–1877, December 1986. Reprinted from Physical Therapy with the permission of the American Physical Therapy Association.)

been completed. In this way both contractile and noncontractile tissues can be stressed and will reproduce symptoms. The screening examination will indicate whether specific examination of a particular area is necessary.

Indications for specific examination of the shoulder complex include postural abnormality of the shoulder girdle or glenohumeral joint; deformity or wound in the area; abnormal response to upper limb elevation;

238 / Sports Medicine

TABLE 2.—Interpretation of Pattern of Responses to Resisted Testing

Combined Test Results	Status of Nervous System	Status of Muscular System
Strong and painless	no abnormality	no abnormality
Strong and painful	no abnormality	contractile lesion present
Weak and painless	nerve compression or peripheral neuropathy	longstanding rupture or tendon avulsion
Weak and painful	serious pathological condition (fracture, tumor)	serious pathological condition (fracture, tumor, recent severe tear)
All tests painful	acute inflammation or psychogenic condition	

(Courtesy of Bowling, R.W., et al.: Phys. Ther. 66:1866–1877, December 1986. Reprinted from Physical Therapy with the permission of the American Physical Therapy Association.)

symptoms on resisted shoulder girdle elevation or on resisted glenohumeral joint abduction; and pain on resisted elbow flexion or extension which is localized to the shoulder region. If these features are lacking, referred pain should be suspected.

Following subjective evaluation and determination of the site of pain and of its nature, the posture of the head, spine, and upper extremity is noted. Active range of motion is studied to identify adhesive capsulitis. A so-called capsular pattern may not, however, be an indication for joint mobilization (Table 1). A capsular motion barrier is the normal end feel for most glenohumeral joint motions.

TABLE 3.—Interpretation of Resisted Test Results* at Glenohumeral Joint for Common Contractile Lesions

Muscle	Abduction	Adduction	External Rotation	Internal Rotation	Elbow Flexion	Elbow Extension
Deltoid	+		+/−	+/−		
Supraspinatus	++		+/−			
Infraspinatus			++			
Subscapularis				++		
Pectoralis major		+		+		
Teres minor		+	+			
Teres major		+		+		
Latissimus dorsi†		+		+		
Biceps brachii			+/−	+/−	++ ‡	
Triceps brachii						+

*+, muscle performs function but rarely involved; +/−, muscle can produce pain with test but more painful with a different resisted test; ++, muscle usually responsible for positive test results.
†Also produces pain with resisted shoulder-girdle depression.
‡Many false negative test results.
(Courtesy of Bowling, R.W., et al.: Phys. Ther. 66:1866–1877, December 1986. Reprinted from Physical Therapy with the permission of the American Physical Therapy Association.)

Severe pain may produce an "empty end feel." Pain following the motion barrier usually reflects stretching of contracted connective tissue, as in late adhesive capsulitis. Pain occurring before the motion barrier is met indicates an acute condition. Mobility testing is used to examine the range of "joint play" or accessory movements.

Resisted tests (Table 2) are designed to stress the contractile tissues of a joint. Isometric contraction with the joint in neutral position will reproduce symptoms if a painful disorder involves the contractile tissues. False results may be minimized by carefully performing the procedures and by considering the results of other tests. The strength of contraction should be recorded (Table 3). If pain and weakness are noted, a serious disorder may be present. A painless and strong response usually indicates an intact musculotendinous unit. Finally, palpation is done to detect tenderness of involved structures. If indicated, a neurologic examination is carried out.

▶ Many times an athlete will come for an examination with a relatively painless shoulder, describing a pain that occurs only when lifting heavy weights or throwing many times. The authors do suggest that in some overuse syndromes of athletes it may be better to examine the athlete immediately after the condition has been aggravated by activity.

Joint mobilization techniques recently have been attempted by many therapists and trainers treating shoulder injuries. The evaluation of the injury is very important to determine the cause of the pain and to develop a treatment program. We have found mobilization techniques to be very beneficial in our shoulder treatment and shoulder rehabilitation programs.—F. George, A.T.C., P.T.

The Axillary Nerve and Its Relationship to Common Sports Medicine Shoulder Procedures

William Jay Bryan, Keith Schauder, and Hugh S. Tullos (Baylor College of Medicine)
Am. J. Sports Med. 14:113–116, March–April 1986   3–32

Surgical procedures including anteroinferior acromioplasty-rotator cuff repair incision, inferior capsular shift, and posterior entry shoulder arthroscopy were simulated in cadaver dissections, with emphasis on the position of the axillary nerve.

The vertical "saber" incision for anteroinferior acromioplasty (Fig 3–11) was carried out. A deltopectoral incision was used for access in the inferior capsular shift procedure for multiaxial rotary instability. A trocar was inserted via a posterior stab wound in shoulder arthroscopy (Fig 3–12).

The average distance from the anterior acromioplasty incision to the axillary nerve was 0.65 cm, and the average distance with the anterolateral incision was 0.9 cm. Both incisions placed the nerve in jeopardy. The average distance from the inferior border of the shoulder capsule to the main nerve trunk in the capsular shift procedure was 0.3 cm. The arthros-

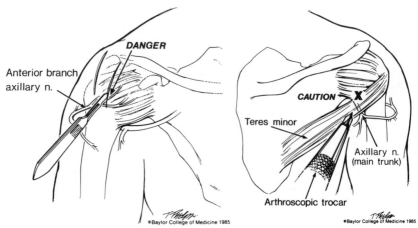

Fig 3–11 (left).—Relationship of anterolateral and more medially placed vertical incision to anterior branch of axillary nerve.

Fig 3–12 (right).—Relationship of standard posterior shoulder arthroscopic stab wound to axillary nerve main trunk. (Courtesy of Bryan, W.J., et al.: Am. J. Sports Med. 14:113–116, March–April 1986.)

copic trocar was 1.9 cm on average from the main trunk of the axillary nerve.

Detailed knowledge of the anatomical relationships of the axillary nerve is necessary to safely perform surgery for disabling shoulder conditions. The axillary nerve, through its deltoid innervation, is important in maintaining shoulder abduction and, to a lesser degree, flexion and extension.

▶ A basic and nicely illustrated article emphasizing the vulnerability of the axillary nerve to surgical misadventure. The fact that Neer and Foster (*J. Bone Joint Surg.* 62A:897–907, 1981) reported three instances of postoperative axillary neurapraxia in 40 patients who had an inferior capsular shift procedure justifies this effort.—J.S. Torg, M.D.

Arthroscopic Surgery of the Shoulder: A General Appraisal
D.J. Ogilvie-Harris and A.M. Wiley (Toronto Western Hosp. and Univ. of Toronto)
J. Bone Joint Surg. [Br.] 68-B:201–207, March 1986   3–33

More than 800 shoulder arthroscopies have been done in the past decade, and 439 patients have had arthroscopic surgery on the shoulder. A 4-mm arthroscope is introduced posteriorly to visualize the anatomic structures (Fig 3–13). Surgery is performed through accessory posterior or anterior portals.

Successful results generally were achieved in treating frozen shoulder by manipulating the joint to break down extrasynovial soft-tissue contracture. In patients with rotator cuff lesions, the best results were achieved when tendonitis was present. Half of patients with partial tears or re-tears had successful results, but those with a complete tear had a poor outcome.

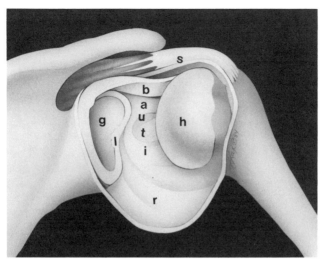

Fig 3–13.—Typical structures that may be visualised routinely at arthroscopy: *g,* glenoid; *l,* glenoid labrum; *b,* biceps tendon; *h,* humeral head; *s,* undersurface of supraspinatus; *t,* subscapularis tendon; *u,* subscapularis bursa; *r,* infraglenoid recess; *a,* superior glenohumeral ligament; *i,* inferior glenohumeral ligament. [Courtesy of Ogilvie-Harris, D.J., and Wiley, A.M.: J. Bone Joint Surg. (Br.) 68-B:201–207, March 1986.]

About two thirds of patients with mild degenerative arthritis had a successful outcome, but only one third of severely affected patients did so. About two thirds of patients with osteoarthritis and a glenoid labrum tear (Figs 3–14 and 3–15) had relief of symptoms.

Biceps tendon lesions also were treated effectively, and loose bodies were successfully removed in several instances. A few patients with rheu-

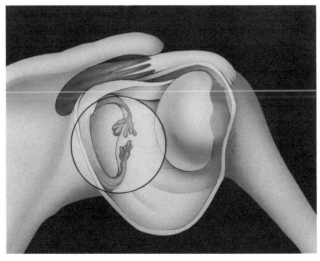

Fig 3–14.—Isolated tear of the glenoid labrum; unstable. [Courtesy of Ogilvie-Harris, D.J., and Wiley, A.M.: J. Bone Joint Surg. (Br.) 68-B:201–207, March 1986.]

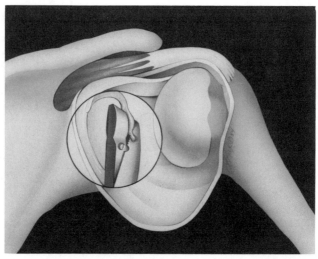

Fig 3–15.—Excising torn portion of glenoid labrum. [Courtesy of Ogilvie-Harris, D.J., and Wiley, A.M.: J. Bone Joint Surg. (Br.) 68-B:201–207, March 1986.]

matoid arthritis underwent arthroscopic synovectomy. Patients with septic arthritis had the joint irrigated and debris removed, but synovectomy was not done in these cases. Percutaneous fixation for anterior instability has been successful in a small number of cases. Complications occurred in 3% of patients having arthroscopic surgery, the most frequent being massive leakage of fluid from the shoulder joint. Articular cartilage was damaged in five cases.

Arthroscopic surgery is a safe and effective approach to some shoulder disorders. Manual traction is preferred over use of an arm holder. Further work is needed on the arthroscopic release of rotator cuff impingement and on the role of arthroscopically controlled stabilization.

▶ The observations of the authors regarding the efficacy of arthroscopic surgery on the glenohumeral joint are in keeping with our own experience. Also, I would agree with the reservations regarding percutaneous fixation for anterior instability.—J.S. Torg, M.D.

Anterior Glenoid Labrum Damage: A Painful Lesion in Swimmers
William C. McMaster (Univ. of California at Irvine)
Am. J. Sports Med. 14:383–387, September–October 1986   3–34

A specific shoulder lesion produces pain and disability in swimmers. The patient with damage to the anterior glenoid labrum presents with shoulder pain and, often, clicking in certain motions. Pain tends to occur at hand entry and during the catch phase of swimming. The initial episode may represent anterior subluxation of the glenohumeral joint. The Kocher

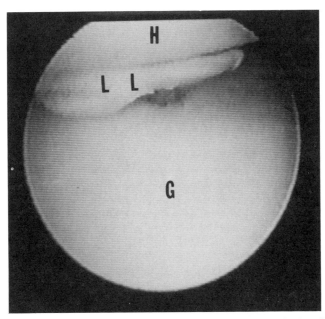

Fig 3–16.—This view from posterior shows the humeral head (*H*) above and the glenoid (*G*) below. A detached fragment of labrum (*L*) is seen incarcerated in the joint. The fragment remains tethered to the glenoid labrum at about 5 o'clock. An associated labral detachment was present anteriorly. (Courtesy of McMaster, W.C.: Am. J. Sports Med. 14:383–387, September–October 1986.)

maneuver may reproduce the click and pain, but the event itself does not recur. Arthroscopy confirms damage to the anterior labrum, involving the arc of labrum between the superior and inferior glenohumeral ligaments. Damaged tissue may or may not be separated from the glenoid. Tethered fragments of labrum may become incarcerated in the joint (Fig 3–16). The anterior edge of the bony glenoid may exhibit cartilage damage, and this may be an early phase of the Bankhart lesion.

Swimmers suspected of having an anterior labral lesion should have CT arthrography. Arthroscopy is then performed, for the damaged labrum does not respond to rest. The motorized debrider is probably the most useful instrument, and TV video equipment should be available. If the labrum remains attached, its frayed edge may be smoothed with the debrider. Adequate debridement will prevent the labral edge from catching as the humeral head glides across it during adduction and internal rotation. Sling support usually is not necessary.

Arthroscopy is a low-risk procedure in patients suspected of having intra-articular lesions. Labral debridement is most strongly indicated in patients having minimal or no apprehension on abduction/external rotation. The glenoid labral lesion may be effectively remedied arthroscopically in properly selected competitive swimmers.

▶ Based on our own experience, the author has presented what appears to be a valid observation regarding lesions involving the anterior glenoid labrum. Unfortunately, the observation is not substantiated by data. Clinical material, length of follow-up, and postsurgical results are lacking. Perhaps in the future this essential documentation will be forthcoming.—J.S. Torg, M.D.

MR Imaging of the Normal Shoulder

Dominik J. Huber, Rolf Sauter, Edgar Mueller, Hermann Requardt, and Horst Weber (State Univ. of New York at Stony Brook, and MR Development Labs., Erlangen, West Germany)
Radiology 158:405–408, February 1986   3–35

A simple method was developed of obtaining high-resolution magnetic resonance (MR) images of the shoulder off-center to depict the anatomy of the glenohumeral joint. Images of the shoulders of a healthy man aged 24 were obtained in the axial, sagittal, and coronal planes, using a 0.5-T imaging system and a specially designed surface coil. Multiple high-resolution spin-echo images were generated utilizing an off-center zoom technique.

The rotator cuff, long biceps tendon, articular capsule, regional muscles, and bones were visualized by MR imaging. The coronal and sagittal views were the most useful for demonstrating the rotator cuff. The long biceps tendon was best visualized on axial sections. Axial scans showed the insertion of the capsule into the glenoid anteriorly, forming the subscapularis recess. Both coronal and sagittal sections showed the subacromial and subdeltoid bursas.

High-resolution MR images of the shoulder obtained with a surface coil and an off-center zoom technique are useful in depicting the anatomy of the joint. Patients with suspected rotator cuff tears might be usefully evaluated by this method.

▶ This examination is limited, since only one patient is presented and we are presuming that this patient has normal shoulders. The insertion of the rotator cuff onto the greater tuberosity was not well demonstrated on their MRI study, and unfortunately this is the "critical zone" for rotator cuff tears. Further investigation and special techniques will be necessary to expand the usefulness of MRI in evaluating the shoulder.—J.S. Torg, M.D.

Shoulder Instability: Impact of Glenohumeral Arthrotomography on Treatment

Georges Y. El-Khoury, Mary H. Kathol, Joseph B. Chandler, and John P. Albright (Univ. of Iowa)
Radiology 160:669–673, September 1986   3–36

Glenohumeral instability is a frequent cause of disability in athletes. Labral pathology may be assessed accurately by double-contrast arthrography followed by either multidirectional tomography or CT. The arthro-

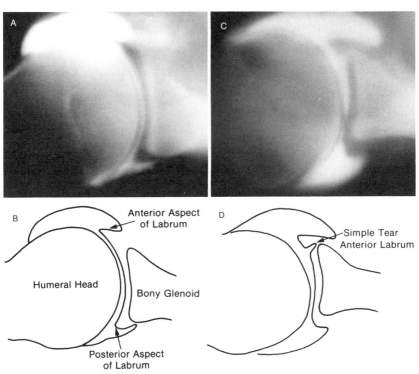

Fig 3–17.—A, arthrotomogram shows normal findings. B, line drawing of A. C, grade I lesion shows contrast material in a tear at the junction of the anterior labrum with the articular cartilage. D, line drawing of C. (Courtesy of El-Khoury, G.Y., et al.: Radiology 160:669–673, September 1986. Reproduced with permission of the Radiological Society of North America.)

tomographic appearances were correlated with the clinical findings in 114 patients seen between 1978 and 1984 with shoulder instability. The patients, with a mean age of 21.5 years, usually were involved in competitive athletics. Anatomical instability was present in 60% of the cases. Double-contrast arthrography was performed with 60% Renografin and air, and pluridirectional tomography at 3-mm intervals followed (Fig 3–17).

Arthrotomography showed labral tears in 86% of patients with anatomic instability of the shoulder, and in 90% of 10 patients with recurrent dislocation. All but 1 of 39 patients with anterior involuntary subluxation had labral tears. Labral tears were present in 40% of patients with functional instability of the shoulder. Anterior labral abnormalities were most frequent. Forty-four patients with anatomical instability and 12 with functional instability were operated on. There were no false-positive arthrotomographic findings in this group. In two cases of functional instability, however, only part of the pathologic condition was demonstrated.

Glenohumeral arthrotomography showed close correlation between labral pathologic findings and anatomical instability of the shoulder in this series. The examination is helpful in cases of both anatomic and functional instability in indicating when conservative management is appropriate. In surgical candidates the study can help in planning a more lesion-specific procedure.

▶ The required patient position is very uncomfortable. The study requires that the arm be extended with the patient lying on the affected side motionless throughout the entire examination. In addition to these technical difficulties, interpretation is dependent on the tomographic quality. A CT examination following an arthrogram is another modality used for demonstrating the glenoid labrum pathology. Although it is more expensive, it can be performed in a more comfortable position and is easily tolerated by the patient.—J.S. Torg, M.D.

Closed Reduction of Anterior Subcoracoid Shoulder Dislocation: Evaluation of an External Rotation Method
Daniel F. Danzl, Salvator J. Vicario, Gregory L. Gleis, Joseph R. Yates, and David L. Parks (Univ. of Louisville)
Orthopaedic Rev. 15:75–79, May 1986   3–37

Shoulder dislocations are the most frequently occurring type of dislocation. This article describes a useful closed-reduction technique for shoulder dislocation and evaluates it.

The patient is placed in the supine position, and the involved arm is slowly adducted against the patient's side. The elbow is kept at 90 degrees. The physician slowly rotates the forearm without longitudinal traction. This is slow, since it is necessary to stop every few degrees until spasms abate. However, no significant force is required. Most patients are reduced after about 5 minutes of external rotation. Painkillers can be administered prior to the start of the procedure.

Of 100 patients who were seen with anterior shoulder dislocations, 78 experienced successful reduction using this method. This method was easy to perform and relatively safe. This method is recommended for the closed reduction of anterior shoulder dislocation.

▶ The external rotation method of glenohumeral dislocation reduction was initially described by Leidelmeyer (*Emerg. Med.* 9:233, 1977) and evaluated by Mirick et al. (*J.A.C.E.P.* 8:528, 1979). This current prospective evaluation of the technique emphasizes its gentle and atraumatic nature. The authors state that the gradual external rotation at the head of the humerus allows relocation without the rim of the head jumping over the glenoid. Without the familiar traction "clonk" they report that initially both the patient and physician may be unaware that relocation has occurred.—J.S. Torg, M.D.

Anterior Dislocation of the Shoulder: Experience With a Modified Clavicular Harness

M. Ishikawa, E. Fujimaki, N. Kobayashi, H. Hirose, T. Katagiri, and A. Nagata
(Showa Univ., Tokyo)
Int. Orthop. 10:127–130, June 1986   3-38

Shoulder dislocation frequently recurs, and no treatment method has proved decisively effective. A modified clavicular harness has been used in high-risk cases following reduction of the dislocation. Of 417 patients seen at two ski clinics between 1972 and 1984, 199 had initial dislocations and 226 had recurrent dislocations. The age peak was in the third decade. Forty-one high-risk patients who were younger than 29 years at initial dislocation, who had capsular detachment, or who had fixation for less than 3 weeks were treated with the clavicular harness. Absence of a tuberosity fracture also was a risk factor. The harness covered the anterior part of the shoulder joint and the lower anterior region over the anteroinferior part of the glenoid (Fig 3–18). The patients were followed for 1 year after initial dislocation, along with 75 patients treated in a conventional harness.

Patients treated in a conventional bandage had a recurrent rate of 29%, but more than half of these patients failed to follow the recommendation for 3 weeks of fixation, chiefly because of disability from restricted arm

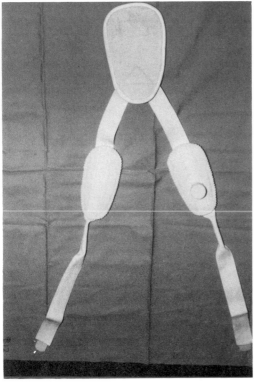

Fig 3–18.—The modified clavicular harness comprises a pad of hard material covering the anterior part of the shoulder joint and a smaller pad, with a diameter of 4 cm and a thickness of 1 cm, placed over the lower anterior part of the joint covering the anteroinferior part of the glenoid. (Courtesy of Ishikawa, M., et al.: Int. Orthop. 10:127–130, June 1986. Berlin-Heidelberg-New York: Springer.)

motion. All patients treated in the modified harness used it for longer than 3 weeks, with mean time of about 4 weeks. There were no recurrent dislocations in this group 1 year after primary dislocation. There also were no complications or neurologic complaints.

Use of a modified clavicular harness for 4 weeks has prevented recurrent anterior shoulder dislocation in patients at risk. No recurrences were observed during 1 year of follow-up in this study, while several patients treated with a conventional bandage had recurrent dislocation.

▶ The concept that the modified clavicular harness enhances primary healing of the anterior capsular detachment is interesting. Also, the use of shoulder arthrography to demonstrate capsular detachment has not, to my knowledge, been studied previously. It should be noted that the group of patients immobilized by "conventional fixation with Desault or Velpeau bandages" is not comparable with the group immobilized with a modified clavicular harness. As noted by the authors, the former group "did not follow recommendations of 3 weeks immobilization whereas the later group were immobilized for 4 weeks."—J.S. Torg, M.D.

Boytchev Procedure for the Treatment of Anterior Shoulder Instability
G.B. Ha'Eri (Kern Med. Ctr., Bakersfield, Calif.)
Clin. Orthop. 206:196–201, May 1986   3–39

The current techniques for the treatment of recurrent anterior dislocation of the shoulder require immobilization of the arm and loss of external rotation. Therefore, a clinical evaluation of a modified Boytchev procedure was carried out.

The patient is placed semireclining at 30 degrees. An anterior deltopectoral approach is used. The coracoid process is predrilled in the long axis. The conjoined tendons are then retracted to the penetration of the musculocutaneous nerve into the coracobrachialis. With the arm held in internal rotation, a blunt dissector is passed between the subscapularis muscle and the capsule of the shoulder joint. Opening the instrument creates a tunnel, through which the detached coracoid process is passed and reattached to its original site with a cancellous lag screw. The arm is placed in a sling for 2 to 3 weeks, during which time physiotherapy is started.

Twenty-six repairs have been performed with this procedure. After an average of 2 years' follow-up, all the results were satisfactory. Eight patients experienced a loss of external rotation of less than 15 degrees. There were no redislocations. This procedure stabilizes the shoulder immediately and allows physiotherapy to begin on the first day following the operation. Further follow-up is necessary to assess the long-term success of this procedure.

▶ It is interesting to note that, in this procedure for anterior glenohumeral instability, the joint is not entered. The wisdom of neglecting to remove loose bodies and torn cartilagenous labrums, which on occasion are bucket handled, should be questioned.—J.S. Torg, M.D.

Treatment of Recurrent Anterior Dislocation of the Shoulder by DuToit Staple Capsulorrhaphy: Results of Long-Term Follow-Up Study
Juluru P. Rao, Alfred M. Francis, John Hurley, and Roman Daczkewycz (Jersey City Med. Ctr., Union City, N.J., Cleveland Clinic Found., and Park Ridge, Ill.)
Clin. Orthop. 204:169–176, March 1986   3–40

Patients with recurrent anterior dislocation of the shoulder generally respond to surgical intervention, but there is still controversy over which procedure to use. The authors present their experience with 80 duToit staple capsulorrhaphies on 79 consecutive patients with recurrent anterior dislocation of the shoulder. Average follow-up period for 65 patients was 9 years (range, 26 months to 10.5 years). The mechanism of injury included excessive rotation in varying degrees of abduction in 35 (64%) patients, hyperextension or hyperabduction in 12 (18%), and direct trauma in 18 (28%).

With the shoulder elevated, an incision is made extending 3 in along the anterior axillary line just lateral to the coracoid process and deepened to the deltopectoral interval. With the shoulder in external rotation, a transverse incision is made in the subscapularis along its fibers at the junction of its middle and lower third, and deepened to the capsule. The humeral head retractor is inserted with the shoulder internally rotated and flexed, with the lower head of the retractor hooking behind the posterior lip of the glenoid. The Bankart lesion is identified when the tip of a hemostat passes freely around the glenoid rim, indicating detachment of the labrum from the anterior rim of the glenoid.

The anterior rim of the glenoid is roughened. Barbed staples are inserted 0.5 cm medial to the anterior rim of the glenoid, parallel to the articular surface of the glenoid. The ideal position of the staples is close to the inferior lip of the glenoid, thus securing the inferior glenohumeral ligament. The capsule is closed with multiple interrupted sutures using O-Ethibond on an OS-4 cutting needle. Postoperative management includes shoulder immobilization for 2 days, pendulum and circumduction exercises on the third day progressing to abduction, adduction, and internal and external rotation by day 12.

Underlying pathologic findings consisted of a Bankart lesion in 94% of patients, a markedly lax and redundant capsule in 6%, and bucket-handle tears of the glenoid labrum in association with a Bankart lesion in 6%. Results were excellent in 94%, good in 4%, and poor in 2%. There was an average loss of 10 degrees of external rotation. Recurrence of dislocation occurred in one patient (1.78%). Of the 70% of patients engaged in sports, 58% returned to athletic activities after surgical repair.

The chief pathologic lesion in recurrent anterior dislocation of the shoulder is the detached labrum. Stapling the glenoid labrum to the glenoid is an effective method of correcting this problem. DuToit capsulorrhaphy can be performed through a limited skin incision with minimal dissection. The procedure results in minimal restriction of shoulder motion and a very low recurrence rate.

▶ In this series of patients with recurrent anterior dislocation of the glenohumeral joint treated by the duToit staple capsulorrhaphy, the redislocation rate following surgery is reported as less than 2%. It is also reported that 70% of the patients in this series returned to athletic activities including pitching, basketball, golf, football, and wrestling. The fact that the patients' shoulders were mobilized on the second postoperative day presumably is responsible for minimal loss of external rotation. Void (*J. Bone Joint Surg.* 47A:1514, 1965) has reported on 49 duToit staple capsulorrhaphies with an average of 5.9 years follow-up and redislocation rate of 4%.—J.S. Torg, M.D.

The Use of the Putti-Platt Procedure in the Treatment of Recurrent Anterior Dislocation: With Special Reference to the Young Athlete
Kenneth A. Collins, Charles Capito, and Mervyn Cross (Royal North Shore Hosp. of Sydney, St. Leonards, Australia)
Am. J. Sports Med. 14:380–382, September–October 1986   3–41

Anterior dislocation is a common, painful, limiting, and often recurrent injury of the shoulder in young adults. The clinical records of 104 young athletes who underwent the Putti-Platt and combined Putti-Platt/Bankart procedures for reconstruction of 107 anterior dislocations of the shoulder were reviewed. Questionnaires were mailed to 74 patients, noting the results of reconstruction. The majority of the patients were young males engaged in contact sports, especially rugby football. The Putti-Platt (n = 59) procedure has been described previously; an additional Bankart procedure (n = 48) was performed when a glenoid tear was found using stable capsulorrhaphy. Patients were strapped for 6 weeks, and thereafter underwent physiotherapy. Average follow-up period was 66 months (range, 22 months to 10 years).

Overall, nine redislocations were noted in the clinical records of all patients. Of the 71 patients who completed the questionnaire, 8 of 74 operations had redislocations. Average time to redislocation was 44 months (range, 19 to 61). There was only one redislocation in the absence of significant trauma. Despite an average loss of external rotation of 20 degrees, 62 of 71 patients were able to play any sport without functional impairment. Fourteen patients reported some pain in the affected shoulder, but only one experienced significant discomfort.

The Putti-Platt procedure provides excellent shoulder stability for active sportsmen without significant loss of performance.

▶ There is a 10.6% redislocation rate in this series. This compares favorably with the two other large series of Putti-Platt procedures which report redislo-

Chapter 3–Sports Injuries / **251**

cation rates of 13.6% and 19.0% (Morrey: *J. Bone Joint Surg.* 58A:252, 1976; and Hovelius: *J. Bone Joint Surg.* 61A:566, 1979). Also, Brav (*J. Bone Joint Surg.* 37A:731, 1955) reported redislocation rate of 7.3% and a resubluxation rate of 41%. One third of the patients in the series of Collins et al. also experienced pain in the affected shoulder.

Despite the fact that there was an average restriction in external rotation of 20 degrees in this patient group, the authors conclude that "The Putti-Platt procedure provides excellent shoulder stability for active sportsmen without significant loss of performance." This is probably accounted for by the fact that there are no football quarterbacks or baseball pitchers in Australia.—J.S. Torg, M.D.

Locked Posterior Dislocation of the Shoulder
R.J. Hawkins, C.S. Neer II, R.M. Pianta, and F.X. Mendoza (Univ. of Western Ontario, London, Ontario, and Columbia Presbyterian Med. Ctr., New York)
J. Bone Joint Surg. [Am.] 69-A:9–18, January 1987   3–42

Locked posterior dislocation of the shoulder is associated with an impression fracture of the articular surface of the humeral head (Fig 3–19), but many of these lesions still are missed. Forty patients seen between 1965 and 1982 with 41 involved shoulders were reviewed. Causative factors included motor vehicle accidents, seizures, alcohol-related injury, and electroshock therapy. The 32 males and 8 females had an average age of 49 years. The average time from injury to diagnosis was 1 year. Patients had problems combing hair, washing, shaving, and even eating. Most patients had received physiotherapy without effect. Motion of the locked shoulder was limited. Axillary roentgenograms consistently confirmed the diagnosis. Twenty patients had an undisplaced fracture of the proximal humerus.

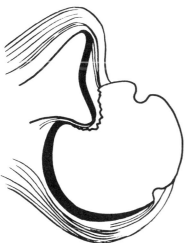

Fig 3–19.—Diagram of a transverse section through the shoulder, showing a locked posterior dislocation. The posterior part of the rim of the glenoid is located within the impression fracture of the humeral head. [Courtesy of Hawkins, R.J., et al.: J. Bone Joint Surg. (Am.) 69-A:9–18, January 1987.]

In seven instances the deformity was accepted. Closed reduction succeeded in 6 of 12 cases. Transfer of the subscapularis tendon was attempted in nine shoulders and succeeded four times. Transfer of the lesser tuberosity succeeded in all four cases so treated. Hemiarthroplasty succeeded in six of nine shoulders; the others required revision. Total arthroplasty was performed on ten shoulders as a primary or secondary procedure. One of these shoulders dislocated postoperatively and was not treated further. The average follow-up was 5.5 years.

An inactive poor-risk patient with locked posterior shoulder dislocation need not be treated. Closed reduction may be attempted in recent dislocations where the defect involves less than 20% of the articular surface. If it fails, transfer of the lesser tuberosity should be carried out. This procedure is indicated primarily in dislocations 6 weeks to 6 months old, with a defect involving 20% to 45% of the articular surface. Older or more extensive cases should be managed by hemiarthroplasty, if the glenoid is normal. Otherwise, total shoulder replacement is indicated, with a bone graft if necessary.

▶ Although extremely rare to occur in the athletic patient population, unreduced posterior dislocation of the shoulder can present a diagnostic problem. The practitioner should be alerted to the possibility of this problem in any patient who cannot outwardly rotate the humerus past neutral.—J.S. Torg, M.D.

Rotator Cuff Tears: Preliminary Application of High-Resolution MR Imaging With Counter Rotating Current Loop-Gap Resonators

J. Bruce Kneeland, Guillermo F. Carrera, William D. Middleton, Nicholas F. Campagna, Lawrence M. Ryan, Andrzej Jesmanowicz, Wojciech Froncisz, and James S. Hyde (Med. College of Wisconsin, Milwaukee, General Electric Med. Systems, Milwaukee, and Jagiellonian Univ., Krakow, Poland)
Radiology 160:695–699, September 1986   3–43

The use of surface or local coils in magnetic resonance (MR) imaging improves the signal-to-noise ratio and therefore image quality, but the need to "decouple" the receiver coil from the transmitted radiofrequency (RF) is a problem. A new type of RF coil for MR imaging and spectroscopy consists of two loop-gap resonators of equal diameter, positioned along a common axis and tuned to the mode in which the current in the loops flows in opposite directions. The coils are "decoupled" from a uniform excitation field of arbitrary orientation by intrinsic decoupling and by means of back-to-back fast recovery diodes.

Measurements made using the new coils and a phantom saline tank showed that the signal-to-noise ratio obtainable was nearly identical to that obtained with single loops. The normal knee, wrist, and shoulder were imaged with a 1.5-tesla MR system using circularly polarized radiofrequency. Eight patients with rotator cuff tears also were examined, and the MR images showed abnormalities in six of them.

The complex internal anatomy of the structure has made it difficult to establish criteria for diagnosing a tear. The low-intensity structure identified as the cuff tendon is discontinuous and appears different on various coronal sections in the AP view.

Refinement of diagnostic criteria may well enhance the clinical usefulness of the new type of RF coil in MR imaging.

▶ Demonstration of the shoulder with MRI is difficult and special coils have been developed for this examination. The preliminary results presented here are promising; however, they are not yet readily available, and correlation of the MRI images with surgical findings is still pending.—J.S. Torg, M.D.

Pitfalls of Rotator Cuff Sonography
William D. Middleton, William R. Reinus, G. Leland Melson, William G. Totty, and William A. Murphy (Washington Univ., St. Louis)
AJR 146:555–560, March 1986   3–44

Several reports indicate that sonographic examination of the shoulder is a reliable, effective, noninvasive means of detecting rotator cuff tears. However, several potential sources of interpretative errors exist. Bilateral shoulder sonograms, performed on 106 patients, were analyzed to identify the causes of scan misinterpretation and to suggest ways to improve the accuracy of the technique.

Errors of sonographic interpretation were classified into four categories: (1) those from failure to recognize normal anatomy, (2) those caused by soft tissue abnormalities, (3) those caused by bony abnormalities, and (4) those caused by technical limitations of the study. Normally, the echogenicity of the rotator cuff was greater than that of the deltoid muscle. However, in older patients, the echogenicity of the rotator cuff was less than or equal to that of the deltoid muscle and was confused for nonvisualization of the cuff. Confusion caused by the normal posterior thinning of the rotator cuff, as well as mild inhomogenities in the rotator cuff, could result in a false-positive diagnosis of rotator cuff tears. These errors were easily overcome by increasing experience and comparison to the normal, contralateral rotator cuff.

Hyperechoic foci caused by calcific tendinitis of the rotator cuff in two patients were misinterpreted as rotator cuff tears; careful evaluation of the conventional roentgenograms was helpful in eliminating false-positive diagnoses from calcific tendinitis. Similarly, review of the plain films prior to sonography could have avoided problems in interpretation resulting from fractures in two patients and inferior glenohumeral subluxation in two other patients.

The major technical limitation of sonography arose from the inability to image the rotator cuff beneath the acromion. Although rotator cuff tears were rarely isolated in this location, passive maneuvers allowed imaging of otherwise hidden parts of the cuff.

Sonography is an effective, noninvasive diagnostic technique for rotator cuff tears. Potential pitfalls in diagnosis can be avoided by thoroughly understanding the anatomy, strictly insisting on proper patient positioning, using the opposite side for comparison, and carefully inspecting the plain films of the shoulder prior to sonographic examination.

▶ This is an excellent review of potential diagnostic errors in ultrasound of the rotator cuff. As with arthrography or any specialized radiographic study, technique, proper equipment, and the experience of the examiner are crucial to the accuracy of the examination.—J.S. Torg, M.D.

Ultrasonographic Evaluation of the Rotator Cuff and Biceps Tendon
William D. Middleton, William R. Reinus, William G. Totty, C. Leland Melson, and William A. Murphy (Washington Univ., St. Louis)
J. Bone Joint Surg. [Am.] 68-A:440–450, March 1986   3–45

The invasiveness, morbidity, and high cost of arthrography prompted a trial of ultrasonography as a noninvasive means of imaging the soft tissue structures of the shoulder. Bilateral studies were carried out on 106 patients referred for shoulder arthrography, 75 males and 31 females with a mean age of 47 years. Thirty-six patients had an arthrographic diagnosis of rotator cuff tear, while 20 had other soft tissue abnormalities. Sonography was done just before double-contrast arthrography, using a real-time 10-MHz high-resolution scanner. Transverse scans of the bicipital tendon groove, distal biceps tendon, and the intra-articular part of the tendon were obtained, along with longitudinal scans of the long axis of the tendon.

The normal rotator cuff was seen as a band of tissue between the humeral head and deltoid muscle. Tears appeared most often as focal thinning of the cuff, but complete non-visualization of the cuff was also observed. A tear was documented in half of ten patients with focal discontinuity in the echogenicity of the cuff without thinning. Sonography detected 91% of rotator cuff tears, and the specificity of the study also was 91%; the predictive value of a positive study was 84%. All but 2 of 20 patients with a sonographic effusion of the biceps tendon sheath exhibited soft tissue abnormality within the joint.

Ultrasound study of the shoulder can be the initial imaging modality in patients suspected of having a rotator cuff tear or abnormality of the biceps tendon. The procedure is more rapid and less expensive than arthrography and involves no risk or discomfort. Arthrography will remain a necessary complementary study in a small number of cases.

▶ Ultrasound, properly performed by an experienced ultrasonographer, is an excellent method of examining the rotator cuff and biceps tendon; however, there are pitfalls and limitations, as pointed out by this author (see Abstract 3–44). These include failure to recognize normal anatomy, soft tissue and bony abnormalities, and technical limitations of the modality.

As the authors indicate, ultrasound and double-contrast arthrography are complimentary studies. Double-contrast arthrography is limited in that partial tears either within the substance of the ligament or confined to the dorsal aspect of the rotator cuff will not be diagnosed arthrographically but are depicted by ultrasound; conversely, ultrasound cannot recognize tears of the rotator cuff hidden by the acromion process. Arthrography should not be regarded as an examination with high morbidity. A. H. Newberg et al. (*Radiology* 155:606, 1985) reported extremely low morbidity in an evaluation of 126,000 arthrograms.—J.S. Torg, M.D.

Chronic Rotator Cuff Tears
Paul S. Rosenberg and Russell P. Clarke (Univ. of Cincinnati)
Orthop. Rev. 15:33–42, May 1986   3–46

Treatment of chronic rotator cuff tears remains controversial. An overview of rotator cuff tear is presented, as well as a discussion of treatment modalities.

Ninety-five percent of rotator cuff tears are initiated by impingement wear rather than by circulatory impairment or trauma. A continuum of stages encompassing the impingement syndrome has been described: stage 1, which consists of edema and hemorrhage; stage 2, of fibrosis and tendonitis; and stage 3, of bone spurs and tendon rupture. This continuum is age dependent and may be treated differently depending on the stage.

A cuff tear can occur after injury to the shoulder without fracture or dislocation, after anterior dislocation of the glenohumeral joint, and after anterior dislocation of the glenohumeral joint with an associated fracture of the greater tuberosity. Roentgenographic abnormalities are common. When suspected clinically and roentgenographically, an arthrogram is usually indicated for (1) patients older than 40 years with an impingement syndrome unresponsive to conservative management for 12 weeks; (2) an injury resulting in sudden, marked weakness of the shoulder; (3) rupture of the long head of the biceps associated with shoulder symptoms; and (4) dislocation followed by shoulder symptoms in patients older than 40 years. Indications for anterior acromioplasty include (1) a complete thickness tear on the arthrogram; (2) a negative arthrogram in a patient older than 40 years with persistent disability for 1 year despite conservative management; (3) patients with stage 2 disease; and (4) patients undergoing other surgical procedures in which the rotator cuff and long-head of the biceps are weak and less effective in preventing proximal migration of the head (prosthesis).

Conservative management includes rest, analgesia or anti-inflammatory agents including steroids, avoidance of painful range of motion, physical therapy, and modification of life-style. Proponents of conservative management argue that with time the inflammatory reaction will subside and that although the integrity of the cuff may not be completely intact, the patients will nevertheless have an excellent functional result.

Surgical approaches are subdivided into 5 basic types: (1) an anteromedial approach with release of the anterior deltoid; (2) an anterior approach with T-incision of the deltoid; (3) a superior approach with partial or total acromionectomy; (4) a posterosuperior approach with osteotomy of the acromion; and (5) combinations of the preceding. Whatever approach is used, several basic surgical principles apply. A full range of motion should be established prior to surgery. The rotator cuff should be adequately exposed. The supraspinatus should be freed of adhesions by finger dissection or periosteal elevator for mobilization. Avoid repairs in abduction and maintain adequate tension on the supraspinatus. Debridement of degenerative tissue should be undertaken.

Postoperative management is crucial to the success of the procedure. Physical therapy should be started almost immediately and should include hand and elbow motion. Codman exercises and passive exercises can be performed on days 10 to 14, isometric exercises on days 14 to 21, and active and active-assisted range of motion, including abduction and external rotation, on days 21 to 28. Reoperations should be avoided.

Surgical Treatment of Tears of the Rotator Cuff in Athletes

James E. Tibone, Burton Elrod, Frank W. Jobe, Robert K. Kerlan, Vincent S. Carter, Clarence L. Shields, Jr., Stephen J. Lombardo, and Lewis Yocum (Kerlan-Jobe Orthopaedic Clinic, Inglewood, Calif.)
J. Bone Joint Surg. [Am] 68-A:887–891, July 1986   3–47

Most athletes with lesions of the rotator cuff of the shoulder respond to conservative measures of rest, anti-inflammatory medication, steroid injections, and physical therapy. If these measures fail, the athlete must consider either surgical intervention or discontinuing the particular sports activity that is aggravating the shoulder. Forty-five athletes with either a partial (n = 30) or complete (n = 15) tear of the rotator cuff were treated with anterior acromioplasty and repair of the tear. All these tears were in the area of the supraspinatus tendon. Minimum duration of follow-up was 24 months (average, 42 months).

Postoperatively, 87% of patients reported improvement of their shoulders, although only 76% reported significant relief of pain. Despite this, 77% still perceived some difficulty with throwing or overhead activities. Overall functional results were good in 56% of patients, which allowed them to return to their sport competitively without significant pain. Among pitchers and throwers, 41% overall returned to their former competitive level, and 32% returned to competition at the professional or collegiate level. Patients with an incomplete tear fared no better than those with a complete tear.

Although it provides satisfactory relief of pain, acromioplasty and repair of the rotator cuff of the shoulder in young athletes should be undertaken judiciously since it does not allow athletes to return to their former competitive status in sports. A long period of rest from the offending activity, combined with stretching and strengthening exercises for the rotator cuff, should be advocated initially, particularly in patients with a partial tear. Surgical intervention may be the only alternative in complete tear of the rotator cuff to prevent progression and disability with aging.

Shoulder-Muscle Strength and Range of Motion Following Surgical Repair of Full-Thickness Rotator-Cuff Tears

D.R. Gore, M.P. Murray, S.B. Sepic, and G.M. Gardner (Med. College of Wisconsin and Zablocki VA Med. Ctr., Milwaukee)
J. Bone Joint Surg. [Am.] 68-A:266–272, February 1986   3–48

Although tears of the rotator cuff are relatively common, the indications for surgical repair are still controversial. Many have reported favorable results in terms of pain relief, patient satisfaction, and range of shoulder motion, but studies quantitating strength of shoulder muscles and functional abilities after rotator cuff repair have not been performed. A retrospective study was conducted to measure strength and range of motion of the repaired shoulder and to assess subjective estimates of pain and function after rotator cuff repair to establish what can be reasonably expected by the patient and the surgeon after such an operation.

Fifty-eight patients (49 men), aged 29 to 75 years, underwent 63 primary repairs of full-thickness rotator cuff tears, including 5 men who had bilateral repairs. Follow-up ranged from 2 to 22 years.

Patients had an average 126 degrees of postoperative active flexion of the shoulder and an average 130 degrees of postoperative active abduction. Passive motion averaged 21 degrees more than active motion. The strength of the shoulder abductors averaged about 86% of normal. Short tears (less than 2.5 cm) were associated with greater strength and range of motion than long tears. Most patients reported marked pain relief and rated themselves as experiencing only mild deficits, or none, in their daily activities. Of 19 patients who had been unable to work before operation, 15 were able to return to work, but not necessarily to the same type of job they had done before their shoulder problems started.

Repair of the Rotator Cuff: End-Result Study of Factors Influencing Reconstruction

Harvard Ellman, Gregory Hanker, and Michael Bayer (Univ. of California, Los Angeles)
J. Bone Joint Surg. [Am.] 68-A:1136–1144, October 1986   3–49

Lesions of the rotator cuff have become well recognized because of publicity surrounding their occurrence in athletes. The authors retrospectively reviewed data on patients who underwent surgical rotator cuff repairs over a 12-year period and correlated the history, physical examination, and preoperative radiologic results with the operative findings, technical difficulties, and prognosis associated with the reconstructive operation.

The study comprised 50 patients (39 men), aged 27 to 85 years, who underwent 50 rotator cuff repairs, including 41 patients (82%) whose dominant shoulder was operated on. Average follow-up was 3.5 years. Conservative treatment and corticosteroid injections had failed to relieve symptoms before operation. All patients had some pain about the shoulder, including 38 (76%) who had long-standing and progressively increasing pain characteristic of a late stage II or stage III impingement lesion.

Surgical results, based on ratings of postoperative pain, function, range of motion, strength, and patient satisfaction, were satisfactory in 84% and unsatisfactory in 16% of the patients. Correlation of preoperative and postoperative findings showed that pain and functional impairment were significantly relieved by operation. There was a direct correlation among the duration of preoperative pain, the size of the cuff tear, and the difficulty of the repair. Preoperative strength of abduction and external rotation were directly related to outcome; results were poorest in patients with the greatest weakness.

Reconstruction of a torn rotator cuff can be successful in a high percentage of shoulders. Careful preoperative assessment is of value in planning the operation and realistically predicting the outcome.

▶ It has been my own experience that rotator cuff tears are unusual in young physically active people. The impression that one draws from the article by Ellman and colleagues (Abstract 3–49) is that good results can be anticipated from surgical repair. However, Gore et al. (Abstract 3–48) and Tibone et al. (Abstract 3–47) clearly demonstrate that although pain relief may be obtained, return to previous functional levels is not to be anticipated. Perhaps arthroscopic cuff debridement and subacromial decompression will yield more favorable results in the athlete (Abstract 3–46).—J.S. Torg, M.D.

Biomechanical Study of the Ligamentous System of the Acromioclavicular Joint
Kimitaka Fukuda, Edward V. Craig, Kai-Nan An, Robert H. Cofield, and Edmund Y.S. Chao (Mayo Clinic and Found.)
J. Bone Joint Surg. [Am.] 68-A:434–439, March 1986   3–50

The ligamentous structures of the acromioclavicular joint were examined by gross study and quantitative measurements in 12 human cadaver specimens from subjects aged 50 to 70 years. The distances between insertions at varying extreme positions of the clavicle were studied by biplane radiography (Fig 3–20). Load displacement tests were done with sequential sectioning of the ligaments. Several modes of joint displacement were used in the study (Fig 3–21).

The acromioclavicular ligament appeared to be a primary constraint to posterior displacement of the clavicle and posterior axial rotation. The conoid ligament primarily constrained anterior and superior rotation, as well as anterior and superior displacement of the clavicle. The trapezoid ligament was less constraining to clavicular movements, except for axial compression motion toward the acromion process.

In many directions of displacement the acromioclavicular joint contrib-

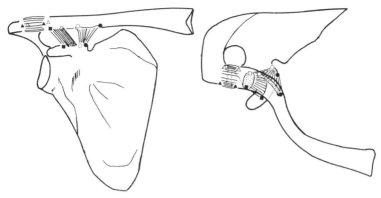

Fig 3–20.—Metal markers inserted at points of attachment of ligaments to bones for biplane radiographic study. *Open circle*, conoid ligament, lateral margin; *solid circle*, conoid ligament, medial margin; *open triangle*, acromioclavicular ligament, anterior margin; *solid triangle*, acromioclavicular ligament, posterior margin; *open square*, trapezoid ligament, posteromedial margin; and *solid square*, trapezoid ligament, anterolateral margin. [Courtesy of Fukuda, K., et al.: J. Bone Joint Surg. (Am.) 68-A:434-439, March 1986.]

uted more to constraint at lesser degrees of displacement, and the coracoclavicular ligaments contributed more to restraint when there were larger amounts of displacement. The conoid ligament was the chief constraining element with larger amounts of displacement.

These findings confirm the importance of the acromioclavicular ligament in maintaining stability between the clavicle and scapula, particularly in daily activities. The trapezoid is the major coracoclavicular constraint to

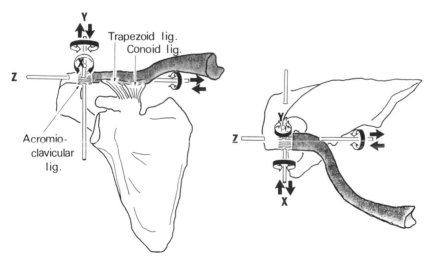

Fig 3–21.—Simultaneous anteroposterior and tangential radiographs were made of ten selected positions of the joint by rotation about three axes (x, y, and z). Anteroposterior displacement and superior-inferior rotation of clavicle take place along and about x axis, respectively. Superior-inferior displacement and anteroposterior rotation of clavicle take place along and about y axis, respectively. Axial rotation and displacement of clavicle take place about and along z axis, respectively. [Courtesy of Fukuda, K., et al.: J. Bone Joint Surg. (Am.) 68-A:434-439, March 1986.]

axial compressive loading of the joint, but the coracoid has a larger role in most other directions of loading.

▶ It is important to note the clinical relevance of this study as stated by the authors: "All of the ligaments supporting the acromioclavicular joint provided substantial contribution to stability of the joint. The contribution changes with the direction and amount of loading. The maximum strength of healing after an injury to the acromioclavicular joint is a goal. All ligaments should be allowed to participate in the healing process. Some repair methods, notably those involving excision of the distal part of the clavicle, may not make this possible."—J.S. Torg, M.D.

Conservative or Surgical Treatment of Acromioclavicular Dislocation: A Prospective, Controlled, Randomized Study
Eilif Larsen, Arne Bjerg-Nielsen, and Poul Christensen (Gentofte Hosp., Hvidovre Hosp., and Bispebjerg Hosp., Copenhagen)
J. Bone Joint Surg. [Am.] 68-A:552–555, April 1986   3–51

To compare the functional results and costs of surgical treatment and short-term bandaging, the authors conducted a prospective study of 84 patients who were seen at three centers between 1979 and 1983 with acromioclavicular dislocations. Forty-one patients were operated on, and 43 had bandaging for 2 weeks, followed by use of a sling for 2 weeks. Similar bandaging was used after reduction of the acromioclavicular joint and wiring. Average follow-up after injury was 13 months.

Initial clinical results were better with conservative treatment, but no significant differences were apparent at follow-up. Two patients had reoperation for residual pain, and three others required resection of the lateral end of the clavicle and transfer of the coracoacromial ligament, two because of pain and one for skin problems. Correct anatomical position was maintained in all but 2 surgical cases. Several complications occurred in the surgical group, but there were none in the conservatively treated group. Sick leave was insignificantly shorter with conservative treatment.

Surgery for acromioclavicular dislocation is warranted only in a thin patient with a prominent clavicle, when function is needed for work, and perhaps if heavy weights are lifted at work. Most other patients are best treated by using a sling until pain resolves, and then by physiotherapy for range of motion and strengthening the shoulder.

▶ This study represents the first prospective, randomized study comparing conservative and operative treatment of acute acromioclavicular dislocations. A modified Phemister procedure was used as the standard operation, with the interarticular meniscus being removed, the acromioclavicular joint reduced and transfixed with two threaded Kirshner wires, and the acromioclavicular and coracoclavicular ligaments as well as any obvious muscle ruptures sutured. Thus, the conclusion to be drawn is that conservative management is as good as this particular surgical procedure, but not necessarily all surgical procedures.—J.S. Torg, M.D.

Surgery for Ununited Clavicular Fracture
Antti Eskola, Seppo Vainionpää, Pertti Myllynen, Hannu Pätiälä, and Pentti Rokkanen (Helsinki Univ., Finland)
Acta Orthop. Scand. 57:366–367, August 1986   3–52

Most fractures of the clavicle are closed and heal well with conservative, nonoperative management. The reported incidence of nonunion ranges between 0.1% and 5%. The authors studied the results of corrective surgery for nonunion of clavicle fractures after conservative management.

The study comprised 16 male and 8 female patients, ranging in age between 22 and 79 years, who were operated on for ununited clavicular fractures over a 12-year period. All patients had disabling pain, including 6 patients who were unable to work. The average time from the accident to operation was 24 months, with a range of 4 to 36 months. Cancellous bone grafts were used in 21 of 24 patients; 18 procedures involved rigid plate fixation.

Four patients experienced postoperative complications, including superficial wound infections (n = 2), loosening of the plate with nonunion (n = 1) and without nonunion (n = 1). Follow-up included rating of subjective outcome, local pain, pain radiating to the extremities, range of motion of the shoulder joint, and roentgenograms of both clavicles.

Seventeen patients had a good subjective outcome, six patients had satisfactory results, and one patient had a poor result. Only one of the patients who had undergone rigid plate fixation and cancellous bone-grafting experienced nonunion of the clavicle. Eight patients experienced pain on exercise. X-ray films demonstrated a shortening of the clavicle in four patients, and six patients had deformed clavicles. All patients were able to return to their previous occupations, but one patient required transfer to lighter work.

Outcome of Clavicular Fracture in 89 Patients
A. Eskola, S. Vainionpää, P. Myllynen, H. Pätiälä, and P. Rokkanen (Helsinki Univ., Finland)
Arch. Orthop. Trauma Surg. 105:337–338, October 1986   3–53

Of all clavicular fractures treated, 82% are located in the middle third, 12% in the lateral third, and 6% in the medial third. Treatment of a broken clavicle generally consists of immobilization with a sling for 3 weeks. Most fractures of the clavicle heal well, with the exception of type-III fractures of the lateral end which have a nonunion incidence ranging from 1% to 4%. The authors studied the outcome of clavicular fractures treated at this institution during 1982.

Of a total of 118 patients who were treated for clavicular fractures, 69 male and 20 female patients, ranging in age between 3 and 81 years, with 40 right-sided and 49 left-sided injuries, were available for follow-up 2 years later. The hand on the fractured side was dominant in 35 patients and nondominant in 54 patients. Causes of the fractures included 22 falls, 38 sports-related injuries, and 29 traffic-related accidents. None of the patients had open fractures. There were 58 middle-third fractures, 27 lateral fractures, and 4 medial fractures. In all, 83 patients were treated with immobilization, and 6 patients were operated on.

Analysis of follow-up data shows that 65 patients had good results, 20 had satisfactory results, and 4 had poor results. The fracture united in 87 of 89 patients, including the 6 patients who had been operated on and who were asymptomatic at follow-up. Two patients had asymptomatic nonunion. Slight pain on exercise was reported by 20 patients, including 4 patients who also experienced pain at rest. Subjective abduction weakness was noted in 11 patients of which 8 showed shortening of the clavicle on radiographs. In three patients, a 20- to 40-degree restriction of abduction was noted. Of 43 patients who showed deformity of the clavicle, 22 considered it cosmetically disturbing. Roentgenographic examination showed a shortening of the clavicle in 47 patients, including 17 who experienced pain. However, all patients were able to return to their previous work.

▶ These two articles (Abstracts 3–52 and 3–53) discuss two problems associated with clavicular fracture: (1) pain and weakness associated with shortening of the clavicle, and (2) nonunion after conservative management. Unanswered are the questions of (1) the association of nonunion with open reduction, and (2) refracture with early return to contact activities. To be noted is the high frequency (38/89) of clavicular fractures resulting from athletic injuries.—J.S. Torg, M.D.

Lower Extremity Injuries

Exercise Pain in the Lower Leg: Chronic Compartment Syndrome and Medial Tibial Syndrome

M.J. Allen and M.R. Barnes (Leicester Royal Infirmary, Leicester, England)
J. Bone Joint Surg. [Br.] 68-B:818–824, November 1986   3–54

Many athletes experience pain in the lower leg precipitated by exercise, but relieved by rest. Symptoms often subside within a few weeks, but some athletes continue to experience pain which becomes more severe with time until exercise becomes extremely painful or impossible. Causes for increasing leg pain include stress fracture, medial tibial syndrome, and chronic compartment syndrome. The authors studied the etiology of pain in the lower leg during exercise.

A total of 110 athletes, including 24 women, ranging in age between 12 and 31 years, and 86 men, ranging in age between 16 and 44 years, had persistent exercise-related pain in the lower leg of at least 6 months' duration. All patients had undergone conservative treatment prior to entering the study. Compartment pressure was measured with a previously described technique. Technetium bone scans were used to exclude stress fractures. Based on test findings, patients were assigned to one of three diagnostic groups: chronic compartment syndrome, medial tibial syndrome, and nonspecific findings.

Chronic compartment syndrome was diagnosed in 105 limbs, including 12 that were treated conservatively, and 73 limbs that were operated on by fasciotomy and for which follow-up data were available 3 months later. None of the patients who underwent surgery experienced complications, and all patients were able to return to full activity between 6 and 8 weeks after their operation. All but three patients had improved.

Medial tibial syndrome alone was diagnosed in 28 limbs, including 6 patients who had bilateral findings, and in another 28 limbs in association with anterior compartment syndrome. Many patients were able to continue exercise despite pain. Only four patients had to discontinue exercising.

Patients with nonspecific findings responded to conservative treatment with physiotherapy.

▶ The authors indicate that subcutaneous fasciotomy of the affected compartments is the treatment of choice for chronic compartment syndrome. We certainly agree with this but emphasize the necessity for accurate determination of the involved compartment. It is further observed that the treatment of patients with medial tibial syndrome, either by operation or conservatively, is unsuccessful. Mubarek (*Am. J. Sports Med.* 10:202–205, July–August 1982) has written that "The available information on the medial tibial stress syndrome supports the theory that it most likely represents a periostitis at this location of the leg and not a compartment syndrome . . . . at this time, the data is not conclusive and we do not recommend fasciotomy for this entity." Rather than a longitudinal fasciotomy, we have had some success incising the insertion of the crural fascia and insertion of the tibialis posticus from the posteromedial tibial ridge.—J.S. Torg, M.D.

Chronic Anterior-Compartment Syndrome of the Leg: Results of Treatment by Fasciotomy
Jorma R. Styf and Lars M. Körner (East Hosp., Göteborg, Sweden)
J. Bone Joint Surg. [Am.] 68-A:1338–1347, December 1986   3–55

Previous studies have shown that nonsurgical treatment of chronic anterior compartment syndrome for 12 months did not relieve symptoms, whereas fasciotomy produced good results in 60% to 100% of all surgically treated patients. However, the value of fasciotomy has been questioned because it reportedly decreases the force exerted by normal muscle which would be an important consideration in treating athletes. The authors evaluated the effects of fasciotomy on chronic anterior compartment syndrome and athletic performance.

The study was done in 14 male and 5 female patients, ranging in age between 17 and 51 years, including 11 patients with bilateral and 8 patients with unilateral compartment syndrome, for a total of 30 affected legs.

Two patients also had compression of the superficial peroneal nerve, and one patient also had lateral compartment syndrome. All patients had participated in athletic events, and all had suffered pain for an average of 30 months. All patients underwent fasciotomy because conservative treatment had failed.

At follow-up 8 months after fasciotomy, 10 patients (20 legs) had no pain and were satisfied with the results of the operation, 8 patients (9 legs) were not satisfied, and 1 patient (1 leg) was worse after surgery than before. Of the nine patients who were not satisfied, two patients had recurrences of symptoms and fasciotomy was again performed. At follow-up 8 months after the second fasciotomy, both patients were asymptomatic. Postoperative intramuscular pressures in the anterior compartment were normal at rest as well as during and after exercise. Functional capacity of the anterior tibial muscle was actually increased after fasciotomy.

Fasciotomy will relieve the pain of chronic anterior compartment syndrome with normalization of intramuscular pressure.

Exertional Tibialis Posterior Compartment Syndrome
C.H. Rorabeck (Univ. Hosp., London, Ontario)
Clin. Orthop. 208:61–64, July 1986   3–56

Surgical decompression has been effective in most cases of exertional deep posterior compartment syndrome with elevated tissue pressures; nevertheless, some fasciotomies have failed, especially with decompression of the deep posterior compartment. The possibility that the tibialis posterior

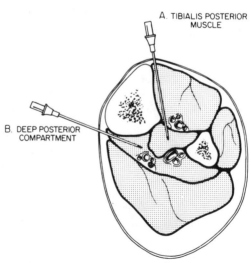

Fig 3–22.—This illustrates the needle position for insertion of the Slit catheter into both the tibialis posterior muscle and the deep posterior compartment to allow simultaneous pressure readings. (Courtesy of Rorabeck, C.H.: Clin. Orthop. 208:61–64, July 1986.)

muscle occupies its own fascial compartment was examined by comparing tissue pressure measurements made simultaneously in the tibialis posterior and the deep posterior compartment. Five patients with clinical features of exertional posterior compartment syndrome participated in the study. All had pain extending distally from the middle third of the posteromedial tibial border, induced by exercise and interfering with athletic activities. Pressures were recorded simultaneously from the two sites (Fig 3–22).

Preexercise pressures were 4 to 11 mm Hg in the tibialis posterior muscle and 7 to 12 mm Hg in the deep posterior compartment. Average peak-to-peak pressure readings at the two sites during the gait cycle were similar in all patients. All patients became symptomatic while running, and all postexercise tibialis posterior pressures were considerably higher than deep posterior compartment pressures. Fasciotomy of the tibialis posterior muscle compartment was performed via a medial approach. All patients were free of symptoms after 6 to 24 months.

Pressure studies should be done in the tibialis posterior muscle in patients with refractory exercise-induced posteromedial leg pain, where nonoperative measures have failed. Pressures should be recorded before, during, and after exercise. Delayed return to normal values after exercise may be the single best sign of tibialis posterior compartment syndrome. Pressures exceeding 10 mm Hg present 20 minutes after cessation of activity call for surgical decompression.

Repeat Compartment Decompression With Partial Fasciectomy
Simon Bell (Prince Henry's Hosp., Melbourne, Australia)
J. Bone Joint Surg. [Br.] 68-B:815–817, November 1986   3–57

Chronic compartment syndrome, a cause of exercise-associated leg pain, is treated by decompression of the involved compartment, performed by making a longitudinal incision in the fascia. The author reports on five patients who had persistent symptoms and positive pressure studies following adequate decompression. A second decompression alleviated their symptoms.

Five healthy males who suffered persistent leg pain for more than 6 months following anterior compartment decompression were evaluated and treated by the author. The fascia had been split through a longitudinal skin incision along its entire length. Intracompartmental pressure was measured using a wick catheter or a slit catheter monitoring system, with the patient at rest or exercising the anterior compartment muscles using a system of weights and pulleys. These patients each underwent a repeated decompression with partial fasciectomy.

The patients were able to walk with crutches 5 days after surgery and eventually could walk and exercise without pain. Three of the patients returned for follow-up pressure studies, results of which all proved to be normal.

The failure of the first decompression was most likely due to the growth of fibrous scar tissue rejoining the two cut fascial edges, resulting in an anterior compartment that was still too small. Following a second operation with fasciectomy, all patients were symptom free. Thus, partial fasciectomy, rather than simply splitting the fascia, appears to be helpful in a second operation to relieve chronic compartment syndrome.

▶ Although not explicitly stated, these two articles (Abstracts 3–56 and 3–57) indicate the necessity for precise determination of the compartment or compartments involved and then implementation of an accurately placed fasciotomy. This certainly seems preferable to routinely performing a four- or five-compartment fasciotomy.—J.S. Torg, M.D.

Isolated Dislocation of the Proximal Tibiofibular Joint
Philip A. Thomason and Marc A. Linson (Baystate Med. Ctr., Springfield, Mass.)
J. Trauma 26:192–195, February 1986   3–58

The second reported case of anterolateral dislocation of the proximal tibiofibular joint involved a soccer player who was attempting to regain balance.

Male athlete, 19, reported injury to the left knee when making a right-to-left

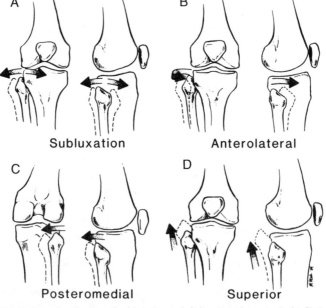

Fig 3–23.—Ogden's classification of subluxation and dislocation of proximal tibiofibular joint. A, subluxation; increased anteroposterior and medial lateral movements of proximal fibula are seen. B, anterolateral dislocation; fibular head is displaced both anteriorly and laterally. C, posteromedial dislocation; fibular head is displaced both posteriorly and medially. D, superior; fibular head is displaced upward. (Courtesy of Thomason, P.A., and Linson, M.A.: J. Trauma 26:192–195, February 1986. © by Williams & Wilkins, 1986.)

pass by a right foot kick, with the left foot planted and the knee flexed. The foot was plantar-flexed and fully inverted, with the leg externally rotated at the hip when the subject fell to his left despite trying to restore his balance. A prominent left fibular head and mild tenderness were noted, and films showed anterolateral dislocation of the proximal fibula. The fibular head was manually reduced and pain quickly resolved. A cast was placed for 3 weeks. After 6 weeks the subject played soccer, and 3 months after injury he skied. Findings at 1 year were normal.

Ogden distinguished four general types of proximal tibiofibular dislocation (Fig 3–23). Most true dislocations are anterolateral and are seen with sudden inversion and plantar flexion of the foot with knee flexion and external rotation of the leg. The subject may report having landed with the flexed knee beneath his body. Acute anterolateral dislocations are managed by closed reduction, followed by casting for 3 weeks. Chronic subluxation or arthritis is best managed by resecting the proximal fibular head.

Posteromedial dislocations are similarly reduced, but are less stable after initial reduction. Superior dislocations are reduced manually, but the fibular head may be resected if chronic pain or instability ensues.

Recurrent Dislocation of the Superior Tibiofibular Joint: Surgical Stabilization by Ligament Reconstruction

Carl R. Weinert, Jr., and Richard Raczka (Univ. of California, Irvine)
J. Bone Joint Surg. [Am.] 68-A:126–128, January 1986   3–59

Recurrent dislocations of the superior tibiofibular joint are rare injuries that occur spontaneously or after acute traumatic dislocation. Most patients are physically active adolescents or young adults. Bracing, rest, arthrodesis of the joint, and resection of the proximal fibula have given varying results. An alternative surgical approach has been designed to restore stability to the joint through ligament reconstruction.

Girl, 15, had had anterior dislocation of the right fibular head 5 months earlier during a gymnastic maneuver. The dislocation reduced spontaneously, but recurrent dislocations ensued when the right knee was flexed beyond 85 degrees. The fibular head was readily dislocated anteromedially, manually, or by voluntary contraction of the peroneal muscles with the foot stabilized. Peroneal nerve function was normal.

The posterior half of the biceps tendon was transected proximally and mobilized to the level of the fibular head (Fig 3–24). A drill-hole then was made from the anterolateral tibial surface through the metaphysis, and a Bunnell-type suture and the tendon graft were used to reduce the dislocation (Fig 3–25). The graft was sutured to the periosteum of the anterior aspect of the tibia under tension (Fig 3–26). A cast was worn for 6 weeks after operation. The patient was fully active a few months after surgery and without symptoms. No dislocations had occurred after 3.5 years. The patient bicycled but had not resumed gymnastics.

The dislocated superior tibiofibular joint may stabilize if the patient can avoid activities that produce dislocation. Otherwise ligament reconstruc-

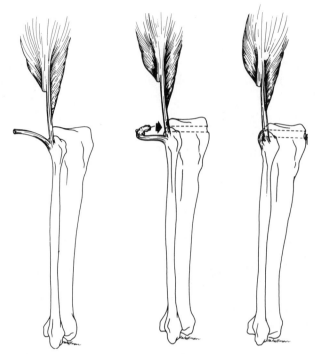

Fig 3–24(left).—Biceps tendon is split longitudinally for approximately 7 cm. Posterior half is transected proximally and mobilized.

Fig 3–25(center).—Free end of graft is passed posterior to anterior through drill-hole in tibia.

Fig 3–26(right).—Tendon is sutured to anterior aspect of tibial periosteum under tension, with fibular head in reduced position.

[Courtesy of Weinert, C.R., Jr., and Raczka, R.: J. Bone Joint Surg. (Am.) 68-A:126–128, January 1986.]

tion is suggested. Arthrodesis should be avoided, but the proximal fibula may be resected as a salvage procedure if pain or instability recurs after ligament reconstruction.

Recurrent Dislocations of the Proximal Tibiofibular Joint: Report of Two Cases

A.A. Giachino (Univ. of Ottawa, Ontario)
J. Bone Joint Surg. [Am.] 68-A:1104–1106, September 1986   3–60

Traumatic anterior dislocation of the proximal tibiofibular joint, resulting in chronic instability, is a rare injury. Ligament reconstruction was performed in an adult athlete and a child with this lesion.

Man, 21, a university football player, felt pain in the lateral aspect of the left knee and heard a pop when tackled from the rear with the knee flexed. Weight-bearing improved over time, but instability was evident 6 weeks after injury. After 5 months the fibula was dislocated anteriorly by moderate finger pressure. Ligament reconstruction of the lax proximal tibiofibular joint was carried out, using part of

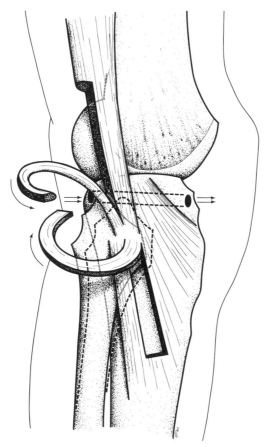

Fig 3–27.—Repair of the capsule using a strip of biceps femoris tendon and deep fascia of the anterior compartment of the leg. [Courtesy of Giachino, A.A.: J. Bone Joint Surg. (Am.) 68-A:1104–1106, September 1986.]

the biceps femoris tendon and a 10-cm rolled strip of deep anterolateral compartment fascia. The new ligaments were placed about the fibular head and through a tibial hole from posterior to anterior and then were anchored in fascia anteriorly (Fig 3–27). After using a plaster cast for 3 weeks and a cast-brace for 3 weeks, the patient returned to football without symptoms. After 22 months he remained competitively active and had normal knee findings. The patient's status was unchanged 3.5 years postoperatively.

Arthrodesis of the proximal tibiofibular joint may produce osteoarthritis and pain, and fibular head resection may be contraindicated in athletes and children. Ligament reconstruction avoids these problems and is a relatively simple procedure. Excellent results were obtained in both cases. A definitive diagnosis of chronic anterior instability of the proximal tibiofibular joint depends on finding an easily dislocatable fibular head.

▶ Dislocation of the fibular head occurs rarely and is difficult to manage (see

Abstract 3–58). This is particularly true of a chronic condition. The practice of resecting the fibular head must be questioned in view of the fact that the arcuate ligament, lateral collateral ligament, capital ligament, and femoral fibular fascia insert into this structure. Mention is not made of the effect of fibular resection on lateral stability of the knee joint. It would appear that the surgical techniques described by Weinert and Raczka (Abstract 3–59) and Giachino (Abstract 3–60) obviate the problems inherent in fibular head resection. Although essentially case reports, it would appear that these particular methods have merit.—J.S. Torg, M.D.

Iliotibial Band Friction Syndrome
Daniel W. Olson (Maitland, Fla.)
Athletic Training 21:32–35, Spring 1986   3–61

Iliotibial band friction syndrome (ITBFS) is an overuse disorder caused by friction between the iliotibial band and the lateral femoral epicondyle in activities involving repeated knee flexion and extension. Often training mileage is inappropriately increased. Excessive internal rotation of the tibia on the femur produces increased tension in the iliotibial band. Hyperpronation theoretically promotes susceptibility to ITBFS. Tibial alignment and lateral femoral condyle size also may be factors in the syndrome, and flexibility must be considered.

The athlete with ITBFS usually has lateral knee pain during distance running, the pain often occurring at a fixed distance. Sprinting does not produce the pain, and varus stress generally does not reproduce it. The diagnosis may be made by applying pressure over the lateral femoral epicondyle with the patient lying on the unaffected side and the affected leg elevated 20 degrees.

Cessation of running might be the most effective measure, but often this is unacceptable. Decreased mileage and a decrease in strike length may be helpful. Stretching of the iliotibial band is effective. Any biomechanical faults should be corrected. The trainer might offer specific graduated guidelines for use in returning to training.

Avoidance of training errors is the most important means of preventing ITBFS. The knowledgeable trainer will be able to help the affected athlete return to full pain-free function.

▶ This is a common injury among distance runners and in those sports requiring a good deal of endurance training through jogging or running. A number of different causes must be examined before a treatment program can be instituted. Training errors must certainly be considered, such as doing "too much, too soon" and abrupt changes in a training program. Distance runners must also avoid running on roads with high crowns or on banked tracks.

This injury usually responds well to a modification in the training program, ice, ultrasound, and appropriate flexibility exercises. The runner with this problem should also be evaluated for orthotics.—F. George, A.T.C., P.T.

Diagnostic and Operative Arthroscopy of the Hip
Ejnar Eriksson, Inga Arvidsson, and Hakan Arvidsson (Karolinska Inst. and Söd-ersjukhuset, Stockholm)
Orthopedics 9:169–176, February 1986   3–62

An anterior approach to hip arthroscopy provides optimal visualization. It is possible to extend the hip up to 10 mm in an unanesthetized subject, which provides good visualization of the joint space. In anesthetized patients a force of 300 to 400 newtons is necessary to extend the hip after joint puncture.

Thirty patients have had hip arthroscopy in the past decade at Karolinska Hospital, most often for unexplained pain in the hip in a young person who had normal findings on films. Synovitis was found in 12 of 14 cases. Several older patients had pain in the hip with only minor signs of degenerative arthritis on films. Lavage of the hip joint was planned for 6 patients.

For arthroscopy patients were placed on a traction table and anesthetized. Extension force then was applied to insert a standard 5-mm arthroscope well below the inguinal ligament. Intensification of the image is necessary if osteochondromatosis is present. A sample of synovial fluid is obtained for x-ray diffraction study, and the joint is irrigated with Ringer's acetate solution before being distended with gas and carrying out arthroscopy. Synovial pathology may be treated arthroscopically, and loose bodies can be extracted. No infections occurred after arthroscopy.

Hip arthroscopy after extension of the joint on a traction table is a useful diagnostic and therapeutic procedure. Partial synovectomy may be carried out and loose bodies can be removed transarthroscopically.

▶ This may be considered basically a methods paper for hip joint arthroscopy. Although the authors document one case of osteochondromatosis successfully treated arthroscopically and six cases of joint lavage for degenerative disease, clear indications for hip arthroscopy are lacking. Also noted is the authors' observation that it is "difficult to move instruments inside the hip joint."—J.S. Torg, M.D.

Conservative Management of Distraction-Type Stress Fractures of the Femoral Neck
H. Aro and S. Dahlström (Central Military Hosp., Turku, Finland)
J. Bone Joint Surg. [Br.] 68-B:65–67, January 1986   3–63

Distraction-type stress fractures of the femoral neck tend to become displaced if symptoms are unrecognized; therefore, immediate internal fixation has been recommended. Experience with four military recruits who had complete distraction-type stress fractures of the femoral neck suggests that these injuries, if not displaced, need not be internally fixed if activity is controlled. One case is described below.

Male recruit, 20, developed a dull ache in his right hip and an increasing limp. Passive hip motion was limited by pain after 2 weeks, and films showed an undisplaced distraction-type stress fracture of the femoral neck with cortical cracks. Absolute bed rest was enforced for 3 weeks, with traction for 1 week to control pain. Increasing sclerosis and formation of endosteal callus were noted after 2 weeks in bed. The upper cortex was reconstituted at 6 weeks, during walking on crutches. Partial weight-bearing then was allowed, and solid union was documented 3 weeks later. The patient began full weight-bearing, and 2 months later he resumed military training.

Distraction-type stress fractures of the femoral neck may heal with conservative management if they are diagnosed before displacement occurs. The injuries stabilize rapidly, but conservative treatment requires close supervision and patient cooperation. Absolute bed rest with traction is necessary until passive movements of the hip cause no discomfort, and films demonstrate formation of internal callus. Weight-bearing should be avoided until bony union is seen, and full weight-bearing should be postponed until the fracture is completely consolidated.

▶ This paper documents the efficacy of conservative management of distraction type stress fractures of the femoral neck. Kaltsas (*J. Bone Joint Surg. [Br.]* 63B:33–37, 1981) has demonstrated the propensity for these lesions to displace. If this displacement occurs, prolonged incapacity, aseptic necrosis and nonunion may complicate treatment which necessarily involves open reduction and internal fixation (Morris in Heppenstall, R. B. (ed.): *Fracture Treatment and Healing,* Philadelphia, W. B. Saunders Co., 1980, pp. 896–911). Stromquist and Hansson (*Acta Orthop. Scand.* 54:687–994, 1983) have reported diastasis of nondisplaced stress fractures with attempted fixation in nonosteoporotic patients. These reports are arguments clearly in favor of the treatment protocol recommended by the authors.—J.S. Torg, M.D.

Knee Injuries

Exercise-Related Knee Joint Laxity
H.B. Skinner, M.P. Wyatt, M.L. Stone, J.A. Hodgdon, and R.L. Barrack (Univ. of California at San Francisco, VA, San Francisco, Children's Hosp., and Naval Health Res. Ctr., San Diego, Tulane Univ., and Kaiser Permanente Grp., El Cajon, Calif.)
Am. J. Sports Med. 14:30–34, January–February 1986   3–64

Currently, knee injuries are the topic of increasingly sophisticated research because of their importance in professional athletics and the increasing participation of the population in recreational sports. However, the role of conditioning and fatigue in these injuries is controversial. It is known that ligaments have a high collagen content, and hence a viscoelastic response to stress would be expected. Some investigators have suggested that there is a relationship between laxity and knee ligament injuries. Highly motivated athletes were used to test the hypothesis that exercise to the point of muscular fatigue may cause laxity of the knee and thereby place athletes at risk for ligamentous injury to the knee.

An exercise protocol was designed to produce muscle fatigue in the hamstring and quadriceps muscle groups, and knee laxity was assessed before and after the exercise protocol. Muscle fatigue was documented by isokinetic testing of right knee flexion and extension power several times during the exercise protocol. Ligamentous laxity was quantitated using a knee arthrometer (KT-1000) before and after exercise. It was found that there was a significant lengthening in knee joint laxity between preexercise and postexercise in the left knee as measured at 15 and 20 lbs of passive displacement force. In addition, maximum manual displacement also revealed a marked increase in joint laxity.

The right knee, which had undergone isokinetic testing, exhibited a similar tendency without a statistically significant difference before and after exercise. Although there was no preexercise side-to-side difference, postexercise measurements showed a left-right difference at 15 lb, 20 lb, and maximum manual displacement.

There is an in vivo increase in the anterior laxity of the knee joint as a result of exercise. The clinical implications of this finding are that more accurate clinical examination of the knee may be obtained after a short cool-down period in the knee with suspected ligamentous injury, and, in addition, athletes should be encouraged to perform vigorous warm-up exercises when entering organized sports activities after cool-down periods of greater than 15 minutes.

▶ The authors make an important point when recommending a short cool-down period when evaluating a knee injury. We are often anxious to do a complete evaluation on the field, immediately after the injury has occurred. I'm sure there are some advantages to this, but the authors' recommendations should be considered. Another good recommendation they make is to include a vigorous warm-up session after a halftime or other long cool-down period.—F. George, A.T.C., P.T.

The Effect of Exercise on Anterior-Posterior Knee Laxity
M.E. Steiner, W.A. Grana, K. Chillag, and E. Schelberg-Karnes (Oklahoma Ctr. for Athletes, Oklahoma City)
Am. J. Sports Med. 14:24–29, January–February 1986   3–65

This is the first report to evaluate the effect of exercise on anterior-posterior (AP) knee laxity. The AP laxity was measured before and after squat power lifting in 24 subjects, basketball playing in 10 subjects, and distance running in 12 subjects. Nine sedentary office workers were used as a control. To assess the role of muscle relaxation in these measurements the effect of general anesthesia was evaluated in 12 knees from 11 patients.

Little difference in laxity was noted before and during general anesthesia. It follows, then, that functionally complete muscle relaxation can be obtained during testing. In sedentary controls there was no significant change in laxity over 2 hours. Squat power lifters exhibited no significant change in laxity following a series of squats at 1.6 times body weight. After 90 minutes of basketball or a 10-km race there was an 18% to 20% increase in mean AP laxity.

It appears that repetitive stress to the knee produces significant increases in laxity, while a few large stresses at a low strain rate do not.

▶ This article, along with the previous article, certainly indicates that there is increased knee joint laxity after repetitive exercise. We should take this into consideration when evaluating injuries and allow for a cool-down period.—F. George, A.T.C., P.T.

1.5-T Surface-Coil MRI of the Knee
D. Lawrence Burk, Jr., Emanuel Kanal, James A. Brunberg, Graham F. Johnstone, Harold E. Swensen, and Gerald L. Wolf (Univ. of Pittsburgh)
AJR 147:293–300, August 1986   3–66

Surface-coil magnetic resonance (MR) imaging can improve the spatial resolution of knee studies when the menisci and articular surfaces are evaluated. Surface-coil MR imaging was performed with reduced fields of view to evaluate 20 patients suspected of having knee abnormalities. Five asymptomatic subjects also were examined. A 1.5-T scanner was used with prototype 14.6- and 7.6-cm round surface coils, and spin-echo pulse sequences. The diagnosis of meniscal tear required areas of increased signal intensity on at least two adjacent images, with a linear appearance or associated with discontinuity of the meniscal surface.

All ten meniscal tears involved the medial meniscus. There were discrepancies with the surgical findings in two cases; in one, later arthroscopy revealed the suspected lesion. Four patients with horizontal degenerative tears had associated abnormalities. Most meniscal tears were detected on T1-weighted images. The T2-weighted images helped provide an "arthrogram effect" in the presence of joint effusion. The study was useful for showing the integrity of articular cartilage over defects in subchondral bone, and also in detecting gross arthritic cartilage lesions.

High-resolution MR imaging of the knee is possible with a reduced field of view using surface coils with small radii. The method is helpful in characterizing the menisci and articular surfaces, and in evaluating surgical and medical treatments without radiation exposure. Magnetic resonance imaging probably can replace arthrography in many circumstances if costs can be reduced.

▶ The potential of MRI as a diagnostic modality for evaluation of internal knee derangement is still in its infancy because of both limited experience and resolution capabilities. Reports of diagnostic accuracy in evaluating the cruciate ligaments and menisci are readily becoming more common, and studies of the normal anatomy and surgically correlated findings will help us understand the abnormal.—J.S. Torg, M.D.

Magnetic Resonance Imaging as a Tool for Evaluation of Traumatic Knee Injuries: Anatomical and Pathoanatomical Correlations

Bert R. Mandelbaum, Gerald A.M. Finerman, Murray A. Reicher, Steven Hartzman, Larry W. Bassett, Richard H. Gold, Wolfgang Rauschning, and Fred Dorey (UCLA School of Medicine)
Am. J. Sports Med. 14:361–370, September–October 1986   3–67

An attempt has been made to correlate multiplanar cadaver cryosections with multiplanar magnetic resonance (MR) images of the knee, and to correlate the MR and arthroscopic surgical findings in knee trauma. Images were obtained using a spin-echo pulse sequence. Three radiologists experienced in MR imaging interpreted the images of 105 patients in a prospective manner. Eighty-three patients underwent subsequent arthroscopic surgical follow-up. Most had medial or lateral meniscal tears or anterior cruciate tears.

The sensitivity of MR imaging for lateral meniscal tears was 75%, and the specificity was 95%. The overall accuracy of the study was 91%. Medial meniscal tears were detected with a sensitivity of 96%, a specificity of 82%, and an accuracy of 90%. Complete agreement was found in cases of anterior cruciate injury. Magnetic resonance imaging was 100% specific in 22 patients without arthroscopic follow-up, and was positive in 3 of 5 patients who had persistent symptoms.

Anatomical detail of the knee is accurately visualized by MR imaging using solenoid surface coils and thin-section, high-resolution techniques. Excellent soft tissue contrast is obtained with no ionizing radiation. The method has multiplanar imaging capability. Costs are expected to decline as MR imaging becomes increasingly popular.

▶ This study emphasizes the importance of MRI as a tool for evaluation of possible knee injuries, although it is limited in that the anatomical sections do not represent the MRI images but are provided only to demonstrate normal anatomy. The degree of pathology necessary for MRI detection is yet to be determined.—J.S. Torg, M.D.

Knee Injuries: High-Resolution MR Imaging
George W. Gallimore, Jr., and Steven E. Harms (Baylor Univ.)
Radiology 160:457–461, August 1986   3–68

Surface-coil magnetic resonance (MR) imaging was performed in thirty patients suspected of having knee injuries and ten normal subjects. Fifteen patients had arthroscopy and, in some instances, arthrotomy. Magnetic resonance studies were done using a 1.5-T magnet and either a 5-in square coil or a saddle coil providing more even signal distribution. A two-dimensional multisection spin-echo technique was employed.

A partial anterior cruciate tear was correctly diagnosed by MR imaging. All 12 surgically confirmed cruciate ligament injuries were considered abnormal on MR imaging. One suspicious ligament was found arthroscopically to be normal. Five of eight meniscal injuries were correctly diagnosed by MR imaging. Three injuries involving the posterior horns were missed on studies that were somewhat motion limited. One false-positive diagnosis of meniscal injury was made. Three medial collateral ligament injuries diagnosed by MR imaging were confirmed surgically.

High-resolution thin-section MR imaging can accurately diagnose soft tissue injuries of the knee. This method holds the potential of becoming very useful in evaluating patients with suspected knee injuries.

▶ The authors demonstrate the cruciate ligaments on a special angled coronal image which correlates with the surgical view of the cruciate ligament. Although the authors do not specify whether the findings on the MRI correlated specifically with the findings at surgery, their accuracy is excellent. The 3-D images produced by the authors should further enhance the accuracy and certainly the expected findings at surgery. Time and research will be necessary to fully evaluate the usefulness of this new modality.—J.S. Torg, M.D.

Radiographic Assessment in Patellar Instability and Chondromalacia Patellae
G.S.E. Dowd and G. Bentley (Inst. of Orthopaedics, Stanmore, England)
J. Bone Joint Surg. [Br.] 68-B:297–300, March 1986   3–69

Several radiographic methods have been tried in evaluating anatomical anomalies of patellar alignment associated with either patellar instability or chondromalacia. A prospective study was undertaken to ascertain the value of the congruence angle, the sulcus angle, and the patellar tendon-patella (PT:P) ratio in identifying minor degrees of malalignment in patients presenting with patellofemoral pain. The knees of 50 asymptomatic subjects were studied, along with those of 35 patients having proved chondromalacia and 33 others with a diagnosis of patellar instability. Tangential knee radiographs were taken with the knee flexed to 30 degrees to measure the sulcus and congruence angles, and lateral radiographs with the knee flexed 30 to 50 degrees were used to determine the PT:P ratio.

The mean sulcus angle in control knees was 139 degrees, the mean congruence angle was -8.1 degrees, and the mean PT:P ratio was 1.03. A high-riding patella was more frequent in females. No significant differences were found in the patients with chondromalacia, but in those with patellar instability both the sulcus angle and the PT:P ratio were significantly increased. The difference in congruence angles was less significant.

Patellar instability is associated with an increased femoral sulcus angle and an increased PT:P ratio, but it is not associated with an abnormal congruence angle in most cases. Patellar malalignment is not radiographically evident in patients with chondromalacia patellae affecting the medial or "odd" facets where clinical instability is absent.

▶ The authors do not indicate why they chose to perform the Merchant view at 30 degrees of flexion instead of 45 degrees as was described by Merchant (Merchant, A. C., et al.: *J. Bone Joint Surg.* 56A:1391–1396, 1974). They also did not comment about the difficulty in the identification of the apex of the patella, which may have contributed to their results of an insignificant congruence angle.—J.S. Torg, M.D.

Anatomy of the Normal Knee as Seen by Magnetic Resonance Imaging
M. Soudry, A. Lanir, D. Angel, M. Roffman, N. Kaplan, and D.G. Mendes (Haifa Med. Ctr. (Rothschild), the Rappaport Inst. for Research in the Med. Sciences, and Elscint MRI Ctr., Haifa, Israel)
J. Bone Joint Surg. [Br.] 68-B:117–120, January 1986   3–70

The use of magnetic resonance (MR) imaging in orthopedic surgery is expanding rapidly, and a knowledge of the normal appearances of the knee is necessary to diagnose knee disorders correctly. Ten young, healthy subjects underwent MR imaging of the knee using various radiofrequency pulse sequences. The best results were obtained by recording spin-echo sequences in the axial and coronal or sagittal planes, with a slice thickness of 5 mm or 7 mm.

The quadriceps and patellar tendons and posterior cruciate ligament are conspicuous in the midsagittal view. The anterior cruciate ligament may be seen in a sagittal slice slightly lateral to the midline. The femoral articular cartilage is well demonstrated in the parasagittal, or condylar, view, as is the medial meniscus. Both menisci are distinguished in the midcoronal view. An axial view through the distal femur shows the channels through which reconstructed ligaments pass as well as the patellofemoral joint. The insertion of the patellar tendon and the tibiofibular joint are visualized in axial views distal to the joint space.

Standard MR imaging of the knee should, with improved resolution, prove invaluable, particularly in the early diagnosis of knee injuries. A reduction in slice thickness will improve visualization of the menisci and the articular cartilage.

▶ The potential of MRI as a diagnostic modality for evaluation of internal knee derangement is still in its infancy because of both limited experience and resolution capabilities. Reports of diagnostic accuracy in evaluating the cruciate ligaments and menisci are readily becoming more common, and studies of the normal anatomy and surgically correlated findings will help us understand the abnormal.—J.S. Torg, M.D.

Prepatellar Bursitis in Wrestlers
M.C. Mysnyk, R.R. Wroble, D.T. Foster, and J.P. Albright (Univ. of Iowa)
Am. J. Sports Med. 14:46–54, January–February 1986   3–71

Experience with prepatellar bursitis in college wrestlers was reviewed over six seasons. Thirteen of 136 wrestlers developed bursitis, 1 of them bilaterally, and these injuries represented about one fifth of all initial knee injuries seen in this period. Three athletes lost no action. Eight had 1 to 7 recurrences, averaging 1.6 per knee. Seven injuries required surgery.

The mechanism of injury was apparent in only four cases and involved direct impact during a takedown maneuver. Treatment was not uniform. Six bursectomies were done for recurrent aseptic bursitis, and one was done for septic bursitis. Septic cases have been more frequent in recent years. Septic bursitis now is treated by repeated aspirations as needed or by bursotomy under local anesthesia.

Either a single traumatic event or repeated trauma may cause acute prepatellar bursitis in wrestlers. The lighter weight classes appear most vulnerable. Many cases have occurred in the off-season. The role of knee pads is uncertain. Prepatellar swelling is a key diagnostic feature. Surgery is done earlier today than in the past. Steroid injections have not proved helpful.

Initial management includes aspiration with culture, compressive wrapping, nonsteroidal drugs, and immobilization for about a week. A second recurrence calls for bursectomy. Septic bursitis generally responds to oral or parenteral antibiotic therapy; surgery rarely is necessary. Antibiotic therapy is begun before culture results are obtained if clinical infection is apparent.

▶ This is an excellent article that deals with a not-so-simple problem, and it is recommended that it be read in its entirety. Management principles proposed by the authors seem applicable to nonwrestlers as well as wrestlers or, for that matter, nonathletes as well as athletes.—J.S. Torg, M.D.

Patellofemoral Pain: A Prospective Study
Carlan Yates and William A. Grana (Univ. of Oklahoma Health Sciences Ctr. and Oklahoma Ctr. for Athletes, Oklahoma City)
Orthopedics 9:663–667, May 1986   3–72

The pathogenesis and frequency of the various causes of patellofemoral (PF) pain syndrome remain confusing. To elucidate further, 67 knees in 49 patients with PF as their primary diagnosis were studied prospectively. Follow-up ranged from 8 to 19 months (mean, 14.9). The average age was 21 years (range, 11 to 48 years). Treatment consisted of a program designed to avoid the flexed, loaded position for the PF joint, non-steroidal anti-inflammatory drugs, and alteration or restriction of activity. An exercise program was aimed at restoring quadriceps strength and normal hamstring-quadriceps strength ratios.

Of the 67 knees, 51 were of females (76%). Patellofemoral malalignment occurred in 17 knees, 88% of which were of females, and 23% eventually had arthroscopic evaluation with lateral release. Of these, 65% improved and 53% were functionally satisfactory. Patellofemoral compression was evident in 17 knees; only 1 knee underwent arthroscopy and lateral release. Only 29% were improved and only 47% were rated satisfactory. Recurrent dislocation was present in four knees; one knee underwent lateral release and patellar chondroplasty. Only one patient improved, and none was rated satisfactory.

Idiopathic and traumatic chondromalacia were evident in six knees each. Only 50% of the former improved and were rated satisfactory, whereas 83% with traumatic chondromalacia improved; however, only 40% were satisfactory functionally. Of the five patients who had symptomatic plica semilunaris, three had surgical correction and all improved and were rated satisfactory. One patient improved without surgery, and one patient became worse. The majority of the patients failed to comply with recommendations for continued knee rehabilitation.

Patellar malalignment and its progression to patellar subluxation can be managed conservatively with improvement in the majority of cases. Arthroscopic lateral release may be necessary for selected patients with patellar malalignment and subluxation, while more aggressive surgical therapy is recommended in patients with patellar compression syndrome and recurrent dislocation. Symptomatic plicae semilunaris can be managed satisfactorily with surgery, whereas chondromalacia patella may be quite refractory to either operative or conservative management. Noncompliance to continued knee rehabilitation can compromise further the successful management of PF disorders.

▶ This excellent article categorizes patellofemoral pain on an etiologic basis and then correlates responses to various treatment modalities. The interested reader is referred to the complete article.—J.S. Torg, M.D.

Thermographic Diagnosis in Athletes With Patellofemoral Arthralgia
M.D. Devereaux, G.R. Parr, S.M. Lachmann, D.P. Page Thomas, and B.L. Hazleman (Addenbrooke's Hosp., Cambridge, England)
J. Bone Joint Surg. [Br.] 68-B:42–44, January 1986   3–73

Pain in front of the knee is common in athletes. It is often referred to as patellofemoral arthralgia, although this diagnosis is difficult to confirm. This study attempts to define the thermographic pattern found in such patients.

Thermograms of 30 athletes considered to have patellofemoral arthralgia were compared with those of a similar number of matched, healthy athletes as controls. In the affected group, 28 athletes had a diagnostic pattern on thermography. The anterior knee showed a temperature rise on the medial side of the patella. The medial knee view demonstrated that this temperature rise radiated from the patellar insertion of the vastus medialis into the muscle itself.

This pattern, inflammation in the vastus medialis muscle that can be demonstrated by thermography, seems to be diagnostic of patellofemoral arthralgia. Thermography is rapid, noninvasive, and inexpensive and can be used to confirm the clinical diagnosis of patellofemoral arthralgia.

▶ An interesting paper of dubious clinical value. The authors' contention that there is an association of quadricep muscle imbalance and patellofemoral arthralgia is not supported by the data.—J.S. Torg, M.D.

Arthroscopic Percutaneous Lateral Patellar Retinacular Release
Peter A. Lankenner, Jr., Lyle J. Micheli, Ruth Clancy, and Peter G. Gerbino (Harvard Univ.)
Am. J. Sports Med. 14:267–269, July–August 1986   3–74

A majority of patients with the patellofemoral stress syndrome respond to conservative management consisting of static quadriceps and hamstring strengthening. For those who do not respond to conservative measures, open and closed lateral releases are proposed. Thirty-four arthroscopic percutaneous lateral retinacular releases performed for unresponsive patellofemoral pain in 26 patients were reviewed retrospectively. Patients were evaluated for residual pain by various physical examination criteria, and objective measurements of quadriceps and hamstring strength with the Cybex II Isokinetic Dynamometer. Average follow-up was 25.6 months.

After a complete arthroscopic examination of the knee through a standard anterolateral portal, Mayo scissors are used to bluntly dissect between the subcutaneous tissue and extensor retinaculum. At the knee joint, the retinaculum, capsule, and synovium are divided at an angle of 30 degrees to the long axis of the femur, taking care to extend the release up to the vastus lateralis insertion into the rectus femoris. The release is inspected with the arthroscope. The portals are closed with absorbable subcuticular sutures. A compressive lateral release brace is kept on for 48 hours. Isometric quadricep exercises are begun on the first postoperative day and active-assisted range of motion at 48 hours. Active-resisted range of motion is begun when a painless arc of 90 degrees is achieved. Statis quadriceps and hamstring exercises are continued for 3 months postoperatively.

Overall, results were excellent in 9% of patients, good in 53%, fair in 26%, and poor in 12%. A total of 64.7% of the knees were improved by the procedure. Wound healing was good. One knee required postrelease aspiration for persistent hemarthrosis.

Arthroscopic percutaneous lateral retinacular release for the patellofemoral stress syndrome has an acceptable success rate. Its merits include decreased hospitalization, rehabilitation time, and scar tissue. Comparably satisfactory results are achieved with both closed and open lateral release techniques.

▶ The assertion of the authors that 65% of the knees were improved by the procedure and that this represented an "acceptable success rate" must be challenged. Perhaps the problem is that the indication for the surgical procedure, "patellar femoral pain unresponsive to a conservative regimen and stretching and strengthening exercises," represented a flaw in the process of patient selection in that no consideration is given to etiologic factors.—J.S. Torg, M.D.

Acute Patellar Dislocations: The Natural History

Richard J. Hawkins, Robert H. Bell, and Garth Anisette (Univ. of Western Ontario and St. Josephs' Hosp., London, Ontario, Canada)
Am. J. Sports Med. 14:117–120, March–April 1986   3–75

The optimal treatment for patients with acute patellar dislocation remains controversial. To elucidate further, 27 patients with primary patellar dislocations were evaluated. Osteochondral fractures were identified in 14 patients. Twenty patients were treated conservatively (group 1): 11 were treated initially with cylinder cast or splint immobilization for an average of 3 weeks, and 9 underwent early aggressive physiotherapy program at about 4 to 5 days following initial injury. The remaining 7 patients underwent immediate surgical stabilization and lateral release (group 2). The results were compared in terms of the incidence of recurrent patellar instability, frequency of persistent anterior knee pain, predisposing signs of patellar femoral malalignment and the incidence of redislocation, and presence of osteochondral fragments.

Redislocation occurred in three group 1 patients and none in group 2. Fifteen patients in group 1 and three in group 2 had persistent anterior knee pain. Feelings of instability were reported by four and two patients of both groups, respectively. Quadriceps atrophy was noted in four group 1 and three group 2 patients. Eight patients in group 1 had lower limb malalignment, as evidenced by femoral anteversion, patellar squinting, genu valgum, increased Q-angle, external tibial torsion, and tibia varum. There was no significant degree of malalignment in group 2 patients.

Patients with predisposing factors, such as patellofemoral malalignment, abnormal patellar configuration, and a history of prior symptoms of instability, are more prone to recurrent dislocation and may benefit from operative intervention. Immobilization and physical therapy are recommended for patients with primary patellar dislocations, in the absence of predisposing factors. Athroscopy is helpful in patients with osteochondral fragments but no predisposing signs to document the size and location; when indicated, excision may be performed or reattachment may be performed. In patients with both predisposing signs and an osteochondral fragment, excision of the fragment and primary stabilization and realignment of the patellar mechanism is recommended.

Overall, despite this treatment program, 30% to 50% of patients will continue to experience instability or anterior knee pain, or both.

▶ It is interesting to note that analysis of the data reveals that actually only 14% of the conservatively treated patients (group I) had an episode of redislocation. The authors suggest surgery which consisted of arthrotomy, excision of osteochondral fragments, repair of the medial retinaculum, advancement of the vastus medialis, and lateral release in the patient with a combination of predisposing signs of osteochondral fragment. They further note that 30% to 50% of the patients, whether treated operatively or nonoperatively, will continue to have symptoms of instability and/or anterior knee pain. It would be interesting to know what effect a distal extensor realignment with immobilization and elevation of the tibial tuberosity would have on these parameters.—J.S. Torg, M.D.

Lateral Retinacular Release in Patellofemoral Subluxation: Indications, Results, and Comparison to Open Patellofemoral Reconstruction
J.H. Henry, T.H. Goletz, and B. Williamson (San Antonio, Tex.)
Am. J. Sports Med. 14:121–129, March–April 1986   3–76

The results of arthroscopic lateral retinacular release were assessed in 96 patients with patellofemoral subluxation, then compared with those previously obtained by open patellofemoral reconstruction. Four of the patients had bilateral releases. The average age was 28 years. Conservative management with specific exercises had failed to control symptoms. Inability to perform daily activities and expected pathology were other indications for surgical release. The procedure utilized the Smillie meniscotome, placed via the inferolateral portal. When release was achieved the patella could be tilted about 90 degrees medially (Fig 3–28). Tenderness was evaluated by palpation on the patellar facets or on the retinaculum and patellar ligament (Fig 3–29), and mobility was evaluated by pushing the patella laterally with the knee flexed 30 degrees (Fig 3–30).

The average follow-up was 3 years. Good results were obtained in 88% of operated knees, with respect to pain, function, stability, and objective signs. Ten patients who did not improve underwent patellofemoral reconstruction with successful results. Sports activities were resumed in about 80% of instances. A majority of patients underwent shaving for chondromalacia. Five of 18 torn medial menisci and 1 of 6 lateral menisci were repaired. One hematoma required open drainage. Reflex sympathetic dystrophy resolved on conservative treatment. There were no infections.

Successful results were obtained by arthroscopic lateral retinacular release in 88% of cases of patellofemoral subluxation in this series. The results are quite comparable to those obtained by open patellofemoral reconstruction, with much less morbidity. Failures may be salvaged by open reconstruction.

▶ The authors emphasize that 12 of the 100 knees operated on did not improve after lateral retinacular release and that 10 of these required further surgery. Also reported was a 13% complication rate involving mostly postoperative hematomas and reflex sympathetic dystrophy. They emphasize "this is not an innocuous procedure."—J.S. Torg, M.D.

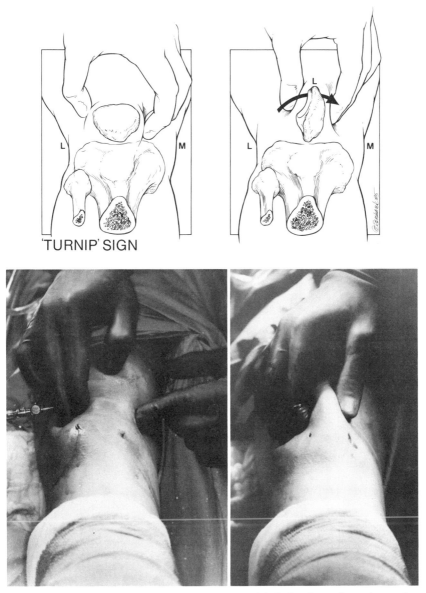

'TURNIP' SIGN

Fig 3–28.—**Top,** complete lateral release has been accomplished when the patella can be turned to its side 90 degrees with the lateral aspect pointing anteriorly and the medial aspect touching the intercondylar notch. This has been called the "turnip sign" by Dr. William G. Hamilton. **Bottom,** the examiner has his fingers on each side of the patella (**left**). The patella is everted and the turnip sign is shown (**right**). (Courtesy of Henry, J.H., et al.: Am. J. Sports Med. 14:121–129, March–April 1986.)

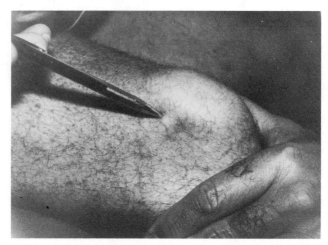

Fig 3–29.—Tenderness was graded by palpating around the patellar retinaculum laterally, medially, inferiorly, and superiorly. It was considered a sign of retinaculitis. Tenderness on the posterior aspect of the patella was suggestive, but not conclusive, of damage to the articular cartilage. (Courtesy of Henry, J.H., et al.: Am. J. Sports Med. 14:121–129, March–April 1986.)

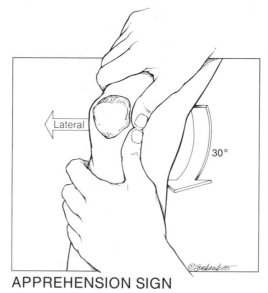

APPREHENSION SIGN

Fig 3–30.—The apprehension sign was described by Fairbanks in 1938. The knee is flexed 30 degrees and the examiner presses the patella laterally with moderate pressure. Apprehension by the patient is considered a positive response. (Courtesy of Henry, J.H., et al.: Am. J. Sports Med. 14:121–129, March–April 1986.)

Factors Predisposing to Patellar Chondropathy and Patellar Apicitis in Athletes

U.M. Kujala, K. Österman, M. Kvist, T. Aalto, and O. Friberg (Sports Med. Research Unit and The Rehabilitation Research Ctr. of the Social Insurance Institution, Turku; and Orthopaedic Hosp. of the Invalid Found. and Central Military Hosp., Helsinki, Finland)
Int. Orthop. 10:195–200, September 1986   3–77

Both patellar apicitis (PA), or jumper's knee, and patellar chondropathy (POC) are frequent and often chronic problems in athletes, and PC is also common in the general population. The anatomical factors predisposing to these disorders were studied in 20 athletes aged 19 to 45 years with PC and 20 others with PA. Twenty athletes with normal knees were also evaluated. A majority of athletes competed at a high level. Jumpers were excluded from the study, and only chronic cases with typical clinical features were included.

Factors significantly associated with PC included an increased anterior drawer sign, an increased passive mediolateral range of motion, and increased hyperextension. Subjects with PA exhibited greater leg length inequality and more patella alta than control athletes. Significant positive correlations were found between various measures of knee laxity in the overall study population. Correlation between the length of the patellar tendon and passive mediolateral patellar motion was 0.82.

Patellar apicitis appears to result from microruptures secondary to jumping on a hard surface. Leg inequality producing asymmetric loading and patella alta both predispose to these ruptures. The intensity of athletic stress is less clearly related to the amount of pain in patellar chondropathy. In addition to cartilage injuries and knee joint laxity, the passive mediolateral range of patellar motion appears to dispose to microtrauma and continued softening of the patellar cartilage.

▶ An interesting study with reasonable conclusions. However, there are several problems. No mention is made of the sex of the subjects in either of the three groups. Placing individuals in the age range of 19 to 45 years in like categories ignores the degenerative changes that occur with particular regard to articular cartilage. I would fully agree with their observations that "the much used lateral release operation, which can increase the hypermobility of the patella, should be done only when the soft tissues at the lateral side of the patella are definitely tight and the patella is laterally positioned, especially in the excessive lateral pressure syndrome."—J.S. Torg, M.D.

Meniscus Tears of the Knee: Prospective Evaluation With CT

Lawrence G. Manco, John H. Kavanaugh, Joseph J. Fay, and Bryan S. Bilfield (Albany Med. Ctr., Albany, N.Y.)
Radiology 159:147–151, April 1986   3–78

The ability of noncontrast axial computed tomographic (CT) scanning to identify and characterize meniscal tears was examined in a series of 209 patients aged 14 to 67 years with unilateral knee complaints. In 59 cases only the symptomatic knee was studied. A total of 359 joints were examined, and 105 were evaluated by arthrography, arthroscopy, or both methods.

The prevalence of disease was 57.5% in this series. The positive predictive value of CT was 96%; CT showed a torn meniscus in 54 of 61 affected knees. Seven false-negative and two false-positive CT results were obtained. More than 80% of meniscal injuries involved the medial meniscus. Nine popliteal cysts, six associated with posterior-horn medial meniscus tears, were seen. Joint effusions did not interfere with meniscal imaging. Tears of both menisci were correctly identified in one case, and chondrocalcinosis was diagnosed in three patients.

Axial CT of the knee is an efficient means of identifying and characterizing meniscal tears. Computed tomography may be slightly less accurate than arthrography or arthroscopy, but it may be the best noninvasive means of detecting meniscal lesions. Prospective studies are needed to assess newer magnetic resonance imaging techniques in comparison with other methods such as CT.

▶ The major disadvantage of the method described here is that the position is extremely difficult requiring the patient to have the contralateral leg elevated for approximately 12 to 15 minutes. The major advantage of the examination is that the surgeon can see the menisci more anatomically than on arthrography. Gross tears can be identified, but partial tears of the undersurface of the menisci would not be identified by their technique. The accuracy obtained by the authors is impressive; however, their results have not been reproduced by other investigators, and CT examination of the menisci should be complimentary to the double-contrast arthrographic examination.—J.S. Torg, M.D.

Clinical Diagnosis of Meniscal Tears: Description of a New Manipulative Test

Allen F. Anderson and A. Brant Lipscomb (Vanderbilt Univ. Hosp. and St. Thomas Hosp., Nashville, Tenn.)
Am. J. Sports Med. 14:291–293, July–August 1986   3–79

A clinical diagnosis of meniscal tears remains difficult in many cases, even for experienced surgeons. A new manipulative test has been developed and evaluated in 93 consecutive patients with 100 suspected or demonstrated meniscal tears. Medial meniscal tears were most frequent.

Along with McMurray's test a medial-lateral grind test was performed by applying valgus stress to the extremity of the supine patient as the knee was flexed to 45 degrees; varus stress was applied as it was extended (Fig 3–31). The test is repeated with progressive stress. A longitudinal or flap tear produces a distinct grinding sensation at the joint line, whereas a complex tear results in prolonged grinding.

From 43% to 63% of patients with meniscal tears had popping, swelling, and pain at the joint line, and 77% had tenderness over the joint line. Results of the McMurray test were positive in 58% of cases, with 5 false-positive results. Results of the medial-lateral grind test were positive in

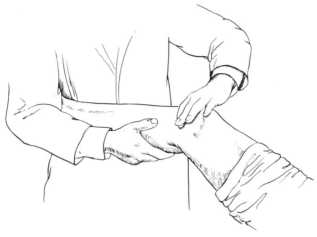

Fig 3–31.—Basic position for examination in medial-lateral grind test. (Courtesy of Anderson, A.F., and Lipscomb, A.B.: Am. J. Sports Med. 14:291–293, July–August 1986.)

68% of patients, with 1 false positive finding and 29 false-negative results. Results of at least one test were positive in 79% of meniscal tears. Both tests were relatively accurate in detecting degenerative and flap tears and less accurate in detecting short longitudinal or displaced bucket-handle tears. Most diagnostic errors involved the lateral meniscus.

The medial-lateral grind test for meniscal tearing requires less flexion than the McMurray test and is applicable to most acute injuries. False-positive findings are infrequent. Both tests should be performed routinely. Neither is pathognomonic for a meniscal tear.

▶ It is certainly refreshing to see a newly described diagnostic modality that does not require an arthroscope, magnetic coil, or computerized roentgenographic apparatus. The authors note that manipulative tests are not pathognomonic of meniscal abnormalities because of the high incidence of false-positive and false-negative results. They further point out that false-positive findings may be produced by "patellofemoral abnormalities, osteoarthritis, snapping of the medial hamstrings, or trapping of a lax normal meniscus." They also point out that when a positive result occurs the contralateral normal knee should be examined in an attempt to rule out a false-positive finding. With regard to the value of the medial-lateral grind test, the test of any test is certainly the test of time.—J.S. Torg, M.D.

Meniscal Tears: The Effect of Meniscectomy and of Repair on Intraarticular Contact Areas and Stress in the Human Knee: A Preliminary Report
Mark E. Baratz, Freddie H. Fu, and Richard Mengato (Univ. of Pittsburgh)
Am. J. Sports Med. 14:270–275, July–August 1986   3–80

Contact pressures were measured in cadaver knee joints in an attempt to determine the effects of partial and total meniscectomies for bucket-

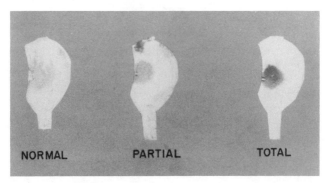

Fig 3–32.—Distribution of pressure on right medial tibial plateau after partial and total meniscectomy. (Courtesy of Baratz, M.E., et al.: Am. J. Sports Med. 14:270–275, July–August 1986.)

handle tears and the differences between repair and segmental resection of a peripheral meniscal tear. Contact distribution was assessed in neutral position and at 30 degrees of flexion before and after removal of the inner one third of the meniscus. Peripheral tears that involved 2 cm of the posteromedial horn of the medial meniscus and the posterolateral horn of the lateral meniscus were created, and studies were done in conjunction with closed repair, open repair, segmental meniscectomy, and total meniscectomy.

Stresses increased by 67% on average after partial meniscectomy and by 236% after total meniscectomy (Fig 3–32). A 110% increase in peak

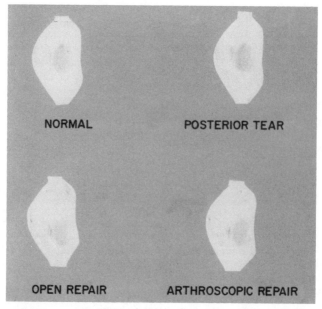

Fig 3–33.—Distribution of pressure on left medial tibial plateau after repair of peripheral tear of meniscus by open and by arthroscopic techniques. (Courtesy by Baratz, M.E., et al.: Am. J. Sports Med. 14:270–275, July–August 1986.)

local contact stress was observed after segmental meniscectomy of the part of the meniscus that was involved in the peripheral tear (Fig 3–33). Contact areas were essentially unchanged after total meniscectomy, but peak local stress increased by 163% over that seen with a normal meniscus.

These preliminary findings suggest that the meniscus is important in weight-bearing, but further work is needed. Contact stresses increase with the amount of meniscus that is removed and the degree to which hoop tension of the meniscus is disrupted. When the knee is loaded in full extension, little difference in weight-bearing characteristics of the meniscus is seen with repair by open or arthroscopic techniques.

Treatment of Osteochondral Defects of the Distal Femur With Fresh Osteochondral Allografts: A Preliminary Report

John C. Garrett (Clinic for Reconstructive Orthopaedic Surgery, Atlanta)
Arthroscopy 2:222–226, 1986   3–81

Osteochondral defects of the femoral condyle may leave a permanent crater. Twenty-four such defects were treated with fresh osteocartilaginous allograft transplants. The 16 men and 8 women had a mean age of 33 years. Grafts from young donors were matched for skeletal size, as estimated from standard roentgenograms, and were transplanted within 12 hours of harvesting.

Ten patients were followed up for 2 years or longer. All 14 patients improved with respect to pain, function, swelling, and buckling. No patient lost more than 10 degrees of motion. Assessment of ten long-term patients with a rating system showed improvement in all instances. Roentgenograms showed osseous bridging of the graft to the surrounding condyle within 6–12 weeks in all but one case, in which a 2 × 5-cm defect occupied nearly the entire posterior aspect of the medial femoral condyle, limiting posterior buttressing of the graft. This defect required 1 year for full circumferential healing. No graft extrusion was seen, and there were no infections or nonunions. Adjunctive Kirschner wires frequently caused pain and hemarthrosis and were removed arthroscopically. All postoperative arthroscopic studies showed a viable graft without collapse.

The early results of fresh osteochondral allograft use in osteochondral defects of the distal femur are promising. Symptoms have been consistently relieved, and overall knee function has improved.

▶ The authors' recognition that "although the use of fresh osteochondral allografts in the treatment of osteochondral defects in the distal femur should be considered investigational, the early results are promising" is appropriate.— J.S. Torg, M.D.

The Anatomy of the Iliopatellar Band and Iliotibial Tract

Glenn C. Terry, Jack C. Hughston, and Lyle A. Norwood (Hughston Orthopaedic Clinic, Columbus, Ga.)
Am. J. Sports Med. 14:39–45, January–February 1986   3–82

The functional anatomy of the iliopatellar band and iliotibial tract is more complex than is commonly perceived. Seventeen fresh or fresh-frozen knee specimens from subjects aged 19 to 72 years and two embalmed cadaver knees were dissected. The six incisions that were used to identify the relevant anatomy included two clinical incisions, one between the iliopatellar band and iliotibial tract and one between the iliotibial tract and the biceps femoris.

The aponeurotic layer consists of arciform fibers which cross the anterior aspect of the patella and the fascia of the vastus lateralis and biceps femoris (Fig 3–34). Superficial, middle, deep, and capsulo-osseous layers were distinguished. Posteriorly the capsulo-osseous layer forms a superficial arcuate whose proximal part is continuous with the plantaris and lateral gastrocnemius fascia (Fig 3–35).

The iliopatellar band connects the anterior aspect of the iliotibial tract and femur to the patella. The lateral patellotibial ligament forms the anterior boundary of the superficial layer and, as such, connects the iliopatellar band and iliotibial tract.

The superficial layer of the iliotibial tract in combination with the deep and capsulo-osseous layers presumably functions as an anterolateral ligament of the knee. The iliopatellar band stabilizes the patella against medially directed forces and is dynamically influenced by the vastus lateralis. Some extra-articular reconstructive operations on the knee act to reconstitute the deep and capsulo-osseous layers of the iliotibial tract.

▶ This article presents an extremely well illustrated description of the ligamentous anatomy of the lateral aspect of the knee. However, the conclusion of the authors that correlation of "variable clinical signs" in patients with antero-

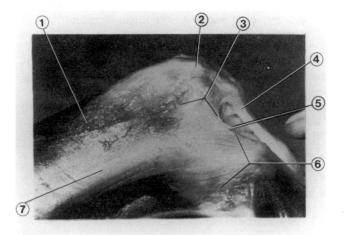

Fig 3–34.—Superficial layer of iliotibial tract and iliopatellar band after aponeurotic layer has been removed: *1,* vastus lateralis; *2,* lateral border of patella where vastus lateralis inserts; *3,* iliopatellar band; *4,* patella tendon; *5,* lateral patellotibial ligament; *6,* iliotibial tract; *7,* proximal portion of aponeurotic layer. (Courtesy of Terry, G.C., et al.: Am. J. Sports Med. 14:39–45, January–February 1986.)

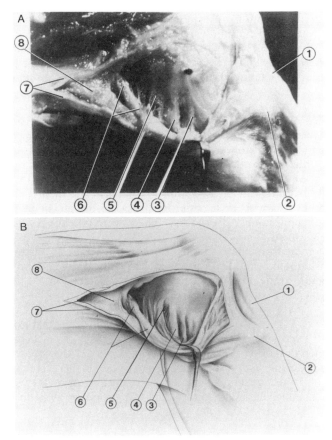

Fig 3–35.—**A,** anatomical relationships seen at dissection of lateral knee: *1*, patella tendon; *2*, Gerdy's tubercle; *3*, fibular collateral; *4*, lateral head, gastrocnemius; *5*, tendon plantaris muscle; *6*, capsulo-osseous layer, iliotibial tract; *7*, cut edges, superficial layer, iliotibial tract; *8*, deep layer iliotibial tract. **B,** artist's enhancement of **A.** (Courtesy of Terry, G.C., et al.: Am. J. Sports Med. 14:39–45, January–February 1986.)

lateral rotatory instability "are not due to anterior cruciate ligmanet rupture alone, but results from associated extra-articular injury as well" is not documented.—J.S. Torg, M.D.

Posterior Instability of the Knee Joint: An Experimental Study
S. Nielsen and P. Helmig (Orthopaedic Hosp., Aarhus, Denmark)
Arch. Orthop. Trauma Surg. 165:121–125, April 1986   3–83

The posterior cruciate ligament (PCL) generally is considered the first line of defense against posterior instability of the knee joint. The stabilizing function of the PCL and of the medial and lateral ligamentous and capsular structures in translational and rotatory instability was examined in 25 normal osteoligamentous autopsy specimens. Anteroposterior tibial displacement and tibial rotation were measured at various degrees of flexion during application of a straight anterior or posterior force of 25 N.

Transection of the PCL increased posterior tibial displacement on flexion to a maximum of 10 mm at 90 degrees of flexion. When combined lesions of the lateral structures were produced, the popliteal tendon appeared to have a major stabilizing function. Posterior tibial displacement in flexion was doubled when all lateral structures were lesioned. Transection of the PCL and all medial structures led to a substantial increase in posterior displacement with flexion. Tibial rotation increased only with combined lesions to either the medial or lateral structures. Combined lateral lesions, including the popliteal tendon, produced a reverse pivot shift. Anteromedial subluxation was released after lesioning of the medial structures. No instability was evident in anteroposterior displacement in extension with any of the lesioning procedures. There were no changes in anterior tibial displacement.

It is apparent from these studies that the tibia must be unconstrained when translational instability is assessed. The clinical detection of complex lesions requires that the posterior drawer test be done at 90 degrees of flexion, with the tibia free to rotate.

▶ The findings of this study support our clinical observations that isolated disruption of the posterior cruciate ligament does not result in functional instability. It is when this lesion is associated with disruption of the medial or lateral supporting structures with resulting two-plane instability that a problem arises. Also, lack of demonstrable posterior laxity in extension coincides with clinical findings, hence the inability to demonstrate PCL deficiency by performing "reverse" Lachman tests.—J.S. Torg, M.D.

Cortical Bone Pegs in the Treatment of Osteochondral Fracture of the Knee
P. Myllynen, A. Alberty-Ryöppy, and A. Harilainen (Univ. Central Hosp., Helsinki, and Jorvi Municipal Hosp., Espoo, Finland)
Ann. Chir. Gynaecol. 75:160–163, 1986   3–84

Patellar dislocation is the most frequent cause of osteochondral or chondral fragments in the knee joint in adolescents. Typically, rupture of the medial fibrous capsule is present, with fracture of either the medial edge or articular facet of the patella or lateral femoral condyle. Both ASIF miniscrews and headless Smillie pins have been recommended for fixation of the fragment. Good function has been achieved after removing the fragment, but union of the fracture may be expected.

Cortical bone pegs were successfully used to fix the loose or loosened fragment in four patients having large osteochondral fractures involving the medial articular facet of the patella and the lateral femoral condyle. Pegs were taken from the proximal anteromedial cortex of the ipsilateral tibia (Fig 3–36). The pegs measured 2 to 4 mm wide and 3 cm long. Holes

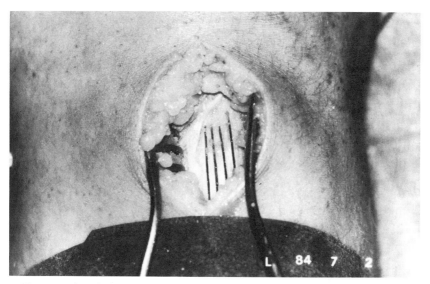

Fig 3–36.—Through a separate incision the tibial cortex is exposed subperiosteally. Bone pegs, measuring 2–3 mm by 3–4 cm are cut with an oscillating saw. The pegs are then elevated with an osteotome and trimmed with a rongeur. (Courtesy of Myllynen, P., et al.: Ann. Chir. Gynaecol. 75:160–163, 1986.)

were drilled through the replaced fragment into underlying bone, and the slightly larger pegs were driven through, incorporating the ends beneath the articular surface with an impactor. The joint was immobilized for 5 to 6 weeks postoperatively. Good results were obtained in all four cases.

Cortical bone pegs are easily obtained and used, and they provide stable fixation without the need for later intervention. Bone pegs may be recommended as a primary means of fixation of large osteochondral fractures of the knee. Further follow-up is needed to determine whether late degenerative changes occur.

▶ Fixation of osteochondral fractures can present a significant technical problem. Both Smillie pins and ASIF miniscrews lack a compression effect and may migrate, bend, or project into the joint. Also, they must be removed later, which imposes a second surgical procedure. Physiologic fibrinogen glue has been used in Germany (*Aktuel Traumatol.* 11:136, 1981) but is not available in this country. Ideally, a biodegradable fixating device is needed but not available. The idea of cortical bone pegs is attractive and seems to obviate most of the aforementioned problems.—J.S. Torg, M.D.

Anterior Cruciate Ligament Injuries: To Counsel Or To Operate?
K. Satku, V.P. Kumar, and S.S. Ngoi (National Univ. of Singapore)
J. Bone Joint Surg. [Br.] 68-B:458–461, May 1986   3–85

Surgical correction of complete rupture of the anterior cruciate ligament, although successful in a majority of patients, is still beset with problems.

Untreated anterior cruciate ligament injuries in 97 knees of 87 patients were reviewed after a mean interval of 6 years to determine the appropriateness of surgical intervention in the management of this injury. Functional ability as well as the incidence of meniscectomy and its timing in relation to any radiologic deterioration of the joint were evaluated.

After recovery from the initial injury, 63% of patients were able to return to their preinjury sport. After a mean interval of 6 years, only 46% were still engaged in their preinjury sports and 27% had deteriorated functionally. A total of 56 knees (58%) had meniscectomy. More meniscectomies were performed in patients who had had their anterior cruciate ligament injury more than 5 years previously than in those who had had their ligament ruptured within the last 5 years, suggesting a risk for meniscal injury even years after ligament injury. Radiologic deterioration was maximal in those who had had a meniscectomy more than 5 years before final review and in those with clinical evidence of meniscal injury but no meniscectomy. Knees with intact menisci were often radiologically normal despite continuing instability.

Based on these results, a program for management after anterior cruciate ligament injury is recommended. Operative stabilization of the knee is recommended in patients with significant instability during activities of daily living. Those who have had partial meniscectomy or meniscal repair, and those with no meniscal injury but who wish to return to strenuous sports, are encouraged to undergo stabilization procedures to protect the meniscus. Patients with anterior cruciate ligament injury and total meniscectomy should refrain from strenuous sporting activities and should undergo a rehabilitation program of muscle strengthening, with agility training and adaptation maneuvers.

Followup of the Acute Nonoperated Isolated Anterior Cruciate Ligament Tear
Richard J. Hawkins, Gary W. Misamore, and Thomas R. Merritt (Univ. of Western Ontario, London)
Am. J. Sports Med. 14:205–210, May–June 1986   3–86

The optimal management of isolated disruption of the anterior cruciate ligament (ACL) remains controversial. The natural course of an isolated tear of the ACL was examined in 40 patients who were followed up for an average of nearly 4 years during nonoperative management. Thirty were first seen within 48 hours of injury. No patient had clinical ligamentous injury other than involvement of the ACL. Examination without anesthesia sufficed in more than one third of the cases. Average age of patients was 22 years. Quadriceps and hamstring exercises were performed under supervision, starting as soon as exercises were comfortably tolerated. Bracing usually was recommended, but was not always used.

Twelve of the 40 patients (30%) required late reconstruction for chronic insufficiency of the ACL at a mean of 33 months after injury. Instability of the knee was a problem for 24 (86%) patients without surgical management. Three patients had "giving way" of the knee with routine daily activities. Most patients, however, had instability only when pivoting on the affected extremity.

Only three patients considered their knee to be as stable and functional as before injury. Few patients were able to successfully compete in athletics as before. Pain usually was not a major complaint, and swelling of the knee was not a concern for most patients. No patient had a subjectively excellent outcome, and only five had a good result.

The prognosis is guarded after an isolated rupture of the ACL, but the question of whether surgery is helpful remains unanswered. The prognosis of the ACL-deficient knee seems to be especially poor in young, active patients who wish to participate in stressful sports activities.

▶ The similar observations and conclusions of the respective authors (Satku, in Abstract 3–85, and Hawkins, in Abstract 3–86) is noteworthy, to wit, the ACL-deficient knee in the young physically active patient does not fare well. Also, noteworthy is the reticence on part of both groups of authors to recommend anterior cruciate ligament reconstruction on routine basis. What is needed is a longitudinal study that will demonstrate whether or not cruciate reconstruction will in fact restore stability, protect the menisci, and prevent development of osteoarthritis. It is hoped that such data will be forthcoming.— J.S. Torg, M.D.

Result of the Insall Procedure (Repair of the Anterior Cruciate Ligament With a Bone Block Iliotibial Band Transfer) in the Treatment of Chronic Anterior Cruciate Instability of the Knee: Analysis of 30 Cases After a Minimum Follow-up of One Year

N. Biga, D. Judlin, J.M. Thomine, and H. Léger (Hôpital Charles Nicolle, Rouen, France)

Rev. Chir. Orthop. 72:115–120, 1986 3–87

The active transfer of ligament grafts has received the least attention of all syndesmoplastic procedures available for the reconstruction of impaired knee ligaments. In 1981, Insall published his technique for the repair of chronic anterior cruciate ligament instability, which involves the active transfer of the iliotibial ligament to the tibial plateau. It is implanted directly on musculoaponeurotic structures of the thigh and the buttocks, which play a major role in the carrying phase of stride. The authors report their results with the Insall procedure.

The study comprised 30 patients who were operated on with the Insall procedure because of a severely disabling chronic instability of the knee that seriously interfered with their daily and professional activities. Average follow-up was 2 years, ranging from 12 to 38 months.

Of 30 operations performed, results of 23 were judged good, 5 were judged fair, and 2 were considered to have had poor results. The lateral stability of the knee was not affected. Of the 22 patients who had participated in leisure sports prior to their operation, 17 were able to practice their sport at their previous level of participation. None of the operated patients was a high-level athlete.

Good results can be obtained with a sufficiently solid and well-vascularized iliotibial ligament transfer in patients who suffer from disabling instability of the knee.

▶ Although Nicholas and Minkoff described this procedure in 1978 (*Am. J. Sports Med.* 6:341–353, 1978) it was Insall who actually devised and was the first to perform the operation (*J. Bone J. Surg.* [*Am.*] 63A:560–569, April 1980). Subsequently, Scott (*J. Bone Joint Surg.* [*Am.*] 67A:532–538, April 1985) has also presented a series of 30 patients with a follow-up of 2 years and longer. In Scott's series results were poor in 20% of the cases; 10% of the patients required additional surgery because of problems with the bone block or screw. In addition to this high rate of poor results and complications, it should be noted that the procedure is difficult to perform technically.—J.S. Torg, M.D.

Combined Anterior Cruciate-Ligament Reconstruction Using Semitendinosus Tendon and Iliotibial Tract
Bertram Zarins and Carter R. Rowe (Harvard Med. School)
J. Bone Joint Surg. [Am.] 68-A:160–177, February 1986   3–88

An intra-articular over-the-top transfer of the iliotibial tract was combined with the transfer of a distally based semitendinosus tendon to treat 100 patients with disruption of the anterior cruciate ligament (ACL). They were among the first 106 patients in a prospective study of this procedure. Average age was 24 years. All but 8 patients had sports-related injuries. Average interval from injury to surgery was 38 months. The specific indication was disabling instability that was reproduced by pivot-shift testing.

Both intra-articular and extra-articular methods are used to route the iliotibial tract and semitendinosus tendon from opposite directions over the top of the lateral femoral condyle and through the same oblique drill hole in the proximal tibia (Figs 3–37 and 3–38). The tendon is sutured to the iliotibial tract laterally, the tract is sutured to the semitendinosus tendon medially below the drill hole, and the capsule is advanced.

Follow-up after 3 to 7.5 years showed a reduction in the positive anterior drawer sign to 1 + or elimination in 80 knees. The positive pivot shift was reduced to 1 + or eliminated in 91 joints. Both strength and tibial rotation were significantly improved. Thirty-five patients were able to return to preinjury athletic activity without limitations and 55 returned to modified athletic activity. Eighty-eight patients were satisfied with the outcome. Only 1 patient considered the operation to have failed. A number of patients had subsequent surgery.

In patients with disruption of the ACL stability of the knee may be improved by a combined reconstructive procedure in which both the iliotibial tract and semitendinosus tendon are used. The best results have

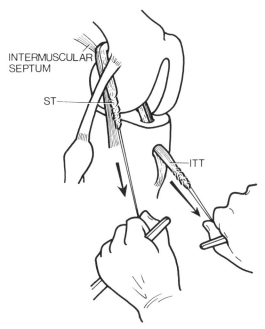

Fig 3–37.—Semitendinosus tendon (*ST*) has been passed through an oblique drill-hole in the antero-medial part of tibia, across the knee, over the top of the lateral femoral condyle, above the lateral intermuscular septum, and deep to the fibular collateral ligament. A strip of iliotibial tract (ITT) that originates on lateral aspect of proximal part of the tibia takes a parallel course and exits through the same drill-hole in the tibia. Both grafts are pulled tight with the knee at 60 degrees of flexion and are held under tension while being sutured to each other. [Courtesy of Zarins, B., and Rowe, C.R.: J. Bone Joint Surg. (Am.) 68-A:160–177, February 1986.]

been obtained in patients without previous operations who are treated within 2 years after injury.

▶ The authors have combined four elements into one operative procedure: (1) there is an intra-articular over-the-top transfer of the iliotibial tract as described by MacIntosh (*J. Bone Joint Surg.* 56B:591, 1974); (2) a distally based semi-tendinosus tendon transfer similar to that reported by Cho (*J. Bone Joint Surg.* 57A:60B, 1975); (3) posteromedial capsular reefing; and (4) lateral capsular reefing. The rationale for this combination of procedures is that it "reconstructs the intra-articular as well as the extra-articular restraints, both of which contribute to knee stability." In that they have not chosen to compare this combination of procedures with simply an intra-articular reconstruction, this rationale remains conjectural. It is noted that the over-the-top replacement precludes an isometric reconstruction. Also, the protracted limitation of knee motion with full extension not occurring until 9 months postsurgery is noted. After ligament reconstruction 35 of the 100 patients were able to return to preinjury athletic activity with no limitation.

I have had no experience with this procedure. However, it appears that the patellar tendon, bone tendon bone graft described by Clancy requires less sur-

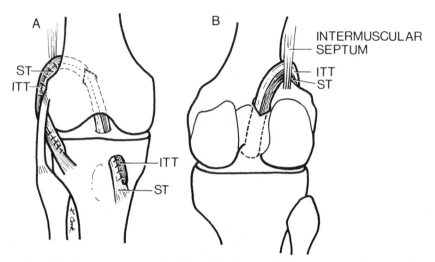

Fig 3–38.—**A,** semitendinosus tendon (*ST*) and iliotibial tract (*ITT*) have been sutured to each other medially and laterally. In addition, both grafts are sutured to arcuate ligament complex posterolaterally to secure the extra-articular component of reconstruction. Grafts are not sutured to the fibular collateral ligament. **B,** posterior aspect of right knee showing final location of both grafts. Semitendinosus tendon and *ITT* both exit the knee through the same small vertical opening high in the posterior part of capsule. Grafts course over the top of the lateral femoral condyle and above the lateral intermuscular septum. If the septum is weak or has been divided, staples can be used to hold the grafts high on the condyle. A groove can be made in the lateral femoral condyle to seat grafts in an over-the-top route. [Courtesy of Zarins, B., and Rowe, C.R.: J. Bone Joint Surg. (Am.) 68-A:160–177, February 1986.]

gery, is isometric, and permits more rapid rehabilitation and a much higher percentage of patients returning to previous activity level.—J.S. Torg, M.D.

Analysis of the Müller Anterolateral Femorotibial Ligament Reconstruction Using a Computerized Knee Model
Michael Gibson, Richard Mikosz, Bruce Reider, and Thomas Andriacchi (Univ. of Chicago Hosps. and Clinics and Rush Presbyterian-St. Luke's Med. Ctr., Chicago)
Am. J. Sports Med. 14:371–375, September–October 1986   3–89

Müller described the use of an anterolateral femorotibial ligament (ALFTL) for reconstructing knees with anterolateral rotatory instability, which is often associated with rupture of the anterior cruciate ligament (ACL). Part of the iliotibial tract complex presumably is injured as well as the ACL in these cases.

In these reconstructions a strip of iliotibial tract is isolated and fixed with one or two screws and special toothed washers at an empirically determined point on the lateral aspect of the femur. Some part of the transplant should be tense in each position of flexion, particularly at 20 to 30 degrees of knee flexion.

A validated computer model of the knee was used to determine the ability of the graft to augment the ACL, its efficacy in resisting loads, and the effects of moving the fixation point 1 cm superior, inferior, and anterior to the predicted neutral surgical attachment. The model predicted that the ALFTL graft is a useful restraint to internal rotation when used with or without an intra-articular reconstruction of the ACL. The ALFTL graft took up more tension at increasing angles of knee flexion and was more effective. Placement of the graft 1 cm anterior to the current surgical attachment site decreased the vector component that lies perpendicular to the long tibial axis, thereby reducing resistance to internal rotation. No ALFTL graft effectively resisted pure anterior displacement at 0 to 30 degrees.

The ALFTL graft of Müller is an effective restraint to internal tibial rotation, with or without intra-articular reconstruction of the ACL. Future studies with the use of this model should be expanded to allow greater degrees of flexion.

▶ Andrews (*Am. J. Sports Med.* 13:112–119, March–April 1986) has been the major proponent of this procedure in this country. It should be noted that in the majority of instances of acute ACL disruption an attempt was made to repair the ligament. Also, on the basis of his experience, Andrews did not believe that the procedure should be used as an isolated procedure on knees where severe, chronic, "complex" instability existed because the stretching of capsular structures placed excessive stress on the iliotibial tendonesis. For more complex instability he suggests a more extensive reconstructive procedure that combines intra-articular anterior cruciate reconstruction and extra-capsular reconstruction as required. Andrews suggests these instabilities be managed by reconstruction of the anterior cruciate ligament using the middle third of the patella tendon combined with extracapsular reconstruction and iliotibial tract tenodesis.

This clinical experience appears to contradict, in part, the observation of Gibon et al. that the anterolateral femorotibial ligament graft is a useful restraint when performed with or without an intra-articular ACL reconstruction.—J.S. Torg, M.D.

The Natural History of the Anterior Cruciate Ligament Autograft of Patellar Tendon Origin
David Amiel, Jeffrey B. Kleiner, and Wayne H. Akeson (Univ. of California, San Diego)
Am. J. Sports Med. 14:449–462, November–December 1986   3–90

Previous studies have shown that autogenous palellar tendon (PT) used in the reconstruction of anterior cruciate ligament (ACL) results in long-term graft viability. However, no studies have been done to follow the evolution of the ACL autograft of PT origin through time. The authors studied the natural history and biology of the ACL autograft of PT origin in a rabbit model.

The study was done with 37 male New Zealand white rabbits who underwent reconstruction of the left ACL with the medial third of the quadriceps/patellar tendon. The rabbits were killed at 2 weeks (n = 5), 3 weeks (n = 5), 4 weeks (n = 5), 6 weeks (n = 17), and 30 weeks (n = 5). At sacrifice, the ACL autograft, the control PT, and the ACL from the right knee were isolated by dissection and processed for histologic and biochemical examination.

When the PT is placed in the anatomical and environmental milieu of the ACL, a process of ligamentization of the grafted tissue results. The autograft depends on synovial fluid for its nutrition prior to revascularization. Cells in the ACL autograft of PT origin originated from a source other than the PT graft. There appears to exist a tissue specificity of fibroblasts whereby PT fibroblasts have different survival needs from those of the graft repopulation fibroblasts. It also appears that the lack of blood supply to the ACL autograft of PT origin does not prevent fibroblasts from migrating into the tissue and establishing the necessary cellularity for the process of ligamentization.

The Phenomenon of "Ligamentization": Anterior Cruciate Ligament Reconstruction With Autogenous Patellar Tendon
David Amiel, Jeffrey B. Kleiner, Richard D. Roux, Frederick L. Harwood, and Wayne H. Akeson (Univ. of California, San Diego)
J. Orthop. Res. 4:162–172, 1986   3–91

The fate of the patellar tendon, which is used to reconstruct knees with a deficient anterior cruciate ligament (ACL), remains uncertain. Morphological and biochemical parameters were evaluated in a rabbit model of autograft replacement and in the normal ACL and patellar tendon. The medial third of the quadriceps-patellar tendon was used in the reconstructions.

The autografts gradually assumed the microscopic appearances of the normal ACL. Ligamentous cellular morphology was noted by 30 weeks after reconstruction. The concentration of type III collagen, not normally present in the patellar tendon, gradually increased in the grafts, and at 10% was the same as in the normal ACL by 30 weeks. The level of glycosaminoglycans also increased to that ordinarily found in native ACL.

Analysis of collagen-reducible cross-links showed that the graft tissue shifted from the usual patellar tendon pattern of low dihydroxylysinonorleucine (DHLNL) and high histidinohydroxymerodesmosine (HHMD) to the high-DHLNL, low-HHMD pattern seen in normal ACLs.

These findings suggest that a process of "ligamentization" takes place when the patellar tendon is placed in the milieu of the ACL. The autograft is dependent on synovial fluid for its nutrition before revascularization occurs at 6 weeks.

▶ This work (Abstracts 3–90 and 3–91) was the recipient of the American Orthopaedic Society for Sports Medicine Basic Science Research Award in 1986. The observation that the lack of blood supply to the ACL autograft of patellar tendon origin does not prevent fibroblasts from migrating into the tissue and establishing the necessary cellularity for ligamentization is significant even though it only pertains to rabbits.—J.S. Torg, M.D.

Reconstruction of the Anterior Cruciate Ligament by Allogeneic Tendon Graft: An Operation for Chronic Ligamentous Insufficiency

Konsei Shino, Tomoatsu Kimura, Hitoshi Hirose, Masahiro Inoue, and Keiro Ono (Osaka Univ., Japan)
J. Bone Joint Surg. [Br.] 68-B:739–746, November 1986   3–92

Results obtained in dogs encouraged a trial utilization of allogeneic tendon as a replacement for the anterior cruciate ligament (ACL) in 31 patients seen between 1981 and 1984 with chronic ACL insufficiency. The mean follow-up was 31 months. The mean time from initial injury to surgery was 2 years. The usual chief complaint was multiple episodes of giving way. Exploration showed an absent or severely attenuated, non-functioning ACL. The medical meniscus was torn in 16 cases, and the lateral meniscus in five. Allogeneic tendon was harvested from fresh cadavers or amputation specimens. A trial ligament of woven Dacron was used to ensure that the reconstructed ligament would be tight. Staples were used in addition to Tevdek sutures to secure a long graft (Fig 3–39).

No patient had episodes of giving way during daily activities or sports activities at follow-up, and all but one had returned to full sports activity. Eighteen patients considered their knee to be normal, and 12 improved; 1 reported a worse status than before operation. No patient had evidence of rejection of the allogeneic tendon. The functional results were graded excellent in 24 cases, good in 6, and fair in 1. Roentgenograms showed

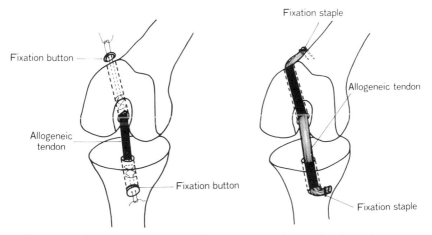

Fig 3–39.—Techniques for reconstruction of the anterior cruciate ligament by a free tendon allograft. **Left,** if the graft is between 6 and 11 cm long, thick Tevdek sutures are placed in both free ends and tied over buttons at the correct tension. **Right,** if the graft is more than 11 cm long, it is secured with staples near its exit from each drill-hole. [Courtesy of Shino, K., et al.: J. Bone Joint Surg. (Br.) 68-B:739–746, November 1986.]

no evidence of abnormal bone responses. At arthroscopy the synovium appeared normal, and the grafts functioned well against anterior drawer stress. No deep infections occurred.

Reconstruction of the ACL with allogeneic tendon graft provides functional stability in cases of chronic ACL insufficiency, without the need to sacrifice autologous tissue. Successful results have been obtained in first-class competitive athletes.

▶ The results, as reported by the authors, are impressive. In addition they have attempted to answer a number of questions. Regarding which patients with ACL insufficiency require reconstructive procedure, they conclude that the active young athlete with a strong desire to continue vigorous sports which include jumping, sudden turning, or body contact will benefit from surgery. They further state that intra-articular reconstruction is necessary in these patients because extra-articular procedures do not always correct the instability fully. However, they augment the repair in the presence of anterolateral instability with a modification of the Ellison procedure.

As to the best substitute, they suggest frozen allogeneic tendon providing there is no risk of contamination. They further state that freeze-drying was not used because of the fear it would reduce mechanical strength of the tendon. Follow-up arthroscopic examination showed that the grafts were thick, taut, and adequately revascularized. This is an important study that attempts to answer many of the questions involved with allogeneic tendon replacement in the ACL-deficient knee.—J.S. Torg, M.D.

Anterior Cruciate Ligament Allograft Transplantation: Long-Term Function, Histology, Revascularization, and Operative Technique
Pantelis K. Nikolaou, Anthony V. Seaber, Richard R. Glisson, Beth M. Ribbeck, and Frank H. Bassett III (Duke Univ.)
Am. J. Sports Med. 14:348–360, September–October 1986   3–93

It is well known that the anterior cruciate ligament (ACL) plays an important role in maintaining stability of the knee. A tear of the ACL often leads to immediate and permanent instability of the knee, which, if left untreated, will result in substantial disability. Since past efforts at repairing the injured ACL have shown that its complex structure makes it extremely difficult to reconstruct, the authors designed an experimental dog model for testing the feasibility of cryopreserved ACL allotransplantation.

The effect of cryopreservation on ligament strength was tested by implanting cryopreserved unilateral autograft and allograft ACL transplants and comparing their relative performance. The ligaments were tested for mechanical integrity for up to 18 months after implantation. Histologic specimens from fresh and cryopreserved ligaments and microvascularization were also studied.

Cryopreservation and duration of storage did not affect the biomechanical or structural properties of the ligaments. Mechanical integrity tests showed that autografts and allografts obtained similar results of nearly 90% of control ligament strength by 36 weeks after implantation. By 24 weeks both autograft and allograft ligaments showed near-normal revascularization. No structural degradation or immunologic reaction was observed during the study.

The promising results of this experimental study and the favorable results obtained in earlier clinical and laboratory studies of deep-frozen allografts suggest future clinical trials.

Replacement of the Anterior Cruciate Ligament Using a Patellar Tendon Allograft
Steven P. Arnoczky, Russell F. Warren, and Melissa A. Ashlock (Hosp. for Special Surgery, affiliated with the New York Hosp.-Cornell Univ., New York) J. Bone Joint Surg. [Am] 68-A:376–385, March 1986   3–94

Autogenous patellar-tendon grafts are widely accepted as suitable replacements for the anterior cruciate ligament following injury. While these grafts are completely revascularized by 20 weeks, they are avascular at the time of transplantation and hence are essentially free grafts. This concept raises the possibility of using a free patellar-tendon allograft as replacement for the anterior cruciate ligament. In 25 adult dogs, the anterior cruciate ligament was replaced by fresh or deep-frozen patellar-tendon allografts. Histocompatibility testing of class-I antigens was performed. No immunosuppressive agents were used. For the deep-frozen allografts, the grafts were placed in sterile saline solution containing penicillin G and streptomycin sulfate and rapidly frozen to − 100 C. The grafts were stored in liquid nitrogen at − 196 C for 4 weeks to 4 months. The morphology of the transplanted allografts was studied at various intervals from 2 weeks to 1 year postoperatively using routine histologic studies and a vascular-injection (Spalteholz) technique.

Fresh patellar-tendon allografts demonstrated marked inflammatory and rejection response after transplantation into the knee joints. This reaction was manifested by perivascular cuffing and lymphocyte invasion. Deep-frozen patellar-tendon allografts appeared to be benign within the joint and underwent changes similar to those observed in autogenous patellar-tendon grafts. Avascular necrosis was noted 1 month after transplantation. The vascular tissues of the infrapatellar fat pad and synovial tissue provided a vascular synovial envelope around the graft and supplied the origin for the intrinsic revascularization and cellular proliferation within the allograft. Revascularization was complete at 5 months, and by 1 year, the graft resembled a normal anterior cruciate ligament. Although all the knees demonstrated some degree of anterior-posterior laxity, the patellar-tendon allograft remained intact in all knees.

Deep-frozen patellar-tendon allografts can be preserved and successfully transplanted to replace the anterior cruciate ligament.

▶ Anterior cruciate ligament allograft transplantation presents two problems, one discussed and one not discussed by the authors. They point out that "one of the key requirements for the use of an allograft transplant is the ready availability of quality material for the surgical procedure. The concept and theoretical aspects of allotransplantation have little meaning if the ACL graft is not available in sufficient quantity. An efficient and reliable tissue bank is required which can provide a selection of graft sizes with guaranteed structural integrity." Second, the potential transmittability of the auto-immuned deficiency syndrome virus with allograft transplantation is not discussed.—J.S. Torg, M.D.

Replacement of the Anterior Cruciate Ligament Using a Synthetic Prosthesis: An Evaluation of Graft Biology in the Dog
Steven P. Arnoczky, Russell F. Warren, and Joseph P. Minei (Cornell Univ.)
Am. J. Sports Med. 14:1–6, January–February 1986   3–95

The biologic effects of a knitted Dacron velour prosthesis were studied when such prostheses were used to replace the anterior cruciate ligament in 21 adult mongrel dogs. Tissue ingrowth and vascularization were assessed at intervals up to a year after surgery.

A prosthesis 4 mm in diameter was used to replace the ligament. It was placed through a hole that was drilled transversely through the proximal tibial crest and sutured on itself after the absence of anteroposterior instability was demonstrated. The infrapatellar fat pad was wrapped about the prosthesis before the joint capsule was approximated.

Synovial tissue began to envelop the prosthesis 1 month after surgery, and the entire graft was covered by 2 months. Vessels were seen through the graft interstices at 3 months, when fibroblasts surrounded the Dacron fibers. Parts of the graft were encapsulated by 6 months. Little further encapsulation occurred in the next 6 months. Inflammation was minimal. Degenerative changes were consistently present after 3 months.

Revascularization in this study resembled that seen with biologic graft materials. The use of infrapatellar fat and synovial tissue optimizes the ingrowth of tissue into the prosthesis. Exposure of newly formed connective tissue to joint forces is necessary if a functional new ligament is to be formed. In the present model the collagen was not functionally aligned.

The Relationship of Vascularity and Water Content to Tensile Strength in a Patellar Tendon Replacement of the Anterior Cruciate in Dogs
Edward G. McFarland, Bernard F. Morrey, Kai N. An, and Michael B. Wood (Mayo Clinic and Found.)
Am. J. Sports Med. 14:436–448, November–December 1986   3–96

There is much controversy over the proper techniques and materials to be used in intra-articular reconstruction of the anterior cruciate ligament (ACL). A variety of autograft tissues have been investigated over the years. Synthetic materials, including carbon fiber, carbon fiber with polylactic acid polymer, polyethylene, and Dacron, are currently being investigated as ACL replacements. Allografts have most recently been suggested as an alternative for ACL reconstruction. An autograft with the patellar tendon is considered the graft of choice by many investigators. The authors tested the biologic and biomechanical characteristics of a patellar tendon autograft used for ACL reconstruction in dogs.

The study was done with 16 mature, mongrel dogs weighing more than 20 kg. The ACL replacement with a patellar tendon was performed on one knee in seven dogs and on both knees in five dogs, and four dogs served as controls. The dogs were studied at 37, 57, and 120 days for vascularity of grafts, measured with technetium-labeled erythrocytes, and for tensile strength with an MTS machine.

After 4 weeks, the grafts had become more vascular, more hydrated, less stiff, and less strong than the controls. The vascular response subsided by 16 weeks, but the grafts remained only 40% as strong as the controls. There was a significant increase in percent water over controls for all time periods. The decrease in strength correlated poorly with vascularity, but correlated well with the increase in percent water. This may be a useful parameter for further study as the most sensitive measure of graft competency.

The model developed in this study can serve as a basis for further studies.

▶ The authors have presented an ingenious method for indirectly determining the strength of patellar tendon autografts in the canine model. The potential clinical relevance of their findings, if any, remains obscure.—J.S. Torg, M.D.

Long-Term Results of Nonoperative Treatment of Isolated Posterior Cruciate Ligament Injuries in the Athlete
James M. Parolie and John A. Bergfeld (Cleveland Clinic Found.)
Am. J. Sports Med. 14:35–38, January–February 1986   3–97

Isolated injury to the posterior cruciate ligament (PCL) is not common, and the treatment remains somewhat controversial. The nonoperative approach to these injuries was examined in 25 athletes, as well as their ability to return to their sport without handicap. All patients were assessed by questionnaire and by clinical examination, x-ray films, dynamometer, and knee arthrometer. The mean follow-up period was 6.2 years.

At follow-up, 80% of the patients were satisfied with their knees. Eighty-four percent of these patients had returned to their previous sport, but 16% had a decreased level of performance. Among the satisfied patients, mean torque dynamometer values for 45 degrees/second, 90 degrees/second, and 180 degrees/second was greater than 100% of the value for the uninvolved knee. Among those not satisfied with their knees, all had values less than 100% of the uninvolved knee for this parameter. The instability of the knee as measured by arthrometer was related neither to patient satisfaction nor to the patients' ability to return to their sport.

It appears, then, that the majority of athletes with isolated PCL injuries who are treated without surgery can return to sports without functional disability, if they maintain muscular strength.

▶ A very good article to support the need for proper rehabilitation after posterior cruciate ligament injury and the importance of rebuilding muscular strength. The authors point out that all of those who were not satisfied with their knee had less than 100% strength of the uninvolved knee. All those who were satisfied had strength greater than 100% of the uninvolved knee. A very "telling" figure.—F. George, A.T.C., P.T.

Knee Arthroscopy

Arthroscopy-"No Problem Surgery": An Analysis of Complications in Two Thousand Six Hundred and Forty Cases
Orrin H. Sherman, James M. Fox, Stephen J. Snyder, Wilson Del Pizzo, Marc J. Friedman, Richard D. Ferkel, and Michael J. Lawley (S. Cal. Sports Med. and Orthopedic Group, Van Nuys)
J. Bone Joint Surg. [Am] 68-A:256–265, February 1986   3–98

Complications associated with open surgery for intra-articular lesions of the knee have been reported frequently. With the advent of athroscopic surgery of the knee, hospitalization time, length of sick leave, hospital costs, time required to return to sports, and time to muscular functional return all have been reduced. However the reported overall complication rate from arthroscopy remains high (4% to 15%). Complications of arthroscopy were reviewed in a large series of knee arthroscopies performed by one orthopedic group.

A retrospective review was made of 3,261 arthroscopies performed by four of the authors between 1976 and 1983. There were 216 complications overall (8.2%), 126 being designated as major and 97 as minor. The major complications that were evaluated were infections, hemarthroses, adhesions, effusions, cardiovascular, neurologic, reflex sympathetic dystrophy, and instrument breakage; the minor complications were difficulties with wound healing and ecchymosis. Patients with an industrial injury had a higher rate of neurologic complications and of reflex sympathetic dystrophy. Diagnostic arthroscopy had the lowest overall complication rate. Partial medial meniscectomy was associated with the highest rate of instrument breakage. Abrasion arthroplasty had the highest rate of complications of wound healing, and subcutaneous lateral release was associated with the most adhesions. Two factors were found to be predictors of complications: age and, if a tourniquet was used, the tourniquet time.

Certain complications may be preventable to some degree and are under the control of the surgeon, while others are unpreventable, and reduction of risk factors becomes the only control the surgeon has. A predictive model has been developed that shows that age and tourniquet time are the most significant risk factors. The use of a tourniquet in itself had no effect on the complication rate, but if a tourniquet was used, a tourniquet time of longer than 60 minutes placed the patient at high risk for the development of complications.

▶ An interesting comparison can be made regarding the complication rates reported by the authors with those reported by the Committee on Complications of the Arthroscopy Association of North America (*Arthroscopy* 1:214–222, 1985). The latter group, using a retrospective survey technique, reported 930 complications occurring in a total of 118,590 arthroscopic procedures with a complication rate of 0.8%. The data of Sherman et al., representing their own experience and with an overall complication rate of 8.2%, would appear to be more accurate and should alert the arthroscopic surgeon to potential problems.—J.S. Torg, M.D.

Knee Arthroscopy With Local Anesthesia in Ambulatory Patients: Methods, Results and Patient Compliance
Ejnar Eriksson, Tom Häggmark, Tönu Saartok, Ahmed Sebik, and Börje Ortengren (Karolinska Hosp., Stockholm, and Astra Pharmaceutical, Södertälje, Sweden)
Orthopedics 9:186–188, February 1986   3–99

Patients who have knee arthroscopy under local anesthesia receive atropine and diazepam as premedication. The skin at puncture sites is injected with 0.5% prilocaine with epinephrine; lidocaine or mepivacaine also may be used. From 4 to 5 ml is injected at each site, and 50 to 60 ml of anesthetic solution is placed in the suprapatellar pouch and joint cavity via the upper lateral puncture site. The knee then is flexed a few times, and arthroscopy is begun after 5 to 10 minutes; the anterolateral approach is used. The joint cavity is distended with 50 to 100 ml of a 1:10 mixture of local anesthetic and physiologic saline or Ringer's acetate.

Data were reviewed on 278 ambulatory patients who had knee arthroscopy at Karolinska Institute on an outpatient basis during a 2-year period. General anesthesia was used in 27% of cases, spinal anesthesia in 51%, and local anesthesia in 22%. More than three fourths of the patients in the local anesthesia group were satisfied. None had to be put to sleep. Fewer patients in the local anesthesia group had postoperative complaints. Nearly half of all patients were able to return to usual work within 2 days of arthroscopy, and all resumed their usual work within 1 week. In no case was more than 500 mg of prilocaine used for local anesthesia.

General anesthesia is best accepted by ambulatory patients who have knee arthroscopy, but local anesthesia is a good alternative. The safety and simplicity of the latter method probably will widen its use in this setting. No toxic complications have occurred in more than 600 arthroscopies done under local anesthesia.

Arthroscopic Surgery Performed Under Local Anesthesia as an Outpatient Procedure
M.I.B. Besser, and S. Stahl (Rambam Med. Ctr., Technion-Faculty of Medicine, Haifa, Israel)
Arch. Orthop. Trauma Surg. 105:296–297, September 1986   3–100

Diagnostic and operative arthroscopy of the knee under general or epidural anesthesia is a well-established procedure. Because of the increasing demand for arthroscopic procedures of the knee, several authors have advocated the use of local anesthesia. In a period of 36 months, 875 patients underwent arthroscopy, either diagnostic ($n = 352$) or surgical ($n = 523$), under local anesthesia as an outpatient procedure. The technique and results are presented.

An intravenous infusion is set up for administration of diazepam if the patient is anxious. A tourniquet is not used. The area where the arthroscope is to be introduced, as well as the anteromedial joint space, is infiltrated with bupivacaine 0.5% and adrenaline. The knee is irrigated with normal saline contained in a bag under pressure. After surgery, the knee is dressed with a small amount of plaster wool and elastic bandage. The patient goes home 30 minutes after the procedure, with instructions to perform SLR exercises and to limit activity for 1 week.

Meniscal surgery was straightforward using the double-puncture method. In many instances, combined procedures were performed, i.e., double meniscectomy or meniscectomy with shaving. Acute locked knees were treated speedily, using intravenous diazepam and pethidine. The lateral suprapatellar portal was also used for removal of loose bodies or excision of the medial shelf or other plicae. In cases of chondromalacia or other chondral lesions of the femoral condyles, the cartilage was shaved to bleeding bone, usually without discomfort to the patient. Complications included septic arthritis in one patient, effusion in 10% of patients, and synovitis. Bleeding was limited by efficient irrigation, and lack of patient relaxation was overcome with intravenous diazepam with or without pethidine, and reassurance.

Arthroscopic surgery under local anesthesia is a safe and reliable method, which not only decreases morbidity associated with general anesthesia but also lowers hospital and patient cost. Results are comparable to those obtained under general anesthesia.

▶ These two papers (Abstracts 3–99 and 3–100) describe the technique and feasibility of performing surgical arthroscopy of the knee under sedation and local anesthesia. This experience parallels that described by Clancy (Snowmass Orthopaedic Conference, March 17, 1986) as well as ourselves. The day has arrived when both diagnostic and surgical arthroscopic procedures will be performed routinely under local anesthesia on an outpatient basis.—J.S. Torg, M.D.

Arthroscopy Update #1: Treatment of Osteochrondrosis Dissecans of the Knee by Arthroscopic Curettage, Follow-up Study
Paul M. Denoncourt, Dinesh Patel, and Penagiotis Dimakopoulos (Massachusetts Med. Ctr., Worcester, Mass., and Harvard Univ.)
Orthop. Rev. 15:652–657, October 1986   3–101

Since the etiology and natural history of osteochondrosis dissecans of the knee are not well understood, the treatment of this disorder has not been standardized. Whereas children and adolescents with nondisplaced lesions will usually heal with restriction of activity alone, the treatment of adults frequently requires surgery. However, there is no agreement on which surgical technique is the procedure of choice at each stage of the disease. The authors conducted a prospective study to determine whether arthroscopic excision of loose fragments in the knee and arthroscopic curettage of the bed to bleeding bone would promote healing of detached and partially detached osteochondral fragments in adult patients.

The study comprised 37 patients with arthroscopically confirmed osteochondrosis dissecans of the knee, involving either the medial or the lateral femoral condyle, who were treated on an outpatient basis as described above. Postoperatively, all patients were instructed to perform active and passive range-of-motion exercises. Ten patients agreed to undergo follow-up arthroscopy 5 to 15 months after undergoing their first procedure.

Follow-up arthroscopy showed that all ten lesions had filled in with fibrocartilage which was firmly attached to its surrounding wall. The junction of the normal hyaline cartilage and the fibrocartilage was smooth in most cases. All patients were asymptomatic at follow-up and had regained full range of motion.

▶ Follow-up evaluation, which averaged 9 months (range, 5 to 15 months), is short and precludes any meaningful conclusion regarding the long-term efficacy and effects of this means of treating osteochondritis dissecans. Also, the authors did not indicate the location of the lesions, i.e., weight-bearing or non–weight-bearing surfaces of the femoral condyle. A prospective randomized study in which some patients had the defect reattached and others had osteochondral allografts would be interesting.—J.S. Torg, M.D.

Arthroscopic Meniscus Repair: A Safe Approach to the Posterior Horns
Craig D. Morgan and S. Ward Casscells (Wilmington, Del.)
Arthroscopy 2:3–12, 1986   3–102

Meniscal tears are serious injuries in young persons. Seventy tears in 67 patients were repaired arthroscopically on an outpatient basis between 1983 and 1985. The average age of the patients was 26 years, and they were followed up for an average of 18 months. Only single vertical longitudinal tears in the outer third of the meniscus were included in the series. Nearly 80% of the tears were chronic. Medial tears were present in 70% of cases. Medial suturing is performed by passing a "loaded" 18-gauge spinal needle from outside to inside (Fig 3–40). Suturing is continued until the tear is completely stabilized (Fig 3–41). Inside-to-outside suturing also is used to repair large peripheral lesions, such as displaced peripheral bucket-handle tears. A similar technique is used for placing sutures laterally.

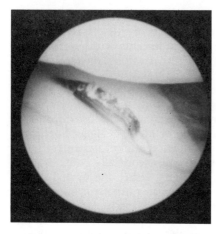

Fig 3–40.—Intra-articular visualization of a "loaded" 18-gauge spinal needle far posterior in the posterior horn seen during a lateral meniscal repair. (Courtesy of Morgan, C.D., and Casscells, S.W.: Arthroscopy 2:3-12, 1986.)

One second tear developed, but the area of the previous meniscal repair appeared intact at repeat arthroscopy. Uneventful healing occurred, with excellent results in 99% of cases. Symptoms resolved completely, and patients were able to resume their previous level of activity. Repeated arthroscopy for evaluation or for anterior cruciate ligament reconstruction showed complete, stable healing in the area of the meniscal repair. No suture material was seen in the region of the tear by 6 months. There was one deep infection and one transient saphenous nerve injury, but no serious neurovascular complications occurred.

Use of the outside-to-inside arthroscopic suturing method for posterior horn lesions reduced the risk of injuring posterior neurovascular structures about the knee. Sutures can be placed in all areas of the menisci. Careful debridement of the tear and local synovial abrasion are important in creating a proper environment for healing.

► The authors report an ingenious method for effecting meniscal repair. Troublesome is the fact that follow-up is short (average, 18 months), the method and criteria for evaluation are ambiguous, and one third of the knees were observed to be anterior cruciate ligament deficient. In view of this, results reported as 99% excellent must be put into perspective.—J.S. Torg, M.D.

Arthroscopic Meniscal Repair Evaluated With Repeat Arthroscopy
Thomas D. Rosenberg, Steven M. Scott, David B. Coward, William H. Dunbar, J. Whit Ewing, Charles L. Johnson, and Lonnie E. Paulos (Univ. of Utah, Univ. of California-Davis, Northeastern Ohio Univ., and Ochsner Clinic, New Orleans)
Arthroscopy 2:14–20, 1986   3–103

About 10% of meniscal tears seen in the past 3 years and one third of longitudinal tears have been repaired arthroscopically. Twenty-nine menisci were repaired in 27 patients, who underwent arthroscopy again 3

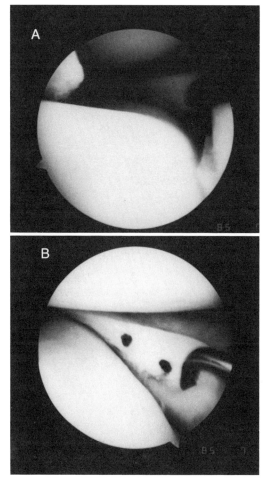

Fig 3–41.—A, acute anterior central tear of the medial meniscus. **B**, same tear as seen in A with the knot sutures in position and the tear reduced. (Courtesy of Morgan, C.D., and Casscells, S.W.: Arthroscopy 2:3-12, 1986.)

months later. Only displaceable longitudinal tears at least 1.5 cm long were included in the series. There were 27 peripheral tears and 2 midsubstance lesions. More than half the lesions were chronic.

During treatment the suturing needle entered the knee from the contralateral portal and exited away from popliteal structures (Fig 3–42). Horizontal mattress sutures were placed from either the superior or inferior surface as needed to optimally approximate the structures (Figs 3–43). Six patients underwent anterior cruciate reconstruction at the same session.

Healing was complete in 24 of 29 repaired menisci and in 22 of 23 stable knees. Only two of six repairs in unstable knees healed completely. Four failures occurred in anterior cruciate-deficient knees. Two knees had decreased motion postoperatively, and one patient developed reflex sym-

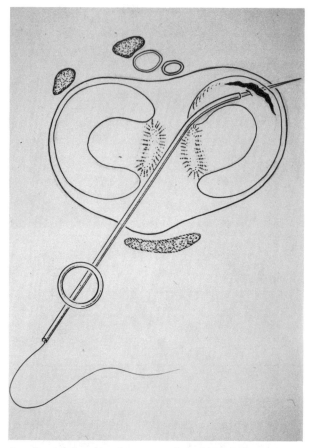

Fig 3–42.—Curved cannula is positioned posterior to the ipsilateral tibial eminence. The needle enters the knee from the contralateral portal and exits away from popliteal structures. (Courtesy of Rosenberg, T.D., et al.: Arthroscopy 2:14-20, 1986.)

pathetic dystrophy. Both former patients required manipulation to gain acceptable knee motion.

Arthroscopic meniscal repair is effective in stable knees with either intact or reconstructed ligaments. Successful repair is possible in all parts of the meniscus without resorting to arthrotomy. Meniscal healing consistently occurs within 3 months in stable knees. Successful repair is less likely in the anterior cruciate-deficient knee.

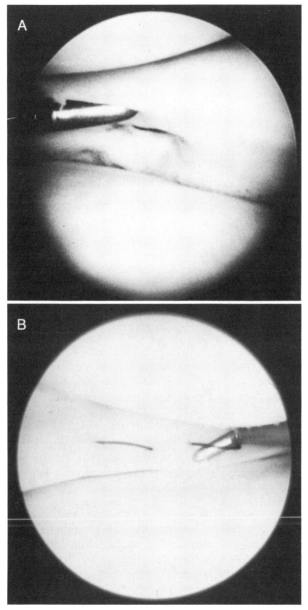

Fig 3–43.—**A,** horizontal mattress sutures placed from the inferior surface of the meniscus. **B,** horizontal mattress sutures placed from the superior surface of the meniscus. (Courtesy of Rosenberg, T.D., et al.: Arthroscopy 2:14-20, 1986.)

Arthroscopic Review of Meniscal Repair: Assessment of Healing Parameters
Robert G. Stone and Gregory N. VanWinkle (Univ. of Texas Helath Science Ctr.)
Arthroscopy 2:77–81, 1986   3–104

This study involved repeated arthroscopy an average of 7.5 months after 16 meniscal repairs to document the state of healing and to discover the fate of nonabsorable suture material in 14 patients. Nonabsorbable suture material was used in 14 of the repairs.

Of the 16 repairs, 56% had healed, 25% had healed partially, and 13% had not healed. These results reflect the fact that repeated arthroscopy was only performed when problems continued to occur. There was no damage to articular surfaces due to the use of nonabsorbable sutures. These sutures were incorporated into the meniscus.

Meniscal repairs at risk for healing problems, derived from this analysis, included repairs of multiple longitudinal tears, tears greater than 40 mm in length, and tears in unstable knees, as well as those that were stabilized with absorbable sutures. These numbers are too few for statistical significance, but they do suggest a trend. Repeated arthroscopy may be necessary in those repairs that are at risk for problems.

▶ The most important point emphasized by these articles (Abstracts 3–103 and 3–104) is that meniscal repair in the anterior cruciate ligament deficient knee is in jeopardy of failure.—J.S. Torg, M.D.

Combined Posterior Incision and Arthroscopic Intra-Articular Repair of the Meniscus: An Examination of Factors Affecting Healing
Gary A. Scott, Ben Lee Jolly, and Charles E. Henning (Univ. of Kansas)
J. Bone Joint Surg. [Am] 68-A:847–861, July 1986   3–105

Surgical management of meniscal injuries remains controversial. An intra-articular suture technique with arthroscopic visualization, combined with a posterior incision, has been developed for the repair of meniscal lesions. The results of 178 meniscal repairs using this technique in 167 patients are presented, with emphasis on factors affecting healing of the meniscal repair. The patients were followed by arthroscopy or arthrography for an average duration of 100 weeks (range, 28 to 231 weeks).

Three important steps in the technique need to be emphasized: stable fixation of the sutures, visualization of the medial meniscus, and dissection of the perimeniscal synovial membrane. Stable fixation of the sutures is achieved by using multiple nonabsorbable sutures (2-0 Ethibond) on the apposed superior and inferior margins of the meniscal tear. The first suture is placed typically at a point 5 to 10 mm anterior to the attachment of the posterior horn of the meniscus. Visualization of the medial meniscus is achieved by using a joint-distractor with the knee maintained in approximately 30 degrees of flexion. Dissection of the perimeniscal synovial membrane is a modification of the technique designed to produce synovial proliferation and neovascularization at the repair site. A biopsy needle and a small nasal-septum rongeur were used previously, but currently only intra-articular rasps are used. The rongeur is introduced into the joint to abrade and roughen the perimeniscal synovial membrane superiorly, and the needle is introduced to penetrate the synovial membrane and coronary ligament inferiorly along the length of the tear.

At follow-up, 61.8% of the menisci had healed, 16.9% had healed incompletely, and 21.3% showed no evidence of healing. Ninety-two percent of the menisci were classified as clinically stable, and 80% of the patients returned to their preinjury sports level. Healing was significantly associated with a narrow peripheral rim (0 to 2 mm) and repair that was associated with reconstruction of the anterior cruciate ligament. A single-longitudinal tear, particularly in the medial meniscus, was associated with a significantly higher rate of healing than was a double longitudinal tear. Although the difference was marginally insignificant, the overall rate of healing increased after the introduction of the technique for dissection of the perimeniscal synovial membrane. Age did not affect healing. There were no vascular or neurologic complications.

Meniscal repair is a logical alternative to restore the normal kinematics of the knee. A narrow peripheral meniscal rim, as well as dissection and stimulation of the perimeniscal synovial membrane, can influence the rate of healing.

▶ Eighty percent of the 167 patients in this series had an associated tear of the anterior cruciate ligament. The meniscal repair was performed concomitantly with reconstruction of the anterior cruciate ligament, with arthroscopic meniscal repair being performed before undertaking reconstruction of the ligament using an arthrotomy. To be noted, 38% of the patients' menisci healed incompletely or not at all. This is somewhat worrisome in view of the fact that the average duration of follow-up was an average of 2 years with some follow-up being as short as 28 weeks. I would suspect that the failure rate will increase with time.—J.S. Torg, M.D.

A Technique for Arthroscopic Reconstruction of the Anterior Cruciate Ligament
Richard B. Caspari, John F. Meyers, and Terry L. Whipple (Med. College of Virginia)
Contemp. Orthop. 12:49–57, March 1986   3–106

Although numerous operations for repair of a torn anterior cruciate ligament (ACL) have been described, no single technique has stood the test of time, because the problem is so complex. The authors describe a technique for arthroscopic reconstruction of the ACL.

Traditional procedures for repair or reconstruction of the ACL involve extensive dissection of the knee and result in significant short-term or long-term morbidity. Many procedures make use of autogenous graft material, which requires further dissection. Sometimes ancillary incisions need to be made, further increasing morbidity and resulting in cosmetic deformity. As a result, there has been much interest in the use of allograft and synthetic materials as substitutes for the ACL, but no ideal substitute has as yet been developed. With the advent of diagnostic arthroscopy it has become possible to inspect the ACL carefully and to define the extent and level of the tear. Reconstruction of the ACL under arthroscopic control is an extension of such diagnostic procedures.

The authors' technique requires absolute precision for optimal results, but it is not particularly difficult and can be learned easily by accomplished arthroscopists. An experienced surgeon should not need to spend more time in performing this operation than would be required for similar open intra-articular ACL substitution operations.

Arthroscopic techniques for ACL substitutions do not solve all aspects of the problem associated with repair of an ACL. It is hoped that continued research will result in more sophisticated implant techniques that will ultimately provide a better solution for this vexing problem.

Arthroscopic Anterior Cruciate Reconstruction Using the Semitendinosus and Gracilis Tendons: Preliminary Report
Raymond A. Moyer, Randal R. Betz, John Iaquinto, Paul Marchetto, Philip D. Alburger, and Michael Clancy (Temple Univ.)
Contemp. Orthop. 12:17–23, January 1986   3–107

Arthroscopic reconstruction of the anterior cruciate ligament (ACL) holds many advantages, including markedly less postoperative pain, a shorter hospital stay, and improved return of normal knee function. The patient's own semitendinosus and gracilis tendons may be used for reconstruction, following arthroscopic inspection of the entire joint and debridement of the intercondylar notch and the medial aspect of the lateral femoral condyle. The reconstruction is accompanied by an extra-articular iliotibial band tenodesis. Return of full extension usually requires about 6 months.

Sixteen patients underwent transarthroscopic reconstruction of the ACL, while 15 others had open surgery. Twenty-two patients were treated for chronic anterior cruciate instability, and nine were treated for acute ACL disruption. The time for arthroscopic surgery averaged 2 hours—30 minutes longer than open surgery—but presently the surgical times are comparable. Proper placement of drill holes is critical to obtaining isometric fixation points for the tendons. The cosmetic appearances were significantly better after arthroscopic surgery. These patients also had considerably less pain than those having open surgery.

The postoperative hospital stay averaged 2 days in the arthroscopy group and nearly 4 days in the open surgery group. No patient has developed patellofemoral symptoms after arthroscopic surgery, but four patients have had significant symptoms following open operation.

The early results of arthroscopic reconstruction of the ACL using the semitendinosus and gracilis tendons are encouraging, but longer follow-up is needed to document long-term stability. Problems associated with the arthroscopic operation have been minor, and no infections have occurred.

▶ These articles (Abstracts 3–106 and 3–107) must be considered technique descriptions in that neither reports the results of the procedures. Specifically, there is no mention of the duration of follow-up, effect of the procedure on joint function and stability, or complications. We trust that such information will eventually be forthcoming.—J.S. Torg, M.D.

Foot and Ankle Injuries

Diagnostic Dilemmas in Foot and Ankle Injuries

James S. Keene and Richard H. Lange (Univ. of Wisconsin Clinical Science Ctr., Madison)
JAMA 256:247–251, July 11, 1986   3–108

Foot and ankle injuries are common in athletes. However, several disabling injuries often go undetected during initial evaluation. These include (1) stress fractures of the great toe sesamoids, the fifth metatarsal, and the tarsal navicular bone, (2) transchondral talar-dome fractures, (3) fractures of the os trigonum, and (4) dislocating peroneal tendons. The evaluation and treatment of these injuries are presented.

Stress fractures of the great toe sesamoids present insidious pain in the area of the first metatarsophalangeal joint, often aggravated by athletic activity. A runner's roentgenographic view of the foot should be taken at 3-week intervals and the diagnosis confirmed by a bone scan. Prolonged immobilization is recommended, but should the athlete decide otherwise, excision of the fractured sesamoid will allow the athlete to return to his preinjury activity level within an average of 10 weeks. Fracture of the diaphysis of the fifth metatarsal (Jones' fracture) is due to repetitive trauma, resulting in insidious onset of aching lateral foot pain. Initial x-ray films often demonstrate an incomplete fracture of the shaft of the fifth metatarsal, with the fracture widening and spreading medially with continued activity. Depending on these x-ray findings, a short-leg cast and nonweight-bearing for 6 to 8 weeks will be successsful in acute fractures. Operative management is recommended for those that show nonunion and medullary sclerosis adjacent to the fracture site.

Stress fracture of the tarsal navicular presents as a vague pain along the medial, longitudinal arch, or as a cramping sensation in the foot that is aggravated by vigorous activity. Special studies for diagnosis include a supinated view, interval x-ray films, and bone scan. Treatment consists of short leg cast and non–weight-bearing for 6 to 8 weeks for fractures that are incomplete or are complete and undisplaced. Displaced fractures are best treated with open reduction, internal fixation, and bone grafting.

Transchondral talar-dome fractures occur with inversion and eversion injuries of the ankle. The athlete may complain of intermittent pain, persistent stiffness, instability, and/or catching and locking of the ankle. Interval x-ray films, tomograms, and stress x-ray films of the ankle are often helpful. Operative treatment is recommended. Fracture of the os trigonum results from a forced plantar flexion of the ankle and presents with a persistent posterior and posterolateral ankle pain, swelling, and giving way of the ankle. A bone scan is often diagnostic. Acute injuries should be treated with a short leg cast for 6 to 8 weeks, but excision is indicated if symptoms persist after 4 to 6 months of conservative management. Dislocating peroneal tendons result from recurrent inversion ankle sprains associated with pain in the area of the peroneal tendons. On examination, particularly on dorsiflexion and eversion of the ankle, the tendons will dislocate lateral and anterior to the lateral lip of the fibula. Operative management is recommended.

▶ This is a well-written, general review article dealing with five distinct problems. It adds nothing new or unexpected and is intended for the general practitioner rather than the surgeon or sports medicine specialist.—J.S. Torg, M.D.

Injuries to the Metatarsophalangeal Joints in Athletes
Thomas O. Clanton, James E. Butler, and Allen Eggert (Univ. of Texas and Rice Univ., Houston)
Foot Ankle 7:162–176, December 1986   3–109

Injury to the metatarsophalangeal (MP) joints, ranging from mild sprains to dislocation or fracture-dislocation, is on the increase among athletes wearing flexible shoes on artificial playing surfaces. The wide range of injuries to these joints necessitates a thorough understanding of the anatomy and biomechanics of the injured area by the physician, who then can prescribe the appropriate therapy. This retrospective study analyzes metatarsophalangeal joint injuries and their long-term consequences among athletes.

Sixty-two cases of injury to the MP joint were treated by the authors. The first MP joint was injured 56 times; the second and third joints were injured twice, the second through fifth MP joints once, and the fifth joint alone was injured 3 times. In 32 cases, the injury occurred by a hyperextension mechanism; in 2 cases it occurred by plantarflexion, and in 1 case it resulted from a contusion. The mechanism in the remaining cases was unknown. All accidents occurred on artificial turf or track surfaces.

After the injury has occurred, ice, compression, and rest, followed by contrast and joint immobilization, is the recommended treatment. An oral nonsteroidal anti-inflammatory agent can also be prescribed. Upon resuming play, the athlete should protect the feet by taping them and wearing stiffer shoes or an orthotic device. Former athletes who suffered MP injuries have shown progressive hallux valgus deformity, early hallux rigidus, and arthritic changes. The relationship between these conditions and their MP injuries is not yet known.

Injury to the MP joints in athletes is both preventable and treatable. The first MP joint is the most vulnerable and, as with the other MP joints, is best protected from injury by a stiff, highly supportive shoe. This type of injury can be successfully treated; nevertheless, further study is warranted, for the long-term consequences of this injury are as yet unknown.

▶ This lesion was first observed to involve the first metatarsophalangeal joint in football players playing on artificial surfaces, thus the term "turf-toe" described by Bowers and Markin (*Med. Sci. Sports Exerc.* 6:326–334, 1978). Presumably, the highly flexible, light-weight shoes used on artificial surfaces permit hyperextension and injury to the plantar portion of the metatarsophalangeal capsuloligamentous complex. The authors suggest that the injury also involved a compression injury to the articular cartilage and underlying bone on the metatarsal head. Also, the authors note that they did see this injury in football players wearing the cleated shoe used on grass with a metal forefoot shank. Recommendations for preventative therapy include stiffening the forefoot in athletic shoes or the use of orthotic devices.—J.S. Torg, M.D.

Results of Surgery in Athletes With Plantar Fasciitis
Robert E. Leach, Mitchell S. Seavey, and Daniel K. Salter (Boston Univ.)
Foot Ankle 7:156–161, December 1986   3–110

Plantar fasciitis is the fourth most common cause of pain in runners, but heel pain is also frequently seen in tennis players, basketball players, dancers, and nonathletes. Many cases are a direct result of recent or markedly increased training intensity, or of participation in a new sport. The authors discuss the etiology of this syndrome and report their experience with surgical treatment in a small group of competitive athletes.

The cause of plantar fasciitis appears to be repetitive trauma that produces microtears in the plantar fascia near its attachment which results in chronic inflammation. Flat feet have been suggested as a predisposing cause of plantar fasciitis. Most patients with plantar fasciitis respond well to conservative treatment of 6 weeks' duration, but symptoms may persist for as long as 3 to 6 months. Plantar fasciitis can be prevented by performing heel cord and plantar fascia stretching exercises. Special athletic shoes with energy-absorbing heel cushions are also recommended. Steroid injections may be indicated in patients with acute, severe pain.

Surgery may become necessary if patients do not respond to conservative treatment and if they wish to continue to compete in athletic events. Of 15 competitive athletes who had a total of 16 operations to release the plantar fascia from the os calcis, 14 athletes were able to return to their previous level of activity after surgery. Only one athlete felt that he had not been helped by the procedure to the extent that he would be able to meet his personal goals.

Most patients with plantar fasciitis will recover with conservative treatment, but surgical treatment offers good results to those who do not respond well to conservative management.

▶ Conservative management of plantar fasciitis in the athlete is not complete without a trial of continuous low Dye strapping for 3 weeks (*Clin. Sports Med.* 6; 291–294, April 1987). I would agree that, in the competitive athlete who does not respond to conservative treatment, release of the plantar fascia from the os calcis is indicated. The authors have observed that ability to return to sports varies considerably, with the majority of patients returning 9 weeks after surgery and most patients continuing to improve up to 6 months following surgery.—J.S. Torg, M.D.

Osteochondritis Dissecans of the Midfoot
Richard C. Lehman and John R. Gregg (Univ. of Pennsylvania)
Foot Ankle 7:177–182, December 1986   3–111

Osteochondritis dissecans is characterized by the development of an osteochondral fracture involving articular cartilage and the underlying subchondral bone. The most common sites for this entity are the femoral condyle, the talus, and the capitellum. In the literature, there has been only one reported case of osteochondritis dissecans in the midfoot; this article reports two more cases.

CASE 1.—Girl, 16, basketball and volleyball player, who for 1 month experienced acute pain when putting weight on her right foot. She then was involved in a car accident. Six months later, she developed right lateral ankle pain, which worsened with exercise. She had no point tenderness or ankle motion abnormalities; however, x-ray films revealed a nonunited "sprain or fracture" of her navicular, probably predating her accident. An osteochondritic lesion of the navicular was revealed by tomography. The fragment was excised and the cavity drilled 2 months after the diagnosis of nonunited osteochondral fracture. She was able to continue her athletic activities without restrictions.

CASE 2.—Boy, 13, cross-country runner had pain in his left foot, which was aggravated by running, jumping, and prolonged walking. He had a semirigid cavus foot with pain and tenderness medially over the insertion of the posterior tibialis tendon. Low Dye strapping across the foot relieved some pain. Radiographs were normal, but the naviculocuneiform articulation showed increased uptake in bone scans, and on tomograms, the first cuneiform showed an osteochondritic lesion. The fragment was surgically removed and abrasion arthroplasty of the bone was performed. Fourteen weeks postoperatively, the patient resumed running.

Osteochondral fractures probably result from compaction, shearing, avulsion, or repetitive microtrauma and are prevalent in young patients with pain exacerbated by exercise. Radiographs and radionucleotide uptake bone scans permit localization of the pathologic condition. Specific diagnosis is made with a CT scan or tomogram. If conservative treatment is unsuccessful, surgery is suggested. The results from these cases demonstrate that surgery was highly successful and that up to 5 years postoperatively no arthritic changes and no resumption of pain had occurred.

▶ It should be noted that the authors recommend conservative rather than surgical treatment in the skeletally immature with this lesion.—J.S. Torg, M.D.

Arthroscopic Treatment of Transchondral Talar Dome Fractures

Champ L. Baker, James R. Andrews, and John B. Ryan (Tulane Univ. and Keller Army Hosp., West Point)

Arthroscopy 2:82–87, 1986

3–112

Transchondral talar dome fractures are flake fractures involving the cartilaginous surface and subchondral bone of the talar dome. Seven men and two women, with an average age of 29 years, were seen between 1982 and 1984, for a total of ten affected ankles. Symptoms had been present for 6 to 16 months. All patients had a history of trauma and had been treated conservatively for sprained ankle. Eight posteromedial and two anterolateral lesions were present. The patients were treated arthroscopically by removal of the loose fragment and curettage of the osteochondral bed. The anterolateral and anteromedial portals (Fig 3–44) are used for both diagnostic and operative ankle arthroscopy. All lesions were readily reached through the anterior portals. It is possible to identify posteromedial talar lesions through the anterolateral portal with the ankle plantar-flexed (Fig 3–45). Surgery usually is performed on an outpatient basis.

Nine patients had good results after an average follow-up of 12.5 months, with no pain, normal physical and radiographic findings, and a full return to activities. One patient had a fair result, because of mild ankle swelling after vigorous activity. One patient had decreased sensation over the dorsum of the foot, and another had transient mild synovitis.

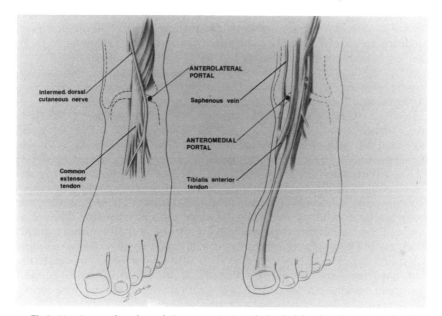

Fig 3–44.—A, anterolateral portal. Entrance point is at the level of the tibiotalar joint just lateral to the peroneus tertius and the extensor tendons. **B**, anteromedial portal. Entrance point is just medial to the tibialis anterior tendon. (Courtesy of Baker, C.L., et al.: Arthroscopy 2:82-87, 1986.)

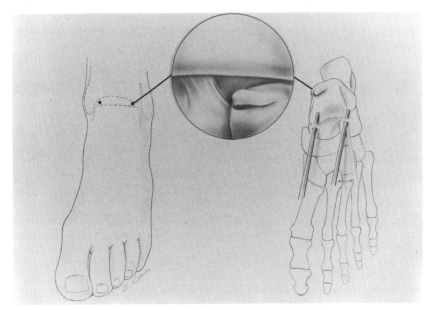

Fig 3–45.—By looking through the anterolateral portal, posteromedial talar lesions can be identified. (Courtesy of Baker, C.L., et al.: Arthroscopy 2:82-87, 1986.)

Operative arthroscopy of the ankle is a reliable means of treating transchondral talar dome fractures in symptomatic patients. Pathologic abnormalities are directly visualized, and adequate débridement is carried out with minimal iatrogenic trauma.

Arthroscopic Treatment of Osteochondral Lesions of the Talus

M. Pritsch, H. Horoshovski, and I. Farine (Chaim Sheba Med. Ctr., Tel-Hashomer, Israel)
J. Bone Joint Surg. [Am.] 68-A:862–865, July 1986   3–113

Twenty-four patients seen between 1981 and 1984 with symptomatic osteochondral lesions of the talar dome had arthroscopy of the ankle joint. Twenty patients were symptomatic for up to 6 months before surgery, and four for longer than 1 year. The 19 men and 5 women had an average age of 28 years. Eighteen patients had a history of trauma. Four patients with grade I injuries and intact, firm cartilage were managed by restriction of sports activities. Six with grade II lesions, characterized by intact but soft cartilage were treated by arthroscopic drilling of the involved area. Fourteen patients had grade III lesions, with frayed cartilage. These lesions were managed by arthroscopic curettage.

Three of the four patients with grade I lesions improved gradually and were free of symptoms after 18 months. One patient had a poor outcome and was found to have a radiographically advanced lesion which was curetted. Two patients with grade II lesions had a good outcome after drilling, two had fair results, one failed to improve, and one had recurrent symptoms and underwent curettement of a grade III lesion. All but 1 of the 14 patients with grade III lesions regained full ankle function after curettage, but 5 had recurrent symptoms that subsequently resolved gradually. One patient had a fair outcome.

Arthroscopy is helpful in planning treatment of osteochondral lesions of the talus, since the radiographic findings do not correlate with the quality of the overlying cartilage. Frayed cartilage calls for curettage. Initial relief of symptoms may sometimes reflect only joint lavage. The longterm success of arthroscopic surgery remains to be established.

Arthroscopic Treatment of Osteochondral Lesions of the Talus
J. Serge Parisian (Hosp. for Joint Diseases Orthopedic Inst., New York)
Am. J. Sports Med. 14:211–217, May–June 1986   3–114

Surgical removal and curettage is the accepted treatment of choice for transchondral fractures of the talar dome. A retrospective study of the arthroscopic treatment of osteochondral lesions of the talus in 18 patients is presented. There were 13 posteromedial and 5 anterolateral lesions. Of these, 16 were due to an inversion type injury of the ankle, one had a bimalleolar fracture of the ankle sustained in a car accident, and one had a bilateral fracture of the os calcis from a job-related falling accident. All patients underwent conservative treatment for at least 4 months prior to referral. Follow-up ranged from 3 months to 3 years.

TECHNIQUE.—General or spinal anesthesia is used. The patient is positioned in the lateral decubitus with the body slightly tilted posteriorly for access to the anterior and posterolateral arthroscopic portals. The supine position is used for access to the anteromedial and anterolateral portals. For posteromedial lesions, a spinal needle is inserted medial to the tibialis anticus tendon to inflate the anterior pouch of the joint, followed by insertion of the smooth obturator of the arthroscope. A drainage needle is inserted into the joint laterally through the anterolateral portal. After complete appraisal of the lesion, the scope is placed laterally and the drainage needle medially. A partial synovectomy of the medial aspect of the joint is performed to facilitate introduction and manipulation of surgical instruments. After gentle probing, elevation and scooping out of the lesion is done with a banana knife. Excision of the lesion is completed with a hemostat clamp. In some cases, the lesion may be fragmented into two pieces. Curettage and abrasion complete the procedure. For anterolateral lesions, the scope is placed medially and the surgical instruments laterally. After excision of the lesion, drilling of the bed may be performed.

Of the ten patients followed up for an average of 2 years, all were fully ambulatory after being kept non–weight-bearing for 6 weeks. Eight patients were followed up for an average of 6.5 months, and all were ambulatory 2 weeks postoperatively. All patients had full range of motion at the time of suture removal (1 to 10 days). Excellent or good results were obtained in 88% of patients. The patient with bimalleolar fracture had a poor result. Complications included a broken ring curette which was easily retrieved, and a suture abscess that cleared up with removal of the suture.

Arthroscopic surgery for osteochondral lesions of the talus, even for chronic lesions, can yield a high percentage of excellent or good results with minimal morbidity, brief hospitalization, and a rapid recovery time for the patient. When performed by experienced surgeons, arthroscopic excision is a reasonable alternative to an open procedure. However, arthroscopic excision is not simple, and it is worth stressing that a technically well-performed arthrotomy is preferable to a poorly performed arthroscopy.

▶ These three articles (Abstracts 3–112, 3–113, and 3–114) document the feasibility (but not necessarily practicality) of dealing with osteochondral lesions of the dome of the talus by surgical arthroscopic methods. Lacking in all three instances is the comparison of results of this particular technique with those obtained by open arthrotomy. Parisien concludes, "arthroscopic excision of the lesion is a reasonable alternative to an open procedure in the hands of a surgeon experienced with the closed technique. The arthroscopic excision is not simple and it is worth stressing the point that a technically well-performed procedure through arthrotomy is preferable to a poorly performed arthroscopic procedure." He also notes that he is "confident that long-term follow-up results will not differ appreciably from these relatively short-term results."—J.S. Torg, M.D.

Talar Compression Syndrome
Alexander E. Brodsky and Momtaz A. Khalil (St. Luke's Episcopal Hosp. and Baylor College of Medicine, Houston)
Am. J. Sports Med. 14:472–476, November–December 1986   3–115

Talar compression syndrome, which is compression of the posterior structures of the ankle during repeated plantar flexion of the foot, is common to ballet dancers, who frequently stand on the tips of their toes. Pain and tenderness occur at the posterolateral aspect of the ankle behind the peroneal tendons, and is a result of the impingement of the os trigonum or the Stieda's process between the calcaneus and the posterior edge of the tibia. The authors describe the anatomy, the diagnosis, and the treatment of this syndrome.

The posterior border of the talus has a groove where the flexor hallucis longus tendon lies. If the talus lateral to the tendon is long, it is called Stieda's process, and if it is a separate bone, it is known as the os trigonum. The patient with talar compression syndrome experiences tenderness over the posterolateral aspect of the ankle, often caused by forceful plantar flexion. The diagnosis is confirmed by lateral roentgenograms, with the plantar flexed.

Of the six dancers that were treated for this syndrome, nonsteroidal anti-inflammatory agents, physical therapy, injection of corticosteroids, and immobilization in plaster for as long as a month were unable to cure the problem. The patients all underwent surgical removal of the os tri-gonum or Stieda's process. All six dancers returned to professional ballet within a few months and remained asymptomatic.

The authors suggest that if conservative treatment of this syndrome is unsuccessful and the patient continues to suffer pain while dancing, surgical removal of the os trigonum or Stieda's process should be considered. A posterolateral incision, with care taken to avoid injuring the sural nerve, is the best site of entry. In cases of coexisting stenosing tenosynovitis of the flexor hallucis longus, a posteromedial incision might be the best site of entry.

► The authors' observations are similar to our clinical experience. The term *talar compression syndrome* is perhaps a misnomer. There appear to be three distinct pathologic conditions that can effect this posterior talar projection: (1) a symptomatic os trigonum, (2) symptomatic Stieda's process, or (3) a symp-tomatic delay/nonunion of Stieda's process. In any instance surgery is curative in cases refractory to conservative means. With regard to the surgical ap-proach, we find a medial incision preferable to the lateral approach recom-mended by the authors.—J.S. Torg, M.D.

Ankle Sprains Classification Based on Anatomical Structures: Winning Entry of the 1986 Student Writing Contest
Janelle Thomas (Old Dominion Univ., Norfolk, Va.)
Athletic Training 21:254–257, Fall 1986   3–116

Ankle injuries make up 20% to 25% of all time-loss injuries in running or jumping sports. It is therefore important for an athletic trainer to be able to assess ankle injuries accurately. Standard classification of ankle injuries is based on the degree of ligamentous damage incurred. The author proposes a two-part classification system that incorporates the standard classification system for ankle sprains.

Ankle sprains may be classified into four general types: lateral, medial, tibiofibular syndesmosis, and intertarsal. Specific ligaments may be in-volved within each of these classes. Within each specific type of injury, the classic grading system of degrees of injury may then be applied. This two-phase approach to classification provides a clear diagnosis from which an appropriate course of management and rehabilitation can be chosen.

Lateral ankle sprains account for about 85% of all ankle sprains. The lateral ligaments comprise three structures: the anterior talofibular liga-ment, the calcaneofibular ligament, and the posterior talofibular ligament. Any of these ligaments may be sprained, but injuries to the latter are rare. Medial ankle sprains account for about 2% to 3% of all ankle sprains. The medial ligament consists of the four-part deltoid ligament. Sprains of the tibiofibular syndesmosis account for about 5% of all ankle injuries. Structures that may be involved include the anterior and posterior tibio-fibular ligaments and the interosseous membrane. Intertarsal ligament sprains can occur in any of the numerous small ligaments that anchor the seven tarsal bones. Most often involved are the bifurcated ligament and the calcaneonavicular ligament.

▶ A standardized classification system for injuries has long been sought after. I'm sure that the term *moderate ankle sprain* does not mean the same thing to all clinicians or evaluators. As the author has described, the more specific we are in our classification, the more likely we are to understand the description of the injury.

I was glad to see the author state that medial ankle sprains occur only 2% to 3% of the time. I had read a number of studies indicating that this inquiry occurs as much as 10% of the time, and I just couldn't match it with my own statistics, which are well below 5%. I thought perhaps we were missing a good number of these in our evaluations.—F. George, A.T.C., P.T.

High-Resolution Magnetic Resonance Imaging of the Ankle: Normal Anatomy
Paul C. Hajek, Lori L. Baker, Ann Bjorkengren, David J. Sartoris, Christian H. Neumann, and Donald Resnick (VA Med. Ctr. and Univ. of California, San Diego, and French Hosp. Med. Ctr., San Francisco)
Skeletal Radiol. 15:536–540, October 1986   3–117

Magnetic resonance (MR) imaging has proved a useful diagnostic tool for evaluating the musculoskeletal system. The potential use of MR imaging in the ankle region was examined in six healthy adults ranging in age from 20 to 33 years with no history of ankle trauma and with normal range of motion. Imaging also was done on six normal ankle specimens from fresh cadavers of individuals ranging in age from 40 to 60 years. Spin echo pulse sequences were obtained, with 3- and 5-mm slice thicknesses and respective interslice gaps of 1.5 and 2.5 mm.

Anatomical detail was well shown on T1-weighted images obtained using high-resolution technique and the surface coil. A 12-cm field of view and slice thickness of 3 mm best delineated normal anatomical structures. A TR of 2,000 ms was optimal. Ligaments and tendons were readily distinguished from muscles. Cancellous bone was clearly outlined on T1-weighted images. Coronal plane images clearly demonstrated the collateral ligaments of the ankle. Sagittal images demonstrated the articular surfaces, especially those of the talocrural joint. Magnetic resonance imaging in the axial plane delineated the flexor and extensor musculotendinous units and their relation to the tibia and fibula.

Magnetic resonance imaging holds great potential for evaluating ankle joint disorders. Contrast studies may help demonstrate the joint capsule, articular cartilage, and the smooth margins of the collateral ligaments.

▶ This study is an excellent demonstration of the MRI appearance of the normal ankle and the potential of this diagnostic modality for evaluating the soft tissues surrounding the ankle. Confirmation of the ability to diagnose pathologic abnormalities will require further research and surgical correlation. The development of contrast agents for MRI is proceeding rapidly and may enhance the usefulness of MRI for evaluating ankle injuries. The potentials are as yet unknown; however, once contrast injection is recommended, the noninvasive quality of MRI is lost.—J.S. Torg, M.D.

Recurrent Dislocation of the Peroneal Tendons: Results of Rerouting the Tendons Under the Calcaneofibular Ligament

Marc A. Martens, Jan F. Noyez, and Josef C. Mulier (Univ. Hosp., Katholieke Universiteit, Leuven, Belgium)
Am. J. Sports Med. 14:148–150, March–April 1986   3–118

Dislocation of the peroneal tendons over the lateral malleolus is rare, but when it becomes recurrent and symptomatic, secondary repair is the treatment of choice. Nine patients with recurrent dislocation of the peroneal tendons, including two with bilateral dislocation, were treated surgically by rerouting the tendons under the calcaneofibular ligament.

A straight incision parallel to the peroneal tendons is made 8 cm above the lateral malleolus, curved over the tip of the malleolus and extended 4 cm over the lateral aspect of the foot. The tendon sheath is opened longitudinally and incised in a Z fashion just distal to the musculotendinous junction. The tendons are then mobilized distally and brought under the calcaneofibular ligament from distal to proximal and repaired following the section plate. The tendon sheath, as well as remnants of the superior peroneal retinaculum, are closed with resorbable sutures. The ankle is immobilized for 6 weeks.

At a mean follow-up time of 30.5 months, good to excellent results were obtained in all patients. All patients regained their preinjury sports activity level at average time of 15 weeks. Numbness or paresthesia over the lateral aspect of the foot in two patients was the only complication encountered.

Rerouting of the peroneal tendons under the calcaneofibular ligament after division of the tendons, as previously described by Sarmiento and Wolf in 1975, is an effective yet simple treatment for recurrent dislocation of the peroneal tendon.

▶ There are several different approaches to surgical management of dislocation of the peroneal tendons. Zoellner and Clancy (*J. Bone Joint Surg.* [*Am.*] 61A:292–294, March 1979) have reported excellent results with a groove deepening procedure. A tendon sling using a slip of the achilles tendon has been described by Escalas et al. (*J. Bone Joint Surg.* 62A:451–452, 1980). Pozo and Jackson (*Foot Ankle* 5:42–44, July–August 1984) have described a rerouting procedure in which the peroneal tendon is placed under the calcaneofibular ligament after osteotomy of the lateral malleolus, the lateral malleolus then being reattached with a screw. Poll and Duiyfjes (*J. Bone Joint Surg.* [*Br.*] 66B:98–100, January 1984) rerouted the tendons by mobilizing a bone block under the calcaneofibular ligament from the calcaneus. The tendons are then relocated, the ligament transposed, and the bone block fixed back into position. Although all authors report satisfactory results, it would appear that a procedure in which the continuity of the tendons are not disrupted would be preferable.—J.S. Torg, M.D.

Early Mobilizing Treatment in Lateral Ankle Sprains: Course and Risk Factors for Chronic Painful or Function-Limiting Ankle
Frank Linde, Inge Hvass, Uwe Jürgensen, and Frank Madsen (Central Hosp., Esbjerg, Denmark)
Scand. J. Rehabil. Med. 18:17–21, 1986   3–119

Early mobilization of lateral ankle ligament lesions is recommended. However, residual symptoms can occur in 25% of patients treated by early mobilization. To determine the course and risk factors for chronically painful or function-limiting ankle following early mobilization, 150 patients with lateral ankle ligament lesions treated with early mobilization without any fixation of the ankle were observed prospectively. The foot was kept elevated during the first 24 hours after injury, and motion and weight-bearing exercises were performed thereafter, according to ability.

After 8 days, 67% of patients were free from pain on ordinary walking and 81% had resumed work. After 1 month, 90% were free from pain and 97% had resumed work. Sports were resumed by 70% of athletes after 1 month and 90% after 3 months. Of the 137 patients available for follow-up after 1 year, 18% had residual symptoms, 14% experienced pain, 7% had functional instability, and 7% had not resumed sports at their normal level. However, only 8% found the condition inconvenient. The only significant prognostic factors for increased risk of residual symptoms were sports activity at a high level and male sex. Athletes accounted for 77% of the patients with residual symptoms compared with 55% of the group without, and residual symptoms occurred in 32% of top athletes (athletes training ≥ 3 times a week) after 1 year.

The incidence rate of residual symptoms after early mobilization of lateral ankle sprains in this study is comparable to that of other studies (between 16 and 39%). Sports activity at a high level is a significant risk factor for chronically painful or function-limiting ankle following early mobilization.

▶ The authors state that the "aim of the study was to describe in a prospective series a course of early mobilizing treatment in ankle sprains and to demonstrate any risk factors of a chronic painful or function-limiting ankle." They note that 90% of the patients in the study returned to painless normal walking and 97% to previous working ability after 1 month of mobilizing treatment. However, they further note that 77% of the athletes in this study had residual symptoms and 32% of what they described as "top athletes" had residual symptoms 1 year after a first sprain. The fact that they did not define either the degree or anatomic site of injury is a problem. Also, they did not compare their results with other forms of treatment in a randomized manner. On the basis of this study it does not appear that early mobilization of lateral ankle sprains in the athlete is necessarily the preferable method of treatment.—J.S. Torg, M.D.

Surgical Repair of Chronic Lateral Instability of the Ankle With a Periosteal Ligament Transfer
R. Roy-Camille, G. Saillant, G. Gagna, J.P. Benazet, and Ch. Feray (Hôpital de la Pitié, Paris)
Rev. Chir. Orthop. 72:121–126, 1986   3–120

Accidental sprains of the tibiotarsal ankle joint occur frequently in active sports. Such sprains, if not treated properly, often become a handicap in active sports as well as in everyday life since one of the most frequent aftermaths of such sprains is a chronic weakness of the tibiotarsal external ligament. Surgery is often the only solution after conservative treatment has failed. The authors report a new technique for repairing lateral instability of the ankle.

With this technique, the fibroperiosteal flap is dissected and pulled through a small tunnel that is made by drilling two holes through the bone at the level where the flap will be attached to the astragalus (Fig 3–46). After pulling the flap through the tunnel, it is attached to the lateral malleolus, either to the talus alone or to the talus and the calcaneum in cases of severe talar tilt. The medial ligament is then passed under the peroneus brevis tendons (Fig 3–47). This technique preserves the peroneus brevis muscle and leaves the mobility of the subtalar joint intact.

During a 4-year period, 23 patients were operated on with this new technique for lateral instability of the ankle. Most patients had sustained their disability during sports events. Of 23 patients, 20 were reexamined after an average of 27 months. Outcome of the surgery was rated perfect

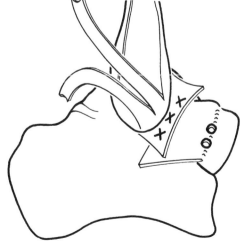

Fig 3–46.—Capsular sheath and perosseous tunnel drilled at the level of the astragalar collar. (Courtesy of Roy-Camille, R., et al.: Rev. Chir. Orthop. 72:121–126, 1986.)

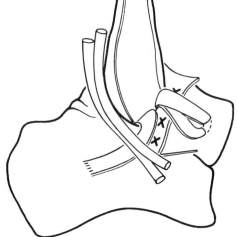

Fig 3–47.—Diagram of the operation showing the capsular sheath and two aspects of the repair: anterior ligament entering and exiting the tunnel and medial ligament passing under the peroneal tendons. (Courtesy of Roy-Camille, R., et al.: Rev. Chir. Orthop. 72:121–126, 1986.)

in ten patients, very good in six patients, acceptable in one patient, and poor in three patients.

Uncomplicated instability of the tibiotarsal ligament in young, active persons who have not responded to conventional physical therapy can be repaired with this relatively simple technique.

▶ What the authors report is the development of an autogenous collagen graft utilizing the fibroperiosteal covering of the distal fibula and lateral malleolus. This appears to be a technique that is certainly worthy of further investigation.—J.S. Torg, M.D.

Ankle Injuries: Clinical Observations
Lester W. Rebman
J. Orthop. Sports Phys. Ther. 8:153–156, September 1986   3–121

Inversion sprains of the ankle are frequently seen by physical therapists. A frustrating by-product of these injuries is the chronic sprain seen in up to 31% of the reported cases. Many treatment regimens have been studied, including cryotherapy, compression, elevation, galvanic stimulation, muscle stimulation, external support, and controlled exercise. However, for the patient with chronic ankle instability, these treatments are frequently incomplete. A simple protocol to improve ankle function after injury is presented.

In step 1, the patient marches in place while resisting the pull exerted by a heavy surgical tubing, and spends 1 to 3 minutes facing in each direction. This forces stabilization from multiple angles as well as during transition from one angle to the other. In step 2, the patient runs in place rather than marching. This step is only carried out when the patient can execute step 1 without pain and without a tendency to roll over. Step 3 involves the patient running and pivoting on each of four 10-degree inclines. In order to progress to step three the patient should be able to carry out step two without pain. In step 3, ankle board exercises are introduced, and patients spend 2 minutes two times per day with their involved foot centered on the board while rolling the board around its periphery in clockwise and counterclockwise directions. Because the goals of this step are to improve proprioception and muscle response, the authors do not allow taping or bracing during rehabilitation.

This program has been found to be subjectively successful in 83% of 29 cases of both acute and chronic ankle problems. Of the 13 patients seen for chronic ankle sprains, all reported a reduction in episode frequency and 9 patients had no recurrence. Of the 16 patients seen for first-time ankle problems, 11 reported no recurrence and 5 showed severe articular involvement and never achieved the level needed to carry out the program. This exercise program is simple, and allows a step-by-step progression in exercise that can be carried out at home.

▶ Functional exercises are a major part of our ankle rehabilitation program. The authors have described a number of different functional exercises which may be incorporated into an ankle rehabilitation regime. We use the ankle balance boards a great deal and feel that restoring proprioception and coordination must be done to prevent chronic ankle sprains from developing. We also take the athletes onto the playing field and run them through a series of agility drills which must be performed satisfactorily before returning to practice or competition.—F. George, A.T.C., P.T.

Miscellaneous Topics

Medical and Public Health Aspects of Boxing
Robert Glenn Morrison (Rockefeller Univ. and Cornell Univ., New York)
JAMA 255:2475–2480, May 9, 1986   3–122

There are an estimated 5,000 professional boxers in the United States and some 25,000 worldwide. In addition, at least 25,000 amateur boxers, many of them teenagers, practice in this country. The number of deaths resulting from boxing is surprisingly low, despite the publicity attending them. Chronic brain damage is recognized as a frequent health hazard associated with boxing. The punch drunk syndrome is characterized by slurred speech, ataxia, impaired memory and dementia, and parkinsonian facial features. Although proponents of boxing have suggested that the syndrome may result from factors in the backgrounds of affected boxers, many studies have indicated a correlation between the number of bouts and the risk of neurologic or psychiatric features of punch drunk syndrome. There is some evidence that amateur boxers do not incur brain damage, but it has proved difficult to analyze the effects of amateur boxing.

Recent reports have confirmed a relation between boxing, even in the modern era, and brain damage; but those who endorse the sport emphasize its benefits in terms of conditioning and personal development. Opponents believe that the risk of brain damage, with its attendant neurological and mental deterioration, outweighs any possible benefits to participants or spectators. Moral arguments against boxing can be made, independent of its medical effects. The AMA has stated that, although it is impractical to attempt to ban boxing, safety reforms are feasible and indicated. Both changes that increase public awareness of the dangers of boxing and those making it safer for participants are desirable. Establishment of a federal regulatory body is a reasonable goal. Professional bouts might be shortened, and boxing form might be emphasized over knockout blows. Physicians must maintain a position of advocating effective reforms while not appearing to approve of the sport.

▶ An excellent review. The original article is highly recommended reading. It reviews the relevant medical literature concerning the health effects of boxing, the contribution by the medical community to the public debate over boxing, and suggests ways the objectives of the medical profession concerning boxing can be best achieved. I would take issue with the statement that "the number of deaths due to boxing is surprisingly low." The reported annual fatality of 13 per 100,000 participants is ten times that of football. The statement that "while head gear would cut down on lacerations and contusions of the face, it has been pointed out that by adding weight and surface irregularities to the head, blows could rotate the head more effectively, which would result in *more* brain damage" must be considered.—J.S. Torg, M.D.

Muscle Fiber Type Changes in Human Skeletal Muscle After Injuries and Immobilization

Tom Haggmark, Ejnar Eriksson, and Eva Jansson (Karolinska Hospital, Stockholm)
Orthopedics 9:181–185, February 1986   3–123

Immobilization of an extremity in a cast after an injury has a pronounced effect on the skeletal muscles of the extremity in question. A rapid atrophy takes place that varies between different muscle groups and even between different muscle fiber types. In earlier studies the authors have found a selective atrophy of the type I fibers after knee surgery and immobilization of the knee in 10-degree flexion. These studies also revealed signs of muscle fiber type changes in the immobilized musculature. Possible fiber type changes after immobilization were studied.

Eight male active athletes operated on for knee injuries were followed with muscle biopsies before and at various intervals after surgery and immobilization. A statistically significant change of the muscle fiber distribution was found. The percentage of type I fibers dropped from an average of 54% to 43%. One competitive cross-country skier showed a dramatic drop from 81% type I fibers at surgery to 58% type I fibers 6 weeks later. After beginning training he returned to 85% type I fibers. One athlete who had undergone surgry and had been immobilized for long periods several times showed a drastic difference in fiber type distribution between his two thighs with 20% type I fibers in the injured leg and 69% type I fibers in his uninjured leg. After 3 years of training, his fiber type composition in the injured leg returned toward the fiber type distribution of the uninjured thigh.

It is evident that muscle fiber type composition can change. The most probable reason for this is that the drastic change from hard sports training to nearly complete immobilization influences both the muscle itself and its innervation and causes this change of fiber types.

▶ An interesting study that the authors recognize "cannot fully prove the idea of transformation of fiber types from one type to another." Other possible explanations are that the changes seen may simply be due to the biopsies not having been taken at exactly the same depth. However, the suggestion that immobilization may be harmful not only by causing atrophy of the muscle but by causing fiber type changes deserves attention.—J.S. Torg, M.D.

Muscle Damage and Endurance Events
R.B. Armstrong (Univ. of Georgia)
Sports Med. 3:370–381, 1986   3–124

There long has been indirect evidence that exercise can injure skeletal muscle. Both soreness and increases in muscle enzymes and myoglobin attest to such damage. Direct histologic evidence of injury to muscle fibers has been obtained in animal studies, although little or no damage is noted in some studies of endurance exercise. The cause of delayed-onset muscular soreness continues to be uncertain.

A demand for adenosine triphosphate in muscle fibers in excess of production may dispose to injury of muscle cells through a cycle that involves impaired ability to extrude calcium ion from the cell. High levels of metabolite in muscle tissue during exercise may lead to injury and pain.

The mechanical strain hypothesis invokes structural damage, especially that which is related to eccentric exercise. Sarcolemmal lesions can explain the initiation of events that lead to necrosis of cells. Because the level of calcium ion is much higher interstitially than in the sarcoplasm of muscle fibers, any structural disruption of the cell membrane could allow calcium ion to move into the cell down its concentration gradient.

Maximal force is attenuated in injured muscles. Injury to fibers generally is considered to be a prerequisite to muscle adaptation in training. There is no direct evidence that medical treatment can prevent exercise-induced muscle injury or hasten the recovery of damaged muscles after exercise. The effect of calcium antagonists will be of interest. Long-term adverse effects from exercise-related muscle injury have not been demonstrated.

▶ An excellent review. The interested reader is referred to the original article.—J.S. Torg, M.D.

Physiological Differences Between Genders: Implications for Sports Conditioning
D.A. Lewis, E. Kamon, and J.L. Hodgson (Pennsylvania State Univ.)
Sports Med. 3:357–369, 1986
3–125

Wide differences in performance are found between the sexes, but many narrow or disappear when male and female subjects are matched for various characteristics. Little difference is apparent in the response to various modes of progressive resistance strength training. The sexes have similar relative gains in strength, and similar composition of muscle fiber types is evident within specific events. Less muscle hypertrophy is seen in women than in men. Conflicting results have been reported in studies of changes in body composition with strength training.

Central and peripheral cardiovascular adaptations to aerobic training are similar in men and women, but women generally have a lower oxygen-carrying capacity. Greater essential fat is a characteristic of women, and percentage of body fat accounts for some differences in comparably trained distance runners.

Men and women are capable of similar performance, and increases in maximal oxygen uptake are similar in men and women who are trained at the same intensity and duration. Menstrual phase is not a prominent factor in performance. The disadvantages associated with female subjects in the heat disappear when the sexes are matched for body fat and peak uptake of oxygen.

Aerobic exercise benefits both men and women, and gender differences should not influence the prescription of exercise. The prescription should be based on the physical work capacity of the individual. Women in general are less strong than men, especially in the upper body, which implies that special emphasis should be placed on upper body strength training for women.

▶ An excellent review. The interested reader is referred to the original article.—J.S. Torg, M.D.

Soft Tissue Fixation to Bone
Daniel B. Robertson, Dale M. Daniel, and Edmund Biden (Dallas)
Am. J. Sports Med. 14:398–403, September–October 1986
3–126

This study compares the strength of various soft tissue-to-bone fixation devices in fresh cadaveric knee joints. Broad and thin, narrow and cordlike, and thick tendinous tissues all were used in the studies, with the distal femur. The barbed and stone staples were compared with suture techniques, the screw with spiked plastic washer, and the screw with spiked soft tissue plate (Fig 3–48). Suture fixation was with No. 2 Mersilene or 0 Dexon suture material, using the Bunnell, modified Kessler, double-weave, and double-loop techniques.

Screws with spiked plastic washers and soft tissue plates proved superior

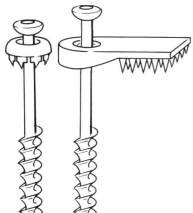

Fig 3–48.—Screw fixation techniques using the spiked plastic washer (*left*) and soft tissue fixation plate (*right*). (Courtesy of Robertson, D.B., Daniel, D.M., and Biden, E.: Am. J. Sports Med. 14:398–403, September–October 1986.)

for all tissue types. The stone staple gave the least desirable results in loading studies. With narrow, cordlike tissues, the screw with soft tissue plate was the best means of fixation. The screw with washer was best for fixing capsular or extensor-mechanism tissue.

If soft tissue fixation sites are exposed to cyclic loading, as in postoperative passive motion exercises, secure fixation is especially important. The best soft tissue fixation is obtained using the screw with spiked plastic washer and the screw with metallic soft tissue plate. Poorer results were obtained using the barbed staple or stone staple.

▶ The more recent practice of early motion after ligament repair and reconstruction makes this study most relevant. It was a well-designed biomechanical effort, the conclusions of which agree with this surgeon's impressions. However, several critical observations are forthcoming. A fifth of the fixation failures were due to the tissues tearing rather than tissue pull-out. The forces used to secure the various devices were not quantified. Also, the possibility of in vivo tissue necrosis was not addressed.—J.S. Torg, M.D.

Acute Soft Tissue Injuries: A Review of the Literature

John Kellett (Australian Inst. of Sport, Chandler, Australia)
Med. Sci. Sports Exerc. 18:489–500, October 1986   3–127

Soft tissue injuries are increasing, with greater participation in a more active life-style and with the use of more intensive training regimens by both men and women. The acute inflammatory phase, which may last for up to 72 hours, has both humoral and cellular components that act concurrently. The latter involve mast-cell degranulation and the release by granulocytes of factors, chiefly prostaglandins, that promote vasodilatation and chemotaxis. The repair phase, lasting from 48 hours up to 6 weeks, is characterized by collagen synthesis and deposition. In the remodeling phase, which may last a year or longer, collagen is modified to increase the functional capacity of tendons and ligaments to withstand imposed stresses.

Cryotherapy has been demonstrated to be useful in reducing pain and the period of disability following soft tissue injury. Heat application has come into disfavor. If possible, cryotherapy is administered within 24 hours of injury. Nonsteroidal anti-inflammatory drugs have been used increasingly, but they have adverse effects, some major. The drugs should be restricted to 3 days after injury. The use of injected steroids in chronic overuse injuries remains controversial, and few physicians recommend steroid therapy for acute soft tissue injuries. Dimethyl Sulfoxide is used less now than previously; definitive studies have proven difficult to perform. Various physical modalities are being used increasingly to treat soft tissue injuries. They include ultrasound application, transcutaneous electrical nerve stimulation, and electrical muscle stimulation.

Early mobilization has many advantages in cases of soft tissue injury. Rehabilitation generally should take place within the limits of pain. Stretching and warm-up are very important aspects of any rehabilitation program. In addition, cardiorespiratory fitness should be maintained. Isokinetic training is useful in promoting muscle strength. The particular rehabilitative measures used should be individualized.

▶ Some type of cryotherapy is the base upon which our treatment program is built. We use cold and compression in the initial stages to combat the effects of hemorrhaging and hypoxia of the uninjured tissue. We continue to use cryotherapy after the hemorrhaging has stopped for its analgesic effect. If pain can be reduced with cryotherapy, more and better exercise can be performed with a resultant increase in circulation with all of the concurrent beneficial effects. If total rehabilitation is achieved, then a reoccurrence of the injury can be avoided.

The author brought up a very interesting point on the use of NSAIDs and why use should be restricted to the first 3 days postinjury, the theory being that the repair process is an inflammatory process and the release of prostaglandins 3 days postinjury should not be interfered with.—F. George, A.T.C., P.T.

Reflex Sympathetic Dystrophy

Pedro Luis Escobar (Univ. of Arizona)
Orthop. Rev. 15:41–46, October 1986   3–128

Reflex sympathetic dystrophy is a disorder of the upper or lower extremities that is characterized by neurovascular disturbances and dystrophic changes of the skin, subcutaneous tissues, bones, and joints. Although early diagnosis and treatment result in prompt elimination of symptoms, reflex sympathetic dystrophies are frequently misdiagnosed or improperly treated. Such patients are then subjected to prolonged and sometimes permanent disability. The author reviews the etiology, clinical manifestations, diagnosis, pathogenesis, and treatment of this disorder.

The etiology of reflex sympathetic dsytrophy, also called shoulder-hand syndrome, remains unknown, but it is associated with multiple medical problems. Its onset can be acute, as observed in patients after trauma to the hand or arm, or delayed, as in patients with myocardial infarction or stroke. Signs and symptoms of the disorder include pain, swelling, reduced range of motion, muscle cramping and muscle atrophy, skin changes, and hyperesthesia. Abnormal laboratory findings include elevated erythrosedimentation rates seen in 70% of all cases, and increased uptake rates in bone scans.

Treatment includes the relief of pain, control of edema, mobilization of the extremity and gain in range of motion, biofeedback, stellate ganglion block with local anesthetics and ultrasound, corticosteroid administration, acupuncture, electrical stimulation, and the use of intravenous regional blocks. Therapeutic measures in late stages of the disorder include capsulotomy and manipulation under anesthesia.

Reflex Sympathetic Dystrophy of the Knee
Ronald Tietjien (Danbury, Conn.)
Clin. Orthop. 209:234–243, August 1986   3–129

Persistent pain around the knee presents a difficult diagnosis, despite careful history, and physical examination, and tests. The syndrome of reflex sympathetic dystrophy (RDS), characterized by excessive physiologic changes in and around a joint following injury, is seldom considered the diagnosis of unexplained knee pain. The author reports on the incidence of RSD in the knee joint and describes how to recognize the syndrome on a clinical basis.

The records of 67 patients with unexplained knee pain were reviewed retrospectively. The patients had undergone x-ray films, bone scans, blood tests, arthroscopy, and biopsy. Several had also undergone arthrotomy. Fourteen patients met the criteria for RSD and had complaints of pain, burning, and numbness sensations, stiffness, mechanical problems, and swelling.

At first, x-ray films were normal, but soon after the symptoms started, roentgenograms showed changes. All patients had osteoporosis in the patellofemoral joint. Bone scans were positive in two thirds of the patients, and were useful for diagnosis. Arthroscopy, but not arthrograms, were also useful.

The 14 patients with RSD were treated with nonsteroidal anti-inflammatory agents or oral steroids. Five received local anesthetic or steroid injections, although they effected only temporary relief. All patients underwent physical therapy, and a few wore braces.

A diagnosis of RSD was made on the basis of clinical examination, roentgenograms, and bone scans. Reflex sympathetic dystrophy is an uncommon and unrecognized source of knee pain brought on by minor trauma. Knowledge of this syndrome and use of arthroscopy to rule out major internal derangement of the knee will reduce the amount of surgery on these knees. Treatment is long lasting and necessitates excellent patient compliance; however, it does improve most knees affected with RSD.

▶ The occurrence of reflex sympathetic dystrophy (Abstracts 3–128 and 3–129) in the postarthroscopy patient has been identified as a problem by Ferkel and Lawley (*J. Bone Joint Surg.* [*Am.*] 68A:256–265, February 1986). In patients with pain without an apparent reason, atrophic changes, decreased bone mineralization, and increased technetium phosphate uptake should be highly suggestive of this problem. To be noted, management of patients with RSD can be exasperating for both patient and physician.—J.S. Torg, M.D.

Psychology of the Injured Athlete
Maureen R. Weiss and Richard K. Troxel (Univ. of Oregon, Eugene)
Athletic Training 21:104–110, 1986   3–130

Recently, the importance of psychological skills for achieving optimal performances in sport has been demonstrated by numbers of athletes at all levels. In the 1984 Olympics, there were many references to the relaxation, imagery, concentration, and confidence skills that were essential to the athletes' training and success. It appears that sport psychology for the elite athlete has taken center stage over the last few years. However, the role of psychology for the injured athlete has received little attention. The goal of the present paper was to discuss how injuries can exert an impact upon an athlete's self-perceptions, and to offer possible solutions in facilitating the rehabilitation process from a psychological perspective.

Injury itself is a stressor. The stress process begins with a situation or sensory stimulus, which can be an environmental (external) event, or it can be produced from internal processes. In the case of an athlete sustaining an injury, the injury itself is a stressor because it places a considerable demand and constraint on the body to adapt. The second step in the stress process is one's cognitive appraisal of the stressor and one's ability to cope with this demand. With regard to the onset of injury, a negative self-talk pattern may emerge in which the person's appraisal may be "What if I don't come back this season?" or "What will the coach think of me?" or "What if my teammates think I'm letting them down?". The emotional response which results from this appraisal is first manifested as physiological arousal, but can also include increased anxiety and worry over the injury. Finally, the fourth step in the stress process is the consequences, which can be performance-, health- or psychology-related. For example, the consequences could be chronic tension in the affected area, loss of appetite or sleep, lack of motivation, and adverse effects on the healing process.

There are multiple common problems among injured athletes, including negative self-talk patterns, negative emotions, somatic complaints, and the overwhelming responses to being unable to cope with the injury. Strategies under the athlete's control are needed to help him or her cope with the natural setbacks that occur during the rehabilitation process, and particularly needed are strategies in dealing with the injury in its early phases. To help athletes cope with injuries the authors recommend the Psychological Skills Training program, which consists of three phases: the educational phase, the skill development phase, and the practice phase. During the first phase, the rehabilitation program should be modified to fit the individual; in order for this to occur, it is necessary for athletic trainers to know their athletes' particular individual qualities, such as their trait anxiety, self-esteem, expectations, and self-motivation. In addition, the trainer should fully explain the effects of the injury to the athlete. During the skill development phase, the authors recommend teaching positive mental attitude, an injury support group, alternative channeling of energy, relaxation exercises. During the practice phase the athletes practice these techniques first under low stress conditions, and then under medium and high stress conditions.

An athletic trainer should become a partner with the athlete in the healing process by utilizing psychological principles and teaching coping skills.

▶ Athletic trainers must treat the mind as well as the body. Many athletes have a difficult time coping with an injury that keeps them from participation. The authors have recommended that we get to know the athlete to determine some of their psychological characteristics. We should also explain the injury and its ramifications to them. We should provide as much positive reinforcement as possible and teach the athlete to cope with the injury.—F. George, A.T.C., P.T.

4 Pediatric Sports Medicine

The Child and Exercise: An Overview
Jan Borms (Vrije Universiteit Belgium, Brussels)
J. Sports Sci. 4:3–20, Spring 1986   4–1

Exercise for children is a controversial and complex topic. On the one hand, organized sports and physical education exert a positive effect on children who are living in an urban environment with an increasingly sedentary way of life. On the other hand, it is thought that children may be harmed by sports competitions designed for and by adults.

The author accepts the premises that there is a need for exercise in our society and that exercise can make an important contribution to health and general well-being and examines the benefits from different types of exercise and the differences between children and adults in adaptive responses to exercise.

Not enough evidence was found to support the view that regular and intense physical training promotes an increase in body size, nor was there any physiologic evidence that severe training has any harmful effect on the body. Exercise capacity and aerobic power increase gradually throughout childhood. Studies have shown that children aged 10 years or younger do not react with the increased $\dot{V}O_{2max}$ that would be expected from endurance activities. In addition, the trainability of endurance seems to depend on the level of biologic maturity of growing children.

After puberty the effects of endurance training have been found to be similar to those observed for adults. However, it is not known how much physical activity is necessary or optimal during the growing years because individual variation is great. Even fewer data are available on the trainability of anaerobic capacity.

It appears that the child differs in some aspects from the adult and is comparable in others. The author recommends that the child should not be considered as an adult in miniature and notes that the same training principles may not always be applied to both. Parents should support their children when the children are ready for sports activities and should differentiate carefully between support and pressure.

Echocardiographic Findings in Children Participating in Swimming Training
R. Medved, V. Facečić-Sabadi, V. Medved (Zagreb Univ., Yugoslavia)
Int. J. Sports Med. 7:94–99, April 1986   4–2

It is well known that increased heart volume is one of the basic effects of systematic endurance training. However it has not been definitely established that systematic sports activities cannot damage a normal heart, and it is not clear at what age a child could be submitted to modern intensive methods of sports training. In adults the efficacy of sports training can be measured by following changes in the heart volume by echocardiography, but in children that is not as easily done because of the combination of growth and training-induced changes in heart volume. The goal of the present study was to determine whether systematic swimming training in children 8 to 14 years of age resulted in echocardiographically measurable changes of individual heart dimensions.

The study consisted of 72 children who systematically trained in swimming for at least one year, or an average of 29.2 months, and who underwent echocardiographic assessment. These results were compared with values obtained from 72 children of the same body area who did not actively engage in sports. It was found that values for left ventriular diameter, left atrium, and heart depth were statistically significantly increased with exercise. Although the values of septum thickness and left ventricular posterior wall were slightly larger, these values were not significant. The contractibility of the myocardium was within the limits of normal values.

Sports training in children results in an increase in echocardiographic dimensions including left ventricular interior diameter in systole, and diastole, diameter of the left atrium, and heart depth. The authors caution that in recording echocardiograms in children, it is necessary to establish whether the child actively engages in sports beforehand, since long-term training leads to changes in some heart structures, which may lead to incorrect conclusions that the finding is pathologic.

▶ Echocardiographic changes in response to sports training are clear in regard to four parameters: left ventricular interior increased diameter in systole; left ventricular increased diameter in diastole; left atrial diameter; and heart depth likewise. This is more pronounced with time. We do not know how long these changes would last in the absence of continued training. The general response is similar to the adult. These changes could be confused with primary congenital heart disease, but an in-depth history of sports participation prior to such studies should be a simple differentiation.—L.J. Krakauer, M.D.

Infant Swimming Classes: Immersed in Controversy
Brian Burd (Santa Barbara, Calif.)
Physician Sportsmed. 14:239–244, March 1986   4–3

Swimming programs that use forced infant submersion have become popular among parents who want their children to learn how to swim at an early age, either to safeguard them from drowning or to give them a head start in competitive events. However, medical authorities are concerned about the safety of this method. The policy statement on infant swimming programs approved by the American Academy of Pediatrics is shown in Figure 4–1.

AMERICAN ACADEMY OF PEDIATRICS
POLICY STATEMENT: INFANT SWIMMING PROGRAMS

There is little justification for infant "swimming" or water adjustment
programs. However, a growing number of programs promoting infant
swimming can be found across the country, and they claim a variety of
benefits such as enhancing parent-child communication and other
"values." Giardiasis transmission and water intoxication with seizures
make these programs somewhat hazardous. It is unlikely that infants
can be made "water safe"; in fact, the parents of these infants may
develop a false sense of security if they believe an infant can "swim"
a few strokes.

RECOMMENDATIONS

The American Academy of Pediatrics, in recognizing the increasing
popularity of swimming programs for infants and the enjoyment of the
parent and infant who share this activity, makes the following
recommendations:

1. A parent who enrolls an infant in a water adjustment program
should understand and accept the risks.

2. To reduce these risks, the programs should follow the national
YMCA guidelines which include prohibiting total submersion, maintaining
an appropriate water temperature, and providing measures to control
fecal contamination.

3. The swimming experience of each infant should be on a
one-to-one basis with a parent or responsible adult. Organized group
swimming instruction should be reserved for children more than three
years of age.

4. Instruction should be carried out by qualified instructors
familiar with infant cardiopulmonary resuscitation techniques in
properly maintained pools.

5. Infants with known medical problems should receive their
physician's approval before participation.

6. Studies of the frequency of risks to infants from water
adjustment programs should be carried out as soon as possible.

Fig 4–1.—Policy statement on infant swimming programs approved by the Council on Child and
Adolescent Health. © American Academy of Pediatrics. Reprinted with permission from AAP News 1985;
1(September):15. (Courtesy of Burd, B.: Physician Sports Med. 14:239–244, March 1986. Reprinted by
permission. A McGraw-Hill publication.)

The main issue in the debate about the safety of infant swimming centers
around the risk of hyponatremia. Although the statistical risk that hyponatremia will develop is not high, children younger than age 9 months
are especially vulnerable to it. Hyponatremia can occur when an infant
swallows excess water to the extent to which the serum sodium concentration is reduced. Symptoms can develop within minutes of a swimming
lesson or may slowly develop hours later. They include lethargy or restlessness, disorientation, weakness, nausea, vomiting, too much or too little
urination, seizures, and coma. In extreme cases, hyponatremia may cause
death.

Besides hyponatremia, infants in swimming classes are at risk of transmission of bacteria, parasites, and viruses through pool water. Acidic water
conditions may well erode dental enamel. Contrary to earlier opinion, it
is apparently safe for children with tympanotomy tubes or grommets to
participate in swimming events.

Several medical practitioners and water safety groups, including the California Medical Association and the YMCA, have taken a stand in favor of restricting or prohibiting forced infant submersion until children are ready to submerge themselves, usually after age 3 years.

▶ There was a great surge of popularity for forced infant submersion within the past few years in an attempt to either teach children early and safe swimming techniques, to make them feel comfortable in the water, or possibly in the sense of training for further competition. Excessive water ingestion, formally called infantile water intoxication, was then recognized as a possible and occasional occurrence, especially in those younger than 9 months. This risk of hyponatremia has caused a change in the official position on such swimming programs, headed by the American Academy of Pediatrics and joined by the YMCA group at the national level. Forced submersion is now not recommended. Fecal contamination is now recognized, with a potential for the spread of giardiasis from fecal contamination in the infant population.—L.J. Krakauer, M.D.

Assessment of Urinary Protein Excretion in the Adolescent: Effect of Body Position and Exercise
Mark T. Houser, Mary Frances Jahn, Ailan Kobayashi, and John Walburn (Univ. of Nebraska)
J. Pediatr. 109:556–561, September 1986   4–4

Postural proteinuria is common among school-aged children, especially adolescents. Identification of isolated proteinuria may lead to expensive

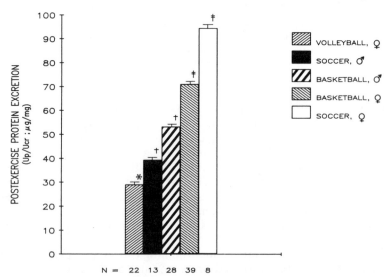

Fig 4–2.—Postexercise protein excretion in male and female student athletes. Values are means ± SEM. Groups with same symbol were not significantly different. (Courtesy of Houser, M.T., et al.: J. Pediatr. 109:556–561, September 1986.)

SENSITIVITY, SPECIFICITY, AND FALSE POSITIVE AND FALSE
NEGATIVE RATES WHEN URINE DIPSTICK WAS USED TO
EVALUATE PROTEINURIA

	Sensitivity (%)	Specificity (%)	False positive (%)	False negative (%)
Group 1*	54.8	93.2	6.8	45.2
Group 2†	73.7	90.7	9.3	26.3

*Calculations based on assumptions that Up/Ucr ≤ 79.4 (95th percentile for recumbent excretion) is normal and that dipstick results of trace or negative are normal.

†Calculations based on assumptions that Up/Ucr ≤ 122.3 (95th percentile for upright excretion) is normal and that dipstick results of trace or negative are normal.
(Courtesy of Houser, M.T., et al.: J. Pediatr. 109:556–561, September 1986.)

and cumbersome investigation, although it has been documented that qualitative and quantitative determinations of protein excretion are prone to significant error due to the problem of obtaining timed urine samples. Moreover, only limited data are available on physiologic proteinuria in the child or adolescent, especially during recumbency.

The authors assessed the effects of body position and exercise on urinary protein excretion in healthy adolescents and calculated reference data for urinary protein to creatinine (Up/Ucr) ratios, which can be used to assess quantitative protein excretion. The adequacy of the urine dipstick as a tool for evaluation of asymptomatic proteinuria was also examined.

The study was performed on 116 healthy adolescents with no history of renal or systemic disease. Random urine samples were examined under defined conditions of recumbency and after both ambulation and exercise during a single day.

The Up/Ucr ratio was significantly higher in girls during recumbency, but no differences in Up/Ucr ratios were found between girls and boys in the upright or postexercise urine samples (Fig 4–2). A progressive increase in protein excretion was found in the upright and postexercise samples. There was wide variability in Up/Ucr ratios, especially in the upright and postexercise samples. The urine dipstick was less sensitive than the Up/Ucr ratio in determining abnormal degrees of recumbent proteinuria (table).

Body position and exercise affect protein excretion significantly. The Up/Ucr ratio in recumbent and upright urine samples is a useful tool for evaluation of proteinuria.

▶ Using the Up/Ucr ratios is a more sophisticated and (I assume) more expensive way of assessing urinary protein excretion, and will provide a quantitative measurement. However, serially negative urinary dipstick immediately following or during recumbency should be sufficient if the presence of urinary protein has been questioned on prior observation. This is a methodical study of the problem.—L.J. Krakauer, M.D.

Pediatric and Adolescent Sports Injuries: Recent Trends

Lyle J. Micheli

Exerc. Sport Sci. Rev. 14:359–374, 1986
4–5

The incidence of sports injuries in young athletes appears to be on the increase. There is no consensus about why this is so or about what can be done to prevent it. The author analyzes the types of sports injury encountered in pediatric practice and discusses ways to prevent such injuries.

Overuse injuries are the result of repetitive work or repetitive sports activities. Formerly, overuse injuries were seen primarily in adults such as construction workers or weekend tennis players who had bursitis or tendinitis. Children used to be mostly involved in recreational play, sometimes resulting in acute macrotrauma injuries such as fractures of the long bones and axial skeleton, sprains of joint ligaments or muscle tendons, and contusions of muscle-tendon units and overlying soft tissue. However, children now increasingly participate in repetitive sports training and frequently incur the same type of repetitive microtrauma injuries as adults.

Overuse injuries of the knee are extremely common and warrant special concern. They usually involve the extensor mechanism, at the site of insertion on the tibia (Osgood-Schlatter disease), the patellar tendon (tendinitis), or the patella itself. Once it has been determined which tissues have been injured, the source of injury should be investigated to prevent recurrence. Injuries can result from such factors as errors in training, poor technique, and type of shoes worn. Overuse injuries of the elbow are frequent in young pitchers as a result of repetitive valgus strain applied to the elbow by throwing.

Many sports injuries in children can be prevented by careful assessment of the child sports candidate. Physical examination should include an evaluation of fitness or lack of it. When a child is not sufficiently fit to participate safely in a particular sport, a prescription of strengthening, stretching, or aerobic exercises may be indicated. Special protective equipment may also be needed in certain cases. Ultimately, it is the quality of adult coaching and supervision that will contribute to a reduction in sports injuries in children.

▶ Sports injuries are increasing in young athletes, and the tenfold incidence of increase in the Boston Children's Hospital experience is impressive. The random injury in sports, regrettable though it may be, has always been more or less accepted. The second type of injury relating to overuse injuries and the consequence of repetitive training and repetitive microtrauma overstressed by training is the important aspect of this review. That it may occur in swimming as well as in direct contact sports is the significant observation. In children there is a greater susceptibility to overuse injury because of the presence of growth tissue, growth cartilage and the growth process itself. The author demonstrated growth cartilage present at three different sites: growth plate, joint surface, and the sites of muscle-tendon insertion, the apophysis.—L.J. Krakauer, M.D.

Iselin's Disease

Richard C. Lehman, John R. Gregg, and Elisabeth Torg (Univ. of Pennsylvania)
Am. J. Sports Med. 14:494–496, 1986   4–6

Iselin's disease is an uncommon disorder occurring in athletic children during the rapid growth period. Sports such as roller skating and ballet may put great stress on the forefoot resulting in inversion injury and swelling in the region of the proximal fifth metatarsal. Pain occurs over the lateral side of the foot with weight-bearing activity. Onset of pain may be chronic or develop insidiously over several months. Radiographs show enlargement of the apophysis or irregular, fragmented ossification patterns and/or widening of the chondro-osseous junction.

Initial therapy consists of rest to reduce the stress reaction and inflammation. A cast may be used in severe cases but crutches or interdiction of activities such as running or jumping can be effective. Ice is applied and oral anti-inflammatory drugs may be prescribed. When the tenderness is resolved, rehabilitation commences with stretching exercises on the uniplanar wobble board followed by progressive resistance exercises. The patient is then put on high-stress activities such as jumping and cutting. If discomfort is tolerable, the child is allowed to participate, but if pain and limping ensue, the activity is temporarily suspended.

In Iselin's disease, there is considerable variation regarding the severity and duration of the syndrome complex. Therapy must be strictly adhered to to prevent recurrent symptoms; however, the symptoms will always resolve when ossification is completed.

▶ For those unfamiliar with the condition, this is a traction apophysitis occurring at the base of the fifth metatarsal and occurring during a period of rapid growth in both sexes where sports tend to put a great deal of stress on the forefoot. The problem relates to the timing of ossification of this apophysis. This is a new syndrome in our literature and is offered as a marker for the future.—L.J. Krakauer, M.D.

Bicycle Helmet Use by Children: Knowledge and Behavior of Physicians

Barry D. Weiss and Burris Duncan (Univ. of Arizona, Tucson)
Am. J. Public Health 76:1022–1023, August 1986   4–7

Bicycle riding causes approximately 1,300 deaths each year in the United States, and nearly half of these deaths occur in children younger than 14 years. Although it is generally agreed that the use of bicycle helmets reduces the incidence of injury and death, less than 2% of elementary, junior high, and senior high students wear them. Therefore, it would seem appropriate that physicians include information on bicycle safety and helmet use in the routine care of their patients.

To assess whether physicians were aware of the importance of bicycle-related head injury and whether they provided education about bicycle safety, 161 pediatricians and family physicians were asked to fill out a questionnaire. Of 106 responses, most seemed well informed on bicycle-related death and injury. Most were aware that less than 5% of children wear bicycle helmets and lack of parental awareness was given as the reason. However, 40% of the physicians said that they never discussed bicycle safety and 29% said that they did not discuss it during well-child care.

The results of this study suggest that many physicians do not educate their patients in bicycle safety. Discussion of helmet use with parents of young grade school children might be appropriate since long-term habits can be instilled at this age. Helmet use could also be discussed with junior high school students as the death rates from bicycle injury are the highest in this group.

► I would guess that peer compliance or a failure thereof is the basic problem in use of bicycle helmets. Until this becomes mandatory law, it is not likely to change as a pattern. Physician participation in the discussion is welcome and may surely be helpful, but I don't think it is the critical factor in the problem, dealing with an activity that has an appalling number of deaths each year in this country, almost half of which occur in the under-14 age group.—L.J. Krakauer, M.D.

Evaluating the Potential Pediatric Scuba Diver
Mark Lawrence Dembert and Julian Faison Keith III (Navy Environmental Health Ctr., Norfolk, Va., and Uniformed Services Univ. of the Health Sciences, Bethesda, Md.)
Am. J. Dis. Child. 140:1135–1141, November 1986   4–8

The authors believe that rigorous standards should be applied to pediatric scuba diver applicants and that minimum age requirements for entry into this course should be over 12 years. The diver is subjected to changes in ambient pressure, the physical demands of swimming in currents, adapting to temperature extremes and situations requiring the use of sound judgment and maintaining composure. If medical problems supervene at sea, the diver is isolated from routinely available emergency services on land.

Two diving problems are barotrauma and decompression sickness. Problems in the middle-ear spaces and paranasal sinuses account for the highest morbidity among divers. If the pressures across the tympanic membrane or sinus ostia cannot be equalized, an entrapment results which can lead to sinus pain and discharge into the middle ear cavity. Pulmonary over-inflation syndromes represent a spectrum of serious barotraumatic medical conditions resulting from overinflation and subsequent alveoli rupture. The latter only occur during ascent, especially while close to the water surface.

Air leakage into the intrapleural, intravascular, or interstitial spaces which can lead to pneumothorax, mediastinal, or subcutaneous emphysema can be treated as for nondiving situations. Air embolism is more serious, since a number of organs can be affected and it requires life support measures with hyperbaric oxygen therapy.

The partial pressure of nitrogen in the compressed air that is breathed by the diver can result in a high amount of nitrogen being absorbed. Slow ascent with several stops are needed prior to surfacing otherwise a tendency toward supersaturation of the tissues with nitrogen can occur, which results in N_2 bubbles that can lead to intravascular or extravascular obstruction of blood flow or pressure on tissue. Symptoms can present from minutes to hours after the dive.

The physician must ensure that the child or adolescent has the basic requisite physical and psychological attributes. The equipment should be appropriately sized. The diver should be in overall excellent health, weigh at least 45 kg, and have a minimum height of 150 cm. The applicant should feel comfortable swimming distances of up to 500 m, have good vision, and be able to use valsalva maneuver techniques.

There should be no sign of obstructive or restrictive disorders such as pulmonary or cardiovascular diseases. Drugs that alter the state of consciousness or the body's response to stress also should disqualify the individual. Hemoglobin, hematocrit, urinalysis, and a baseline chest x-ray are recommended for screening.

▶ Diving, with its open-ended potential for exposure, demands intelligence, sophistication, maturity, and some physical skill. There is a dinosaur school of thought, to which I think I subscribe, that would state that scuba is not a childhood sport and that for the simple reasons of safety, basic certification should come at the age at which one applies to drive an automobile or pilot an aircraft. Unfortunately, this remains a point for philosophic debate alone in a highly unregulated sport activity.—L.J. Krakauer, M.D.

5 Women in Sports

Women in Sports: The Price of Participation
Carol Potera (Ketchum, Idaho)
Physician Sportsmed. 14:149–153, June 1986   5–1

As women have been accepted in new sports and have developed more aggressiveness in participating in the old standbys, they have become increasingly vulnerable to certain types of injury.

It has been found that female athletes have more patellofemoral problems and bunions than male athletes. In part these problems can be attributed to inadequate training of female athletes. Unlike male athletes who start training at younger ages and train year-round, female athletes tend to start later and to train less frequently during the off-season. It is suggested that women are especially vulnerable to injury at the start of the season, when many return to play weighing 5 to 10 lb more than they did at the end of the previous season.

Another prime time for injury is at the transition from high school to college sports, because the intensity, frequency, and duration of training are more intense at the college level. Socialization and lack of skill are also thought to contribute to the female injury rate, partly because women have not yet learned how to be violent in their own defense. However, more basic than sociocultural conditioning is genetic endowment, which may also provide an explanation for some injuries.

Specifically, anatomy and heredity place women at a greater risk than men for bunions and for patellofemoral pain. Bunions are a congenital disorder and can be avoided by wearing wider shoes and spreading a muscle rub on the inflamed toe area. The increased incidence of patellofemoral pain occurs because women have wide hips, which produce a greater Q angle that causes the kneecap to slide laterally (the Q angle measures the relationship between a line drawn down the femur in the direction of the quadriceps pull and another line drawn up the tibia from the tibial tuberosity; the two lines intersect at the midpatellar region).

To prevent injury women need to be more aggressive at training year-round to improve speed, power, endurance, and strength. Only then can the relationship between conditioning and prevention of injury be better examined and the relationship between conditioning and athletic performance be demonstrated.

▶ Maybe more important than year-around training beginning at the high school level for athletes only, our society should spend more time, money, and effort in getting our younger children involved in conditioning type activities at the preschool and elementary school levels. Both boys and girls need this, but the girls will benefit the most.—Col. J.L. Anderson, PE.D.

Should Women Go Easy on Exercise?

Terry Monahan (Minneapolis)
Physician Sportsmed. 14:188–197, December 1986   5–2

Because of recent press coverage, some women may get the idea that exercise is not good for them. The most recent controversy surrounded the release of "Safety Guidelines for Women Who Exercise" by the American College of Obstetricians and Gynecologists. The guidelines are based on the American College of Sports Medicine formula and recommends 15 to 60 minutes of aerobic activity, three to five times per week at 60% to 90% of aerobic capacity.

The guidelines represent minimal levels of exertion to maintain minimum levels of fitness. They were not intended for elite athletes. Certainly, a desire to exercise more than the guidelines suggest should be encouraged, especially since women do not appear to be more likely to experience injury than men. However, elite female athletes often experience amenorrhea. This can contribute to bone loss.

It is important for women to exercise. There is nothing wrong with exercising even beyond the standards set by fitness guidelines.

▶ My concern with this type of article is that it appears that the only exercise that is necessary is aerobic in nature with little regard for maintaining the muscle tone of muscles not normally used in running. The skeletal muscles must be exercised or they will atrophy. For example, many runners have developed low back pain and have been told or determined for themselves that it is as a result of their running. This is only partly accurate. Running itself does not cause low back pain. Failing to strengthen or stretch the muscles of the back most often is the cause of back pain. Runners do not exercise the muscles of the back, and eventually back pain will result. However, this is not only true for runners, but for all of us. At West Point, we have developed an exercise routine, using a "backboard," which we have found to be extremely valuable in treating low back pain. Exercise is valuable for all of us, men and women, but we need to be certain that we are talking about balanced exercise programs if we want to reduce the risk of exercise-related injuries.—Col. J.L. Anderson, PE.D.

Female Athletes: Targets for Drug Abuse
Marty Duda, Assistant Editor of *The Physician and Sportsmedicine*
Physician Sportsmed. 14:142–146, June 1986   5–3

Today, as more female athletes are being recognized and rewarded for their athletic achievements, there is a much greater emphasis on winning than ever before. Drug abuse among female athletes has nearly equalled that of the male athlete, and in fact, more frequent regular use of alcohol, cigarettes, and caffeine is reported in women.

Some of the primary reasons for drug abuse in female athletes are role conflict between femininity and athletic prowess that leads to abuse of anabolic steroids to enhance performance; the "thin is in" body image and ensuing eating disorders; the conditioned desire to please men (the coaches); and the desire to delay maturation to preserve athletic talent. Female athletes have also been drawn into the traditional use of alcohol in victory and defeat.

Discouraging drug abuse in women is important and could begin with implementation of courses designed to help maximize athletic potential. Other courses in subjects, such as imagery, goal setting, and relaxation could be offered as well. The athletes and their coaches should be educated regarding the destructive side effects and long-term effects of drug abuse. Top female athletes, the role models of society, should be encouraged to speak about drug issues. At present these preventive measures are not used extensively, but they show great potential.

▶ As with men, drugs should have no place in athletic competition by women. It is unfortunate that some of them are following the road previously travelled by men. Drug testing must be a part of all major competitions and the users must be disqualified and, if caught a second time, barred for life from competition.—Col. J.L. Anderson, PE.D.

A Comparison of Anterior and Posterior Cruciate Ligament Laxity Between Female and Male Basketball Players
Carol L. Weesner, Majorie J. Albohm, and Merrill A. Ritter (Indianapolis)
Physician Sportsmed. 14:149–154, May 1986   5–4

Several studies have described the type and severity of injuries that basketball players sustain, and it has been shown that female players experience significantly more knee injuries, specifically injuries to the anterior cruciate ligament (ACL), than do male players. Before objective biomechanical testing was available for determining the laxity of knee ligaments several investigators claimed that female players had greater laxity. However, these conclusions were based on subjective flexibility tests.

The authors used an arthrometer to measure the laxity of the ACLs and the posterior cruciate ligaments (PCLs) in the knees of 54 female and 36 male noninjured basketball players and compared the results. With mean leg flexion of 25 degrees and 70 degrees there were no significant differences in laxity of the ACL nor were there significant right-left differences. The differences in the PCL were not observed to be consistent.

Inadequate conditioning rather than laxity may be the major factor in the higher incidence of knee injuries in female basketball players. If this is the case, the authors recommend adequate preseason and in-season conditioning programs to correct this deficiency.

▶ Active women sports participants, including basketball players, do suffer a higher rate of knee injuries than do men who play similar or the same sports. It makes sense that good conditioning programs, off-season and in-season, should be used by coaches who are concerned for the welfare of their athletes. Here at West Point we use isokinetic knee extension and flexion exercises as a part of our "knee spread" program.—Col. J.L. Anderson, PE.D.

Pubic Stress Symphysitis in a Female Distance Runner
James F. Rold and Betty Ann Rold (St. Mary's Med. Ctr., Evansville, Ind., and Indiana Univ., Bloomington)
Physician Sportsmed. 14:61–65, June 1986   5–5

Osteitis pubis is a general term that has been used to describe several disorders of the pubic symphysis. Pubic stress symphysitis, a more specific term, refers to the painful, nonseptic inflammatory condition that occurs in runners and other endurance athletes. The authors describe the diagnosis and management of a female distance runner who had pubic stress symphysitis.

Woman, 30, complained of acute pain in the region of the pubic symphysis that radiated into the adductor muscles bilaterally and into the lower abdomen. The patient had felt some pubic discomfort 6 months before the episode of acute pain, but she had continued her training which included running 75 miles per week and a Nautilis weight-training program. Physical examination revealed marked bilateral focal pubic symphyseal tenderness and pain on abduction and extension of both thighs. Pressure on either side of the pubic symphysis was found to cause pain but no motion or click. Results of all laboratory studies were negative. Approximately 1 year earlier she had been examined for a suspected but nonexistent discrepancy in leg length and at that time a film was taken. The repeat film that was taken on presentation revealed areas of sclerosis on both sides of the pubic symphysis. In addition a radionuclide bone scan showed increased activity on both sides of the pubic symphysis. The patient was treated with indomethacin and complete rest. Approximately 18 months after presentation she resumed light training and has had no recurrence of symptoms.

A clear and precise diagnosis of pubic stress symphysitis can be made with certainty by using physical findings, laboratory analysis, and films and radionuclide bone scans. The correct diagnosis and proper course of therapy are crucial in order to rehabilitate these patients.

▶ The authors make an excellent point that cases of pubic ramus stress fracture and adductor tendon avulsion injury should be clearly differentiated from stress-related osteitis pubis (pubic stress symphysis) because the duration of therapy is substantially longer for stress-related osteitis pubis. At West Point, we have experienced cases of pubic ramus stress fracture with young women who are not competitive runners or endurance athletes, but who have gone from being relatively inactive to participating in a daily exercise program that includes running. We have not experienced the same pubic ramus stress fractures with men participating in the daily conditioning programs.—Col. J.L. Anderson, PE.D.

How I Manage Exercise-Related Menstrual Disturbances

Mona M. Shangold (Georgetown Univ.)
Physician Sportsmed. 14:113–120, March 1986   5–6

Irregular menses and amenorrhea are not uncommon among those women who exercise heavily. All women who stop menstruating for 2 months or who menstruate irregularly should be examined, regardless of exercise status. Anovulation and hypoestrogenism are the two major conditions experienced by such women. Chronic anovulation has been associated with endometrial hyperplasia and adenocarcinoma. Hypoestrogenic women are at increased risk for developing osteoporosis.

All oligomenorrheic and amenorrheic women require a physical examination, including a pelvic examination, and blood tests. Blood tests should measure serum prolactin to screen for hyperprolactemia, thyrotropin, thyroxine, triiodothyronine resin uptake, follicle-stimulating hormone and LH, and beta-human chorionic gonadotropin. Hyperprolactinemia and hypothyroidism require specific evaluation and treatment. Pregnancy requires further care. Ovarian failure in a patient younger than 30 years requires a blood karyotype.

Women who are producing estrogen but not progesterone should be treated with 10 days of medroxyprogesterone acetate, 10 mg per day, every month. Women who produce neither should be treated with a 25-day course of conjugated estrogens in addition to the medroxyprogesterone. Any woman who does not want a pregnancy should be using contraception, even if she has irregular or absent menses.

▶ This author, Mona M. Shangold, has studied, written, and taught more about managing exercise-related menstrual disturbances than anyone else I know of. We should all listen to her and follow her advice.—Col. J.L. Anderson, PE.D.

The Acute Effects of Exercise on Prolactin and Growth Hormone Secretion: Comparison Between Sedentary Women and Women Runners With Normal and Abnormal Menstrual Cycles

Frank E. Chang, William G. Dodds, Marty Sullivan, Moon H. Kim, and William B. Malarkey (Univ. Hosp., Columbus, Ohio)
J. Clin. Endocrinol. Metab. 62:551–556, March 1986   5–7

Menstrual irregularities, such as oligomenorrhea, amenorrhea, and luteal phase deficiencies are often seen in female runners. Physical exercise is known to induce transient changes in peripheral hormone concentrations, and some hormones, including PRL and GH, are known to increase during exercise. Changes in these hormonal concentrations might contribute to the development of menstrual dysfunction.

The responses of PRL and GH to acute exercise were compared in nonrunners, and in women runners with normal and abnormal menstrual cycles. Twenty women (mean age, 25.8 years) participated in the study.

Five of the runners were eumenorrheic, four oligomenorrheic, and six amenorrheic. There were five normal sedentary women. On day 1, the women exercised on a bicycle ergometer. The workload was increased every 2 minutes until exhaustion ensued. On day 2, only submaximal aerobic exercise was given. On day 1, all of the running groups experienced peak PRL levels at 2 and 5 minutes after exercise and the sedentary women showed no increase. On day 2, no significant increase in PRL levels were observed in any of the groups. Levels of GH on day 1 were highest in the running groups at 2 and 5 minutes after exercise. The oligomenorrheic runners had the highest levels, and the nonrunners showed no significant elevation of GH. On day 2, no increase in GH levels were observed in any of the groups with the submaximal exercise. No significant changes were seen in LH, FSH or E_2 levels during either the maximal or submaximal exercises in any of the groups.

We have demonstrated that exercise is not a consistent stimulator of PRL and that a threshold of exertional effort must be achieved to stimualte transient elevations of PRL and GH in well-conditioned runners. It is not known if these elevated levels contribute to menstrual dysfunction in women runners.

▶ The authors have stated that "a threshold of exercise intensity exists that must be achieved before a significant increase in prolactin (PRL) or growth hormone (GH) secretion occurs in women runners and that serum PRL and GH in the nonrunning group did not increase significantly even in response to acute maximal exercise." Therefore the difference appears to be between well-conditioned women and sedentary women. The PRL and GH responses were similar in the running groups regardless whether they were experiencing normal or abnormal menstrual cycles. That is the reason for the last sentence in the abstract as written above. (And the search goes on!)—Col. J.L. Anderson, PE.D.

Amenorrhea in the Adolescent Athlete: Exploration of a Growing Phenomenon

Iris F. Litt (Stanford Univ.)
Postgrad. Med. 80:245–247, 250, 253, October 1986   5–8

As the number of women who participate in athletic activities increases, so does the incidence of menstrual abnormalities, including amenorrhea. Studies have shown that 20% of exercising women and 50% of endurance athletes experience menstrual problems. At present, most of the studies have been conducted in adult women whose menstrual cycles were well established prior to their participation in sports. The few studies conducted in adolescents have revealed delays in pubertal development and menarche.

Although the mechanisms responsible for amenorrhea and delayed puberty in adolescents are unknown, some hypotheses have been suggested. All in some way implicate interference in the mechanisms which control interactions along the pineal-hypothalamic-pituitary-ovarian axis; such interference results in estrogen and progesterone deficiency. Low body fat and weight were thought to delay menses and cause other menstrual abnormalities, but normal menstrual function has been observed in athletes with as little as 4% body fat. Furthermore, a forced period of inactivity in previously amenorrheic athletes prompted return of menses even though neither weight nor body fat increased. Weight loss, anorexia and stress have also been implicated in menstrual disturbances. A characteristic body type such as that seen in runners seems to be associated with vigorous activity and delayed puberty.

Amenorrhea in adolescents resulting from athletic activity is cause for concern, as it may predispose them to ovarian and endometrial cancer, osteoporosis and even pregnancy in those who assume that infertility is associated with amenorrhea. Therapy of amenorrhea and its consequences includes the administration of progesterone as well as calcium supplements. A 10% reduction in exercise frequency and intensity or a rest period of 2 months may also be beneficial.

▶ This report stresses that delay in menarche and other menstrual problems experienced by athletes may result from low body weight or body fat, weight loss, of *emotional* or physical stress. I emphasize "emotional" because we have found that within our population of women at West Point we can rule out all of the other causes except the emotional stress and, except for a few, the physical stress. This report also explains the process of self-selection by young women athletes which seems to make sense. Anyone who is involved with sports medicine or is treating or coaching women athletes, especially adolescents, should read this entire report.—Col. J.L. Anderson, PE.D.

The Effect of Cycle Phase on the Adolescent Swimmers
J. Brooks-Gunn, Janine M. Gargiulo, and Michele P. Warren (Univ. of Pennsylvania; Univ. of Virginia, Charlottesville; and Columbia Univ.)
Physician Sportsmed. 14:182–192, March 1986   5–9

Although the possible effects of the phase of the menstrual cycle on the motor, cognitive, and academic performance of female subjects have been studied extensively, the conclusions are controversial. With the large number of studies on the effect on performance it is surprising that so little information exists on the potential links between the phase of the cycle and athletic performance. The authors hypothesize that cycle phase may be more likely to affect athletic rather than cognitive or psychologic performance because some women experience physical changes, particularly premenstrual water retention and menstrual cramps or breast tenderness, or both.

To examine the relationship between performance and the phase of the menstrual cycle the authors recorded performance times of six postmenarcheal adolescent swimmers who competed on national junior and senior levels during a 12-week period.

The fastest times for the 100-yard freestyle and 100-yard best event occurred during the menstrual phase and the slowest times occurred during the premenstrual phase. The symptoms were assessed biweekly with the Moos Menstrual Distress Questionnaire. The subjects reported feeling better during menstruation than premenstruation, and none reported dysmenorrhea. According to basal body temperature, five of ten cycles were clearly biphasic, 2 were monophasic, and 3 were possibly biphasic with very short luteal phases.

These results, albeit from a small sample, suggest that the phase of the menstrual cycle may affect athletic performance as measured by practice times.

▶ This study raises some excellent questions which need to be addressed by using larger samples and times during actual competition rather than practice times. No doubt the ages and experiences of the athletes must also be considered. Some women athletes are attempting to improve their competitive times by modifying the phase of their menstrual cycle using birth control drugs or other methods. With the knowledge from the available research, they may be wasting their efforts unless they carefully study their performances in relation to their cycles. We also do not know whether there will be long-range medical implications to these attempts to modify the cycle for athletic performance purposes.—Col. J.L. Anderson, PE.D.

Conditioning Exercise Decreases Premenstrual Symptoms: A Prospective Controlled Three Month Trial
J.C. Prior, Y. Vigna, and N. Alojada (Univ. of British Columbia, Vancouver, Canada)
Eur. J. Appl. Physiol. 55:349–355, August 1986   5–10

This study tests the hypothesis that premenstrual symptoms can be decreased during a 3-month program of increasing conditioning exercise in eight women. Six sedentary women composed the control group.

Molimina did not change over the 3 months in the control group. The exercise group showed decreases in overall molimina. Menstrual cycle lengths, body weight, and midluteal estrogen and progesterone levels did not change.

Moderate exercise significantly decreased premenstrual symptoms, without significant changes in weight, hormonal, or menstrual cycle. This study provides preliminary evidence that molimina can be altered by conditioning exercise.

▶ This information should come as a surprise to very few of us. Dr. Evylyn Gendel reported on this in the early 1970s. However, valuable information frequently gets filed away and we forget about it. Here it is again!—Col. J.L. Anderson, PE.D.

Women Athletes With Menstrual Irregularity Have Increased Musculo-skeletal Injuries

Tom Lloyd, Steven J. Triantafyllou, Elizabeth R. Baker, Peter S. Houts, James A. Whiteside, Alexander Kalenak, and Paul G. Stumpf (Pennsylvania State Univ., Hershey, and Jersey Shore Med. Cntr.)
Med. Sci. Sports. Exerc. 18:374–379, August 1986   5–11

Studies have shown a link between intensive exercise and menstrual dysfunction. This article examines the hypothesis that exercise-induced hypoestrogenism might lead to increased musculoskeletal injuries using a retrospective study.

Menstrual and running histories were collected for women running a 10-km race. Of the respondents to the questionnaire, 39% had interrupted their running program for at least 3 months, usually because of injury. These runners were also more likely to have irregular menses and less likely to have been using oral contraceptives than those that had been able to run continuously.

The sports medicine records of 207 women athletes were reviewed. In this group, x-ray–confirmed fractures occurred in 9% of athletes with regular menses and in 24% of female athletes with irregular or absent menses. Data from a larger group of recreational runners confirmed these findings.

The women athletes who are more likely to be injured are those with irregular menses and those who do not use oral contraceptives. Premenopausal women who engage in vigorous exercise programs and do not have regular menses are at an increased risk for musculoskeletal injury.

▶ This is the first time I have seen an attempt to test the hypothesis that exercise-induced hypoestrogenism can lead to an increased risk of bone injury. Most studies have dealt with the potential risks of osteoporosis sometime in the future. The data from this study are interesting and if they can be replicated with other studies may even be compelling. We may have a more immediate problem than we are aware.—Col. J.L. Anderson, PE.D.

Bone Mineral Density After Resumption of Menses in Amenorrheic Athletes

Barbara Drinkwater, Karen Nilson, Susan Ott, and Charles H. Chestnut III (Pacific Med. Ctr. and Univ. of Washington, Seattle)
JAMA 256:380–382, July 18, 1986   5–12

Decreased vertebral bone mineral density among young amenorrheic athletes has been demonstrated when compared to that of athletes with normal cycles. It has been presumed that the factor responsible for the lower bone mineral density is the low level of circulating estrogen observed in these women. Similar effects on bone mass have been observed in other hypoestrogenic states. Whether or not this represents an irreversible loss of bone or a treatable temporary condition is not understood.

Nine athletes were retested after 1 year to determine whether resumption of normal cycles after an extended period of amenorrhea was sufficient stimulus to affect bone mass. Mean duration of amenorrhea in the group was 40.4 months. Seven of the women had regained menses within 1 to 10 months of initial testing, and two remained amenorrheic. They were compared with seven eumenorrheic athletes of similar physical characteristics and training. Single- and dual-photon absorptiometry were used to measure regional bone mass at the distal radius and lumbar vertebrae (L-1 through L-4). The seven women who regained menses showed a significant increase in density of the lumbar vertebrae (.071 gm/sq cm) while the two women who remained amenorrheic showed a further decrease in density. No change was observed at this site in the cyclic group. However, the cyclic women continued to maintain a significantly higher vertebral bone mass density (1.369 gm/sq cm) than the women who regained menses (1.198 gm/sq cm).

The results of this study confirm previous findings that vertebral bone density is highest in cyclic athletes followed by cyclic nonathletes with the lowest scores reported in amenorrheic athletes.

▶ This study is important because it demonstrates that recovery from the effects of secondary amenorrhea cyplors to be possible when menses resumes. The importance of the study goes beyond competitive athletes because the secondary amenorrhea can occur when young women increase their exercise intensity, or experience added stress beyond what they are familiar with. For example, at West Point we have had over 90% of the young women who enter as plebes (freshmen) experience secondary amenorrhea that, for some, has lasted for over a year. Is it possible that many college freshmen women at other schools experience the same thing?—Col. J.L. Anderson, PE.D.

Lack of Influence of the Menstrual Cycle on Blood Lactate
Linda S. Lamont (Cleveland Metropolitan Gen. Hosp.)
Physician Sportsmed. 14:159–163, November 1986   5–13

It has been reported that the performance of female athletes varies with the phases of the menstrual cycle. To determine whether there are changes in energy metabolism that correlate with the phases of the menstrual cycle, the response of blood lactate to 60 minutes of moderate intensity exercise was examined during the early follicular stage and during the midluteal phase of the menstrual cycle in five inactive and four active females.

Lactate increased during exercise in both phases of the cycle in both groups. It did not change significantly between the two phases examined. The menstrual cycle appears not to exert an effect on blood lactate concentration during moderate exercise. A systematic study is required to determine if intensity and duration of exercise may affect blood lactate levels at various stages of the menstrual cycle.

▶ Another study to determine the interaction of the various phases of the menstrual cycle and performance. This one was an attempt to determine if energy metabolism varies across the cycle by examining the response of the blood lactate to 60 minutes of steady-state exercise at about 70% of each athlete's predetermined $\dot{V}o_{2max}$. Although the author found no effect on the blood lactate, she suggests that this may be because of the relatively low exercise intensity. Other investigators have found a lactate difference when graded exercise intensities of 40%, 70%, and 90% were used.—Col. J.L. Anderson, PE.D.

Diet and Bone Status in Amenorrheic Runners
Miriam E. Nelson, Elizabeth C. Fisher, Patricia D. Catsos, Carol N. Meredith, R. Nuran Turksoy, and William J. Evans (Tufts Univ.)
Am. J. Clin. Nutr. 43:910–916, June 1986   5–14

Amenorrheic and normally menstruating athletes were compared to investigate their bone-mineral density, body composition, maximal aerobic power, exercise training, and dietary habits. Twenty-eight women runners participated who were in good health and with regular training involving more than 20 miles of running weekly. Eleven women were amenorrheic and 17 were eumenorrheic.

Physical characteristics and training regimens were similar in the two groups, but the amenorrheic athletes were younger and had reached menarche at a later age. The bone mineral density of the lumbar spine and mean estradiol levels were significantly lower in the amenorrheic women. Bone mineral density was positively correlated with estradiol levels. There was a negative correlation between percent body fat and bone mineral density of the lumbar spine.

A 3-day dietary record showed that amenorrheic women reported a significantly lower intake of energy, carbohydrate, and fat. In 82% of amenorrheic and 35% of eumenorrheic women, protein intake was less than the U.S. Recommended Dietary Allowance. There was no difference regarding the intake of calcium, phosphorus, or fiber. There was also no difference with respect to the relative contribution of carbohydrate, fat, and protein to the total energy intake of the diet.

This study failed to show major differences in body composition between the two groups of women. The lumbar vertebrae showed a significantly lower mineral density in the amenorrheic women. The difference in estrogens, with the average concentration of circulating estradiol in the amenorrheic group at only one third that of the eumenorrheic group during early follicular phase, could significantly affect bone metabolism by changing calcium metabolism or interfering with osteoblast activity.

Data suggest that the amenorrheic women consumed a diet similar to that of the eumenorrheic group but in inadequate amounts. Amenorrhea in athletes may have deleterious long-term health consequences by reducing the mineral content of trabecular bone years before the onset of menopause. The intervention of a dietitian in the evaluation and treatment of this disorder may be advisable.

▶ Over the past 5 or 6 years, there has been a considerable increase in the number of studies about exercise-induced amenorrhea. We are now beginning to understand at least some of the problem better. We have generally found that both amenorrhea and inadequate food intake are not problems that usually concern highly trained women because they have coaches or trainers who understand the interaction between nutrition, performance, and health. However, this is a small percentage of our total athletes and within the majority of our athletic population is where the primary concern lies. Our researchers are also now beginning to discover some of the possible consequences of prolonged amenorrhea, and we are beginning to understand the need for good nutritional counselling for all of our athletes. We do not have all of the answers yet, but we are learning gradually. But is all of this knowledge being disseminated to our young athletes and their coaches and teachers?—Col. J.L. Anderson, PE.D.

Nutritional Intakes and Status of Highly Trained Amenorrheic and Eumenorrheic Women Runners

Patricia A. Deuster, Susan B. Kyle, Phylis B. Moser, Robert A. Vigersky, Anita Singh, and Eric B. Schoomaker (Uniformed Services Univ. of the Health Sciences, Bethesda and Univ. of Maryland, College Park, Md.)

Fertil. Steril. 46:636–643, October 1986   5–15

Women who engage in endurance training may experience disturbances in menstrual function. This study examined the influence of diet on this phenomenon in 80 long-distance runners. Amenorrheic (AM) and eumenorrheic (EU) runners were matched for size, body fat, and training distance for this study.

The serum estradiol level was 104.7 pg/ml in EU runners and 22.5 pg/ml in AM runners. The serum cortisol level was 22.4 μg/dl in EU runners and 26.6 μg/dl in AM runners. Fat intake was significantly lower in AM runners. Amenorrheic runners consumed large amounts of Vitamin A, probably in the form of B-carotene, and dietary fiber. Zinc intake and plasma zinc levels were low in AM runners.

The contributions of dietary fat, B-carotene, and zinc to changes in menstrual function and hormone metabolism merit further investigation.

▶ This study looked at nutritional status of 80 highly trained marathon runners, some of whom were eumenorrheic and some who were amenorrheic, to determine the effect on the development of exercise-related amenorrhea. The investigators examined macronutrient and micronutrient intakes and measured selected blood constituents related to nutritional status and endocrine function. The study has made a valuable contribution to answering the question concerning the effects of nutritional status and exercise-induced amenorrhea. A discriminant function using 11 dietary (8 variables) and nonnutritional (3) variables was formed which correctly classified according to menstrual status approximately 97% of the eumenorrheic and 92% of the amenorrheic runners. The question remains whether this function could be used to correctly classify other lesser trained athletes. My intuition says that it would not work because there is significant evidence which shows that the elite athletes are better informed about nutrition and are better trained.—Col. J.L. Anderson, PE.D.

The Effects of Fitness-Type Exercise on Iron Status in Adult Women
Scott Mead Blum, Adria Rothman Sherman, and Richard A. Boileau (Univ. of Illinois, Urbana)
Am. J. Clin. Nutr. 43:456–463, March 1986   5–16

Several investigators have reported that iron deficiency is more prevalent among highly trained athletes than among sedentary persons. It is well known that iron deficiency, when manifested as anemia, generally decreases physical work capacity and performance. The iron status resulting from milder forms of physical exercise has not yet been studied, even though many individuals presently engage in some form of physical conditioning. Because of blood loss associated with menstruation, women are at the greatest risk for developing iron deficiency. The authors conducted a study in adult women in order to determine whether a fitness-type exercise regimen compromises iron status or iron stores, or both.

The study comprised 24 previously untrained adult female volunteers, ranging in age between 22 and 51 years, who participated in a 35-minute aerobic exercise class four times a week, and 11 adult female volunteers, ranging in age between 20 and 39 years, who served as sedentary controls. All women provided blood samples for study at week 0, 6, and 13.

Hemoglobin levels increased between week 0 and week 6, but decreased between week 6 and week 13. Hematocrit values did not change between week 0 and week 6, but decreased between week 6 and week 13. Iron stores were decreased after 13 weeks of moderate fitness-type exercise, but no iron-deficient anemia developed in the study subjects. The sedentary control subjects showed no changes in hemoglobin or hematocrit levels during the study period. It appears from these findings that the body is able to adapt to the stress of a 13-week program of moderate exercise after a small, but significant compromise in body iron stores. The authors propose a mechanism which may explain the body's response to the depletion of iron stores associated with exercise (Fig 5–1).

▶ This study is important because it deals with a much larger proportion of the population than do the studies of highly trained athletes. The athletes have many people looking after them and studying them. The authors used a model proposed by Cook and Finch for the characterization and classification of iron status from normal to iron depletion to iron deficiency erythropoiesis to anemia. Although they discovered that iron depletion occurred in 20% to 32% of all subjects from both the exercise and control groups, and they found 7% of the exercise group and 22% of the sedentary group experienced iron deficiency

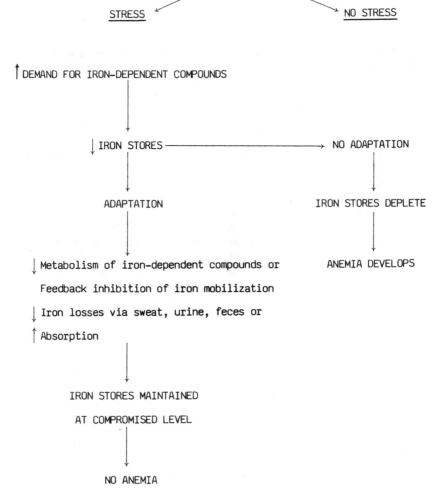

Fig 5–1.—Proposed mechanism for exercise-induced iron cost. (Courtesy of Blum, S.M., et al.: Am. J. Clin. Nutr. 43:456–463, March 1986. © Am. J. Clin. Nutr., American Society for Clinical Nutrition.)

erythropoiesis, none of the exercise group and only one of the control group developed iron deficiency anemia. They have proposed an adaption mechanism to help explain the body's response to the iron costs associated with exercise.—Col. J.L. Anderson, PE.D.

Effects of Physical Training and Competition on the Iron Status of Female Field Hockey Players

D.M. Diehl, T.G. Lohman, S.C. Smith, and R. Kertzer (Plymouth State College and Univ. of New Hampshire)
Int. J. Sports Med. 7:264–270, October 1986   5–17

The cost of physical training in terms of loss or increased need for iron has not been determined. As measurement of serum ferritin levels provides a reliable indication of iron stores, this assay was used to determine the effects of intensive training and competition on iron stores of female field hockey players, both throughout the season and over the course of 3 years of participation.

These female athletes showed a decrease in iron stores in each of the three seasons studied. After the first season, a decrease of 23 to 25 ng/ml was observed. A further significant decrease was seen following tournament play. After several years of play, serum ferritin levels were frequently between 10 and 20 ng/ml. The lowest levels occurred in third- and fourth-year athletes.

Participation in field hockey appears to decrease body iron stores. Iron reserves seem to become progressively depleted with each successive season of play. The stress of tournament play appears to deplete iron stores further.

▶ What is significant about the findings of this study? Serum ferritin, which is proportional to the size of body iron stores, is measured to monitor iron storage. According to earlier work by Clement, serum ferritin levels below 20 ng/ml in women are associated with absent bone marrow iron. Also, Franco has reported that a serum ferritin level of less than 10 ng/ml almost always indicates iron deficiency. The paper represented by Lampe et al. (5–20) reported that because serum ferritin levels were elevated after a marathon run they may not adequately reflect iron stores. The dietary intake of iron for these subjects was not controlled. It was self-reported and the mean reported intake was 10.0 ± 5.6 mg per day as compared to the RDA of 18 mg/day. What would happen if the intake were to be controlled at the RDA level?—Col. J.L. Anderson, PE.D.

Poor Iron Status of Women Runners Training for a Marathon
J.W. Lampe, J.L. Slavin, and F.S. Apple (Univ. of Minnesota, St. Paul, and Univ. of Minnesota, Minneapolis)
Int. J. Sports Med. 7:111–114, April 1986   5–18

The number of women who participate in athletic activities has markedly increased over the past decade. Because the incidence of iron deficiency in menstruating women is thought to be approximately 25%, concern exists over the iron status of women runners. Hemoglobin is the most commonly measured parameter in monitoring the iron status of female athletes, and it is accepted that concentrations of hemoglobin of less than 12 gm/dl are indicative of a late state of negative iron balance. However, before anemia

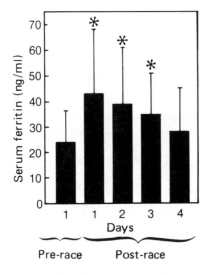

Fig 5–2.—Mean serum levels of ferritin for nine female runners 1 day before marathon race and 1, 2, 3, and 4 days afterward. *Indicates significant difference from prerace value; vertical lines indicate 1 SD from mean. (Courtesy of Lampe, J.W., et al.: Int. J. Sports Med. 7:111–114, April 1986.)

becomes manifest iron balance must become negative and the iron stores in the body must be depleted.

The authors examined the effects of 11 weeks of training for a marathon race and marathon racing on the iron status of female marathon runners by examining the serum levels of ferritin, total iron-binding capacity (TIBC), and iron in nine female runners aged 27 to 34 years. Venous blood samples were obtained at the beginning of the training period, weekly during training, and 1, 2, 3, and 4 days after the race. The subjects completed dietary and menstrual histories, and the diet content of energy, protein, iron, and ascorbic acid was determined.

Serum levels of iron and TIBC and transferrin saturation exhibited no significant change at weeks 1, 7, and 11 during training. Mean serum values of iron and transferrin saturation were noted to be low. During training, eight of the nine women exhibited average serum levels of ferritin that were below 50 ng/ml; one of the eight had values that were consistently below 10 ng/ml. For 3 days after the marathon values of ferritin were markedly elevated (Fig 5–2). None of the subjects noted abnormally heavy menstrual bleeding, and intakes of nutrients were near recommended levels, except for iron.

It is concluded that the iron status of these women marathon runners was poor, suggesting that women runners may have higher dietary needs for iron than sedentary women. The observation that serum levels of ferritin were elevated after the marathon suggests that this measurement may not adequately reflect stores of iron.

▶ This is additional evidence which suggests that the importance of women's iron status is not well understood. While it is true that the iron status of these women marathon runners was poor, it is wrong to assume that this is a problem for only endurance athletes. We have found that many young women, aged 17 to 22 years, who are physically active have serum iron levels lower than recommended.—Col. J.L. Anderson, PE.D.

Marathon Running Fails to Influence RBC Survival Rates in Iron-Replete Women

Irene Steenkamp, Cecily Fuller, John Graves, Timothy D. Noakes, and Peter Jacobs (Univ. of Cape Town Med. School, South Africa)
Physician Sportsmed. 14:89–95, May 1986   5–19

Women endurance athletes have a higher than average rate of iron deficiency, which has been hypothesized to be due to trauma-induced hemolysis. To examine this explanation, hemolysis and RBC morphology and survival were examined in six iron-replete female athletes during training for and running of a marathon.

No significant hematologic changes were found, except that hemoglobin and haptoglobin levels were higher three days following a race. There was also a fall in blood urea at this time. Survival of RBC was normal (i.e., indistinguishable from RBC survival in nonrunning women) in the weeks prior to and following the race and was constant in each athlete.

Mechanical damage in the blood of marathon runners was not found during training or following a race. Therefore, mechanical trauma to blood is not a likely cause of iron deficiency in female marathon runners. The possibility of a nutritional basis for this condition merits further study, as does the idea that the absence of stainable iron in the bone marrow may be an adaptation to endurance exercise, rather than an indication of true iron deficiency.

▶ This study seems to point the finger at the nutritional basis for the iron deficiency noted in many, if not most, women marathon runners. Of course, this study did use only six subjects, and the authors have made no attempt to infer this data to a larger population. Since many endurance runners are using nutritional restriction as a means of reducing body weight it appears that a well controlled research program to determine adequate nutritional needs for endurance athletes should have high priority. The athletes may benefit with better performances and better health.—Col. J.L. Anderson, PE.D.

Sex Differences in Strength and Fatigability

David H. Clarke (Univ. of Maryland)
Res. Q. Exerc. Sport 57:144–149, June 1986   5–20

It is widely recognized that men and women differ in muscular strength; however, it is not known if they also differ in muscle fatigue. It is important to know whether they differ in gross resistance to fatigue (endurance) as well as in relative loss of strength, when maximum levels of strength are not factors. The concept of sex differences in muscular fatigue was examined.

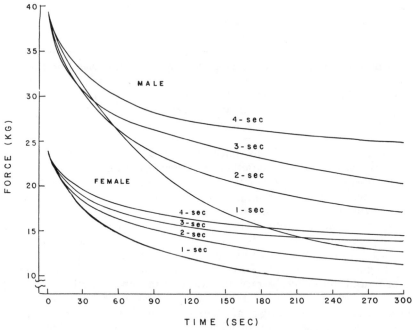

Fig 5–3.—Fatigue curves for male and female subjects at various intercontraction rest intervals. (Courtesy of Clarke, D.H.: Res. Q. Exerc. Sport 57:144–149, June 1986. Reprinted by permission of the American Alliance for Health, Physical Education, Recreation and Dance, 1900 Association Drive, Reston, Virginia 22901.)

The author examined the pattern of fatigue that resulted from systematically varying the intercontraction rest interval in 14 male and 14 female subjects by using a hand-grip fatigue exercise of 5 minutes' duration. The contraction interval was maintained for 3 seconds and the rest interval varied between 1 and 4 seconds. The fatigue trials were separated by at least 1 week, and all testing was carried out on a BLH load cell and recorder.

There were no significant differences in initial maximum strength for either male or female subjects over the four testing conditions, but significant differences did exist in final strength and absolute and relative endurance for both groups. Female subjects were markedly lower than male in initial and final strength and in absolute endurance. However, female subjects had substantially more relative endurance than the male subjects. The fatigue curves were found to be two component exponentials, with a half-time decay for the main component of 116 seconds for the male subjects and 80 seconds for the female (Fig 5–3).

In this study female subjects fatigued at a faster rate than did male subjects throughout most of the exercise. Although male subjects are stronger and have a greater absolute endurance than female subjects, female subjects have more relative endurance than male subjects.

▶ These findings are similar to what we have found at West Point during the 11 years when we have been able to compare the performances of men and women. I personally have not been able to figure out, within the parameters of our program, how to help the women take advantage of the greater relative endurance this study has found.—Col. J.L. Anderson, PE.D.

Gender Differences in Strength
Vivian H. Heyward, Sandra M. Johannes-Ellis, and Jacki F. Romer (Univ. of New Mexico)
Res. Q. Exerc. Sport 57:154–158, June 1986   5–21

Studies have shown that women are about one half (50%) as strong as men in the upper body and two thirds (68%) as strong as men in the lower body. The greater upper body strength in men compared to women was believed to be the result of dissimilar use of the muscle groups or a function of body size and bone diameters.

The upper and lower strength of 103 physically active men and women were measured with the Cybex II isokinetic dynamometer. Statistical analyses were performed using multivariate analysis of variance (MANOVA) and multivariate analysis of covariance (MANCOVA). The results indicated that differences in upper and lower body strength between men and women are due to differences in lean body weight and the relative distribution of muscle and subcutaneous fat in the body segments. Upper body strength is more important than lower body strength in characterizing gender differences. Strength variance in men is more a function of lean body weight than differences in muscle distribution of the limbs. Strength variance in women, however, could not be explained by lean body weight alone. Lean body weight accounts for less than half of the variance in both upper and lower body strength of women. Regarding lower body strength, thickness of the thigh skinfold is a significant contributor and in upper body strength, large arm girth was a significant factor.

Because lean body weight and arm girth combined accounted for only 34% of the variance in upper body strength in women, it is evident that additional factors need to be studied before variations in upper body strength of women are fully understood.

▶ As we study these gender differences in strength, it is important that we think about what is the significance of our findings to understanding and improving performance. I mean not only athletic performance but also work performance. Over time, as women have had more opportunities in sports and at the work place opening up to them, the methods used in training to improve their performances have been those borrowed from men's programs. Perhaps as we have an opportunity to better understand the gender differences, we will want to develop different techniques and programs for training men and women. The idea should be to challenge everyone and to help each other reach our maximum potential.—Col. J.L. Anderson, PE.D.

Electro-Mechanical Response Times and Rate of Force Development in Males and Females
Douglas G. Bell and Ira Jacobs (Downsview, Ont.)
Med. Sci. Sports Exerc. 18:31–36, February 1986   5–22

It is known that generation of muscle force during a maximum voluntary contraction (MVC) is dependent on both "central" and "peripheral" factors. The central factors include the proportion of the available total motor unit pool that is recruited during contraction, excitability of motoneurons, and the type of motor unit that is recruited during contraction. The peripheral factors include the cross-sectional area of the contracting muscle and the biochemical and electric events that are associated with the joining-sliding-relaxation of the contractile proteins.

There have been conflicting reports about the gender-related differences in the central component. It was hypothesized that there would be a difference between genders and that within each gender the stronger subjects would have markedly faster rates of force development and different electromechanical transit times than weaker subjects.

The authors compared total reaction time, premotor time, electromechanical delay, and the rate of force development in 46 male and 40 female

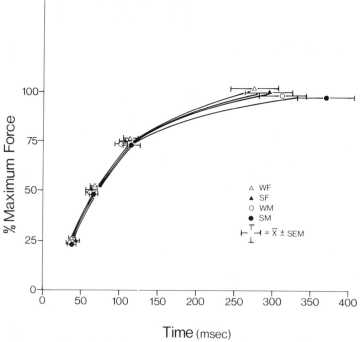

Fig 5–4.—Rate of force development compared to maximum generation of force during isometric, meximum voluntary contraction. WF, weaker female subjects; SF, stronger females subjects; WM, weaker male subjects; and SM, stronger male subjects. Bars, SD. (Courtesy of Bell, D.G., and Jacobs, I.: Med. Sci. Sports Exerc. 18:31–36, February 1986.)

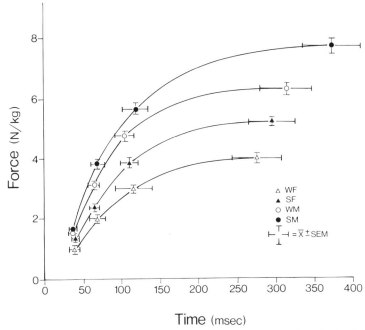

Fig 5–5.—Group comparison of rate of development of force expressed relative to body weight. *WF*, weaker female subjects; *SF*, stronger female subjects; *WM*, weaker male subjects; and *SM*, stronger male subjects. Bars, SD. (Courtesy of Bell, D.G., and Jacobs, I.: Med. Sci. Sports Exerc. 18:31–36, February 1986.)

subjects during an MVC of the elbow flexors. The MVCs were performed against a bar which was attached to a force transducer.

The subjects attempted to flex the elbow with maximal force as rapidly as possible after perceiving a visual stimulus. Subsequently, surface electromyographic activity was recorded from the biceps brachii and was sampled simultaneously with the force transducer data at 2 kHz and stored digitally. The subjects were then separated into four groups, based on the force generated during the MVC: weak female, strong female, weak male, and strong male subjects. It was found that neither reaction time nor premotor time was significantly different across groups (Fig 5–4). However, the electromechanical delay for both male groups was markedly shorter than for both female groups (Fig 5–5). The electromechanical delay was weakly but significantly correlated with rate of force development and maximum force. During a single MVC the times needed to attain 25%, 50%, 75%, and 100% MVC were observed to be similar in all groups.

These results suggest that at least part of the gender difference in maximum strength may be due to differences in electromechanical response times.

▶ Considering the fact that the electromechanical delay may be significantly shorter for men than for women, it appears to help explain the significant differences a number of investigators have found in power measures between men and women, even when strength measurements are equal or nearly equal. We must continue to study this issue to better explain the mechanism behind the apparent electromechanical delay and strength correlation. Some have suggested an alternate interpretation which suggests that the difference in electromechanical delay times could be indirectly related to gender and are a function of the strength differences among the four groups.—Col. J.L. Anderson, PE.D.

Endurance Capacity of Untrained Males and Females in Isometric and Dynamic Muscular Contractions

R.J. Maughan, M. Harmon, J.B. Leiper, D. Sale, and A. Delman (Univ. Med. School, Foresterhill, Aberdeen, Scotland, and McMaster Univ., Hamilton, Ontario, Canada)

Eur. J. Appl. Physiol. 55:395–400, August 1986   5–23

The aim of the present studies was to compare the ability of untrained men and women to perform exhausting exercise of different intensities using both isometric and dynamic contractions. Fifty healthy young adults, 25 male and 25 female, performed a sustained isometric contraction of the knee extensor muscles of their stronger leg to fatigue. These were done at forces corresponding to 80%, 50%, and 20% of the maximum voluntary force of contraction (MVC).

In a second experimental model, 11 women and 12 men were tested using a bilateral elbow flexion weight lifting exercise. Repetitions were performed at loads corresponding to 90%, 80%, 70%, 60%, and 50% of maximum load (IRM), at a reate of 10 min^{-1} to the point of fatigue.

Male subjects were significantly stronger ($p < .001$) than the female subjects in both the static (675 ± 120 N vs. 458 ± 80 N; mean $\pm$ S.D.) and dynamic (409 ± 90 N vs. 190 ± 33N) contractions. There was no difference between the sexes in the time for which forces could be maintained corresponding to 80% or 50% of MVC. Isometric endurance time at a force corresponding to 20% of MVC was greater for women (252 ± 56 vs. 180 ± 51; $p < .001$). Within each sex, correlations between endurance time at different forces were not significant except for a significant ($r = 0.47$, $p < .05$) correlation between endurance times at 50% and 20% of MVC in men.

With the dynamic elbow flexion exercise, men were significantly ($p < .001$) stronger than women. The discrepancy between the sexes was much larger with the men being more than twice as strong as the women. At loads of 80% or 90% of IRM, there was no difference between the number of contractions. Women were able to perform more repetitions at loads of 50% ($p < .005$), 60% ($p < .001$), and 70% ($p < .025$).

The two groups of women taking part in these studies were weaker than the men in both isometric and dynamic exercise modes. In the isometric knee extension task, the men were on the average 47% stronger. Maximum load lifted by the elbow flexors of the men was 2.2 times as great as that lifted by women. But the endurance capacity of the women was greater in both tasks when the work load was relatively low compared to the maximum. At higher forces, no difference was observed between the sexes in endurance performance.

▶ How does one explain the greater endurance capacity of the women in this study at loads of 50% and less of maximum voluntary contraction? How can we interpret the significance of these findings and benefit from them? These questions are important because we must realize that we are dealing with statistics that involve means of samples and not individuals of populations. Some women within the population do fall within the range of performance of men, although the majority fall outside the range at the levels of above 50% MVC.

This information has importance that extends beyond the athletic population into the population as a whole. The opportunity for women to move into non-traditional jobs is a major issue and understanding muscular strength and endurance requirements for various jobs is important. Our sports medicine and industrial engineering researchers should get together and help to answer questions above. Another question we must continue trying to answer is, Can we develop better training programs to help women significantly increase their strength and power levels and improve performances?—Col. J.L. Anderson, PE.D.

The Mechanical Efficiency of Locomotion in Men and Women With Special Emphasis on Stretch-Shortening Cycle Exercises
Ossi Aura and Paavo V. Komi (Univ. of Jyväskylä, Finland)
Eur. J. Appl. Physiol. 55:37–43, April 1986   5–24

It is a commonly accepted finding that men have higher physical performance capacity than women. Women have about 70% of the aerobic capacity of men and, in different performance tests for maximal strength and maximal muscular power, women have reached 68% to 80% of the values obtained by men. The mechanical efficiencies of men and women have not been compared extensively, and it has been suggested that sex differences might be present in isolated negative and positive work and in their combination (stretch-shortening cycle).

Ten men and ten women performed pure positive work, pure negative work, and a combination of negative and positive work (stretch-shortening cycle). For the controlled performance of the various work tasks, a special "sledge ergometer" was utilized. The mechanical efficiency of pure positive work was on average $19.8 \pm 1.2\%$ for female subjects and $17.4 \pm 1.2\%$ for male subjects although the work intensity was equal in both groups. The mechanical efficiency of pure negative work was slightly lower in women than in men ($59.3 \pm 14.4\%$ vs. $75.6 \pm 29.3\%$). The mechanical efficiency of positive work in a stretch-shortening cycle exercise was

$38.1 \pm 6.8\%$ in men and $35.5 \pm 6.9\%$ in the women. In the lower prestretch levels, the women showed a better utilization of prestretch; but with the higher prestretch velocities, the ability of female muscle to store and utilize or to store or utilize elastic energy decreased. Regarding the work due to elasticity, men achieved 46% for "maximal elastic capacity" compared to 41% for the women. This finding demonstrates that female musculature is very elastic, but only at low prestretch levels.

Whether or not basic differences exist between men and women in the reflex control of the muscle as well as in the structure of the entire neuromuscular system is subject to further evaluation.

▶ I repeat that we must always try to determine the importance or significance of the findings as we identify gender differences. The most important finding of this study was that the women showed better efficiency in pure positive work than men, while there were no statistically significant differences observed between the groups in the efficiencies in pure negative work and in the stretch-shortening (negative-positive) cycle exercise. Although the authors cannot explain or account for the significant differences for the mechanical efficiency of the pure positive work, we must continue to search for the significance.—Col. J.L. Anderson, PE.D.

Upper Extremity Strength and Strength Relationships Among Young Women

Richard W. Bohannon (Cape Fear Valley Med. Ctr., Fayetteville, N.C.)
J. Orthop. Sports Phys. Ther. 8:128–133, September 1986   5–25

For hand-held dynamometers to be useful, normal strength values and strength relationships must be calculated with them. This study reports the strength of 10 upper extremity muscle groups in 31 healthy young women and reports on the relationship between the strength of various muscle groups, as assessed by the hand-held dynamometer.

The only antagonistic muscle groups that differed significantly in strength between the left and right sides were the elbow flexor and the extensor muscles. The strength of each muscle group was significantly related to the strength of all other muscle groups on the same body side.

These values should prove useful to clinicians testing the upper extremity strength of young women.

▶ This study may be primarily of interest to clinicians in testing the upper extremity strength of women, but we should all pay attention. One of the outcomes of the "running craze" of the past 10 years has been a reduction in the interest of muscular conditioning, especially of the upper body. Many will read this and think I am crazy for saying such a thing and point to growth of the number of health spas with weight lifting rooms. However, only a very small percentage of our population make use of those facilities. More importantly, running became the darling of the media and the message was not lost on the young children. Today, we see more shoulder injuries at West Point than at any other time in our past. I attribute this to poor muscular development within this 17- to 22-year-old population prior to their arrival here, and the injuries occur before we can correct the problem.—Col. J.L. Anderson, PE.D.

Muscular Power in Young Women After Slow and Fast Isokinetic Training
Richard A. Garnica (Univ. of Southern California, Los Angeles)
J. Orthop. Sports Phys. Ther. 8:1–9, July 1986   5–26

Isokinetic exercise is a type of resistive exercise based on a device that offers constant velocity and resistance. This study was a pilot to determine whether 20 women training at a fast (180 degrees per second) or at a slow (60 degrees per second) isokinetic velocity would have a greater increase in upper extremity muscular power.

The exercise consisted of four bouts of five maximal reciprocal isokinetic contractions of the shoulder muscle groups through 180 degrees, three times per week for 4 weeks. Testing was with a Cybex II® isokinetic dynamometer.

Both groups showed significant power gains after the training period. The two groups showed equivalent power gains in this assay.

These results indicate that neither fast nor slow isokinetic training is more effective at producing increases in power within the 180 degree range of motion of shoulder extension in young women.

▶ Here are some more data to be used in the discussion as to whether fast (180 degrees per second) or slow (60 degrees per second) isokinetic velocity is best in developing muscle power. These findings say it makes either difference, or no significant difference. We have used both the fast and slow isokinetic velocities in our injury rehabilitation programs at West Point. We tend to agree with these findings; it doesn't appear to make much difference.—Col. J.L. Anderson, PE.D.

The Effects of a Strength Training Program on the Strength and Self-Concept of Two Female Age Groups
Rebecca D. Brown and Joyce M. Harrison (Brigham Young Univ.)
Res. Q. Exerc. Sport 57:315–320, December 1986   5–27

This study was undertaken to evaluate the effects of a strength training program on the rate of strength gains and on the self-concept of young and mature women. Participants included 85 sedentary or moderately active women, ages 17 to 26 and 40 to 49 years. Forty-three subjects were in a 12-week program of progressive weight training and 42 control subjects maintained their sedentary life-style. During the first week of the study, psychological inventory was completed prior to strength assessments. Treatment and control groups were randomly assigned for each age group. The mean age of the mature women and the young women were 44.4 and 21.5 years, respectively.

Significant increases ($P < .01$) in mean strength gains on bench press, pulldown, and leg press were found for the mature experimental (ME) and young experimental (YE) groups, compared to the mature control (MC) and young control (YC) groups. Gains in the YE group ranged from 13% in the leg press to 31% in the bench press. Gains in the ME group ranged from 18% in the pulldown to 28% in the bench press. These compared with ranges of 2.5% in the pulldown to 3.8% in the leg press for the YC group and 0% in the pulldown to 8% in the bench press for the MC group.

Participation in a strength training program was effective for increasing strength in both young and mature women. The strength gain was similar in both age groups, although the gain for the ME group in the leg press was twice that of the YE group.

The experimental groups demonstrated significant ($P < .01$) improvements on physical self, self-satisfaction, and global self-concept scores compared to the control groups. Improvement in self-concept was the same for the ME and YE groups. This indicated that the strength program had similar effects on self-esteem regardless of age. Data supported previous literature, indicating that body image and self-perception affect self-concept and that improved fitness, aerobics and anaerobics, can positively affect self-concept. Practical application may be better determined by studies of 15 to 20 weeks with follow-up testing included.

▶ We should not be surprised, but I am pleased, at the findings of this study. We know that women will gain strength if given the opportunity to train properly with a well-conceived training program. The fact that both the young and mature women also experienced positive changes in self-concept, as measured by the Tennessee Self-Concept Scale, tells us that improved strength for women will cause them to not only feel better about themselves, but also will probably help them to perform better at work and play.—Col. J.L. Anderson, PE.D.

HDL-C Concentrations in Weight-Trained, Endurance-Trained, and Sedentary Females

Don W. Morgan, Robert J. Cruise, Barbara W. Girardin, Viola Lutz-Schneider, Deborah H. Morgan, and Wang M. Qi (Arizona State Univ., Tempe, Andrews Univ., Berrien Springs, Mich., and Wayne State Univ., Detroit)
Physician Sportsmed. 14:166–181, March 1986   5–28

Elevated levels of high-density lipoprotein cholesterol (HDL-C) have been associated with a lower level of coronary heart disease. No studies have been published examining HDL-C levels in female weight trainers. This study assessed the serum HDL-C levels in nine female weight trainers, nine female endurance runners, and nine sedentary female controls.

Levels of HDL-C and percent HDL-C were significantly higher in the endurance runners than in the other two groups. There was no difference between weight trainers and sedentary controls along these parameters. Higher HDL-C levels were associated with low alcohol consumption and were more frequently found among subjects who did not use birth control pills.

Levels of HDL-C are associated with specific training methods in females.

▶ The fact that the runner group had higher levels of high density lipoprotein (HDL-C) than the weight trainers should not surprise many people. However, of more interest to me are the facts that nonsmokers, nondrinkers, and non-users of oral contraceptives were also likely to have higher levels of HDL-C.—Col. J.L. Anderson, PE.D.

High-Frequency, Moderate-Intensity Training in Sedentary Middle-Aged Women
S. Johannessen, R.G. Holly, H. Lui, and E.A. Amsterdam (Sportcare, Inc., Pleasanton, Univ. of California, Davis, and Marysville, Calif.)
Physician Sports Med. 14:99–102, May 1986   5–29

It is well established that the intensity, duration, frequency, mode, and progression of endurance training all contribute to the incidence of injury and changes in cardiorespiratory fitness and body composition as a result of exercise training programs. Nevertheless, it can take several weeks for sedentary middle-aged persons to adapt to training, and starting an exercise program without allowing enough time for physiologic adaptation can produce significant orthopedic injury. This article describes the authors' research to determine the effects of high-frequency, moderate-intensity exercise on oxygen consumption, body weight, body composition, and the incidence of orthopedic injury in sedentary middle-aged women.

The study population consisted of 15 women (mean age, 54.7 years; range, 49 to 62 years) who agreed to participate in a conditioning program designed to optimize the training effects without causing excessive orthopedic stress or fatigue. The subjects followed a moderate-intensity program of various aerobic exercises 5 days a week for 10 weeks, and the periods of continuous exercise were lengthened gradually to allow them to adapt physiologically. The subjects showed a 20% improvement in $\dot{V}O_{2max}$, but no change in body weight or composition. Furthermore, none of the women suffered an orthopedic injury.

The authors conclude that this type of program is a safe and effective exercise prescription for sedentary middle-aged women.

▶ The results reported in this study should not surprise anyone, yet the study is very important because of its societal implications. The age group of the subjects is becoming more and more important because of its size. One sure way to cut health care costs is to keep our population within this age group, and those older men and women, healthy. I am certain that this exercise program along with some nutritional guidance would produce reductions in percent body fat over time. We must continue working with our over-55 age group and keep them active and healthy. A sensible approach such as the one used here should help do that.—Col. J.L. Anderson, PE.D.

Physiological Monitoring of the 1984 Canadian Women's Olympic Field Hockey Team

A. Elizabeth Ready and Marina van der Merwe (Univ. of Manitoba, Winnipeg, and York Univ., Toronto, Canada)

Aust. J. Sci. Med. Sport 18:13–18, September 1986   5-30

This study was undertaken to develop a test battery suitable for the assessment of physiologic factors of importance to field hockey and to monitor the physiologic adaptation of Olympic team members during the year prior to the Los Angeles Games. Eighteen Canadian Women's Field Hockey Team members (mean age, 23.4 years) were evaluated on three occasions. Included in the testing protocol were several anthropometric and flexibility measurements, a modified Margaria-Kalamen stair run, the Anaerobic Speed Test (AST), lower body strength as evaluated by the Cybex, and a progressive treadmill run to exhaustion. The results of each athlete on each variable were recorded, and the mean was calculated for the team and by position at each test session.

The average height, weight, and vital capacity of all players at test 1 were 161.7 ± 6.3 cm, 58.0 ± 4.5 kg, and 3.7 ± 0.51 (BTPS) (mean ± S.D.), respectively. Average flexibility testing showed no noticeable changes throughout the year. Average body fat decreased from 18.9 ± 5.0% (N = 16) to 15.7 ± 0.43% (N = 18) between tests 1 and 3. Anaerobic alactic power and vertical velocity, as measured by the Margaria-Kalamen stair test run, decreased slightly during the first training phase. Maximal oxygen uptake ($\dot{V}O_{2max}$) increased by 5.7% and 6.0% during phases 1 and 2, respectively.

The $\dot{V}O_{2max}$ (ml $\cdot$ kg^{-1} $\cdot$ min^{-1}) did not differ significantly between positions and averaged 46.8, 50.8, 54.1, and 57.0 for the goalkeepers, defense, midfield, and strikers, respectively, at test 1. The greatest lower body strength and anaerobic power, and lowest anaerobic capacity as measured by the AST, was demonstrated by the goalkeepers, who were taller, heavier, and had greater body fat than players at other positions. During the stair run, vertical velocity was greatest for the strikers and lowest for the goalkeepers and defense players. The midfield players possessed the highest anaerobic capacity. Peak torque during knee extension was the only parameter that differed significantly by position. A definite trend was observed toward increased maximal aerobic power as positions progressed upfield from the goalkeeper.

The physiologic requirements of field hockey led to development of a training program and a suitable test battery at the High Performance Sports

Centers. Examination of player profiles can provide more insight into the needs of the game, based on identified strengths and weaknesses.

▶ This is the type of scientific testing that we in the West need to do more of to improve the training and development of our athletes who play team sports. We have done pretty well in studying our individual athletes, but have come lately to studying the needs of our team sports athletes. There is still much more that needs to be done.—Col. J.L. Anderson, PE.D.

Physiological Characteristics of Australian Female Soccer Players After a Competitive Season
Derek Colquhoun and Karen E. Chad (Univ. of Queensland, St. Lucia, Queensland, Australia)
Aust. J. Sci. Med. Sports 18:9–12, September 1986   5–31

This study was undertaken to evaluate selected physiologic characteristics of Australian female soccer players after competition. Ten players from state and national levels of competition, aged 15 to 29 years (mean age, 24.4 years), with playing experience of 5 to 11 years (mean, 7.9 years) participated. Parameters investigated included flexibility using the sit and reach test for hip flexibility, percent body fat and lean body weight calculated from body density, Wingate anaerobic power, leg strength using a Cybex 11 isokinetic dynamometer at 60, 120, 180, 240, and 300 deg · sec^{-1}, stepwise incremental maximal oxygen consumption, running economy performed at 9.7, 11.3, and 12.9 km · hr^{-1} for 4 minutes at each speed.

The $\dot{V}O_{2max}$ was 47.9 ± 8.0 ml · kg^{-1} min^{-1}, percent body fat was 20.8 ± 4.7, flexibility was 9.4 ± 7.7 cm, right leg extension was 87.9 ± 14.8 deg · sec^{-1}, right leg flexion was 57.8 ± 14.8 deg · sec^{-1}, left leg extension was 82.4 ± 21.2 deg · sec^{-1}, left leg flexion was 58.0 ± 16.4 deg · sec^{-1}, anaerobic power was 47.8 ± 11.2 watts, and 5-km run was 24.4 ± 2.9 minutes.

The physiologic characteristics of female soccer players following a competitive season was comparable to those of women in other sports. It is important that aerobic and anaerobic energy systems be developed since soccer places heavy demands on both these processes. However, data showed an imbalance of the anaerobic over the aerobic energy system, reflected in low $\dot{V}O_{2max}$ values and percent at which it could be sustained over a prolonged time period. The authors therefore recommend that aerobic training be developed during preseason training and maintained throughout the entire competitive season.

▶ This is another example of the use of scientific testing to develop player profiles and training techniques for sports teams. This study suffers somewhat because of the low number of subjects used. With more players tested, I am certain some of these data would be modified. The authors are correct to be concerned with the mean $\dot{V}O_{2max}$ scores which are rather modest for athletes at national levels.—Col. J.L. Anderson, PE.D.

Comparison of Psychological Androgyny Within a Sample of Female College Athletes Who Participate in Sports Traditionally Appropriate and Traditionally Inappropriate for Competition by Females
Kevin L. Burke (Florida State Univ.)
Perceptual Motor Skills 63:779–782, October 1986   5–32

In this study, female participants in sports traditionally considered inappropriate and appropriate for competition by women were compared on the personality trait of psychological androgyny. Subjects included 49 women university athletes; 11 basketball players, 12 softball players, 17 swimmers, and 9 tennis players. Each team was administered the original Bem Sex-role Inventory on separate occasions. Tabulations of scores classified each athlete as androgynous or nonandrogynous.

A χ^2 test showed no significant difference in androgynous athletes in traditionally inappropriate sports and traditionally appropriate sports plus a phi coefficient of 0.1. A significant difference was indicated from the t test on the masculinity scores between the two groups.

Correlation of traditionally inappropriate sports and androgyny was not supported as there was no significant difference in the number of psychologically androgynous female athletes partaking in sports of both groups. The fact that sports in general attract androgynous women or enhance androgyny may be one reason for nonsupport. Changing attitudes of, and toward women participants may be another reason. Personality characteristics on Bem's scales considered masculine are now ever present in women, as a result of the changing roles of today's women in society.

A significant difference was observed between the masculinity scores in the two sport classifications with inappropriate female sport participants scoring higher. It is therefore suggested that women with higher Bem masculinity scores are more likely to participate in a formerly traditionally inappropriate sport.

Generally, women's sports involve androgynous as well as nonandrogynous women. Evidence is provided that sport teams are not made up of athletes exhibiting the same personality traits. Thus, they must be dealt with as individuals as well as a team. Further studies should consider team vs. individual sports in regard to psychological androgyny.

▶ This is an interesting study, but as pointed out by the author, we cannot be certain that the findings were a result of the athletes choosing the traditional or nontraditional sports according to their psychological androgyny or because those sports which were seen as traditionally inappropriate were team sports, softball, and basketball, and the traditionally appropriate sports were individual sports, swimming, and tennis. In future studies of this type, consideration should also be given to whether the sports are interactive team sports where contact with the opponent is likely and frequently expected, such as basketball, soccer, or noninteractive such as volleyball and to a large extent, softball. Will the more androgynous women select the interactive team sports over the noninteractive team sports or individual sports? At what age does this selection process take place? What is the cause and effect of the self-selection process?—Col. J.L. Anderson, PE.D.

6 Athletic Training

Introduction

The last few years I have introduced this chapter with an editorial on the need for high school athletic trainers. There will be two articles on this subject; however, this year I have selected articles regarding the use of knee braces to prevent knee injuries in football as the lead articles. A most significant study has been published in the January 1987 issue of the *Journal of Bone and Joint Surgery* with an accompanying editorial. This article was written by Teitz et al. and is the first major study on the effects of knee braces. (See Abstract 3–4 for an abstract of this article). Sadly, the study indicates that knee bracing is not beneficial and in fact may be harmful. All three of the articles state that the knee braces tested did not reduce injuries. Two of the articles state that injuries may actually be increased. In my own situation, after using these braces for 3 years, I found no statistical evidence to show that they were either beneficial or harmful. To further confuse the issue, in January 1987 Dr. Paulos presented a paper at the AAOS meeting which indicates that some braces may be more effective than others.

How will this study affect our use of knee braces next year? We will certainly not make the use of these braces mandatory or compulsory as we did in the past. The problem is some of our players have become accustomed to wearing the braces after having used them for 3 years. They like the brace and feel it affords them extra protection. We will probably make the braces available to those athletes who want to wear them. (Is that an indefinite statement, or what?) We will certainly make adjustments in those braces we use on athletes with varum (bowed) knees, to avoid a preloading type of injury, and in fact will discourage those athletes from wearing the braces. I'm sorry that I cannot be more definite on our plans for next fall. We have been unable to agree among ourselves on a definite plan of action.

Perhaps in the future an affordable prophylactic knee brace will be designed.

Frank George, A.T.C., P.T.

Evaluation of the Use of Braces to Prevent Injury to the Knee in Collegiate Football Players
Carol C. Teitz, Bonnie K. Hermanson, Richard A. Kronmal, and Paula H. Diehr (Univ. of Washington)
J. Bone Joint Surg. [Am.] 69-A:2–8, January 1987   6–1

▶ This article is abstracted in chapter 3 (Abstract 3–4). Also of interest is an editorial written by Henry R. Cowell, M.D., Ph.D. (*J. Bone Joint Surg.* [Am.] 69-A:1, January 1987).—F. George, A.T.C., P.T.

Lateral Knee Braces in Football: Do They Prevent Injury?
Lonnie E. Paulos, John P. Drawbert, Paul France, and Thomas D. Rosenberg (Univ. of Utah)
Physician Sportsmed. 14:119–125, June 1986   6–2

Lateral knee braces are being used increasingly by football players in an attempt to decrease the number of valgum knee injuries. The authors review three recent clinical studies and present the results of a biomechanical study of these braces on 14 cadaverous knees to evaluate the effectiveness of these braces.

Three clinical studies comparing football players using and not using lateral knee braces were reviewed. These studies did not show any clear-cut benefit of these braces.

The authors studied the forces and joint opening necessary to disrupt the valgum-restraining ligaments in the unbraced knee and the mechanical properties and protective function of the braces in cadaverous knees. Tests without braces demonstrated that the medial collateral ligament complex is the major restraint to valgum force. The contribution varies with flexion angle. The cruciate ligaments are a secondary restraint. Joint-opening force and ligament tension experiments did not demonstrate any significant benefit from the brace.

These studies indicate that the current types of lateral knee brace do not help to prevent injuries from a valgum force. These braces could actually increase such injuries if they preload ligaments, slip, or cause other stress. Although these results are preliminary, none of the currently available braces can be recommended.

Prophylactic Knee Bracing in College Football
George F. Hewson, Jr., Ricky A. Mendini, and Jon B. Wang (Univ. of Arizona, Tucson)
Am. J. Sports Med. 14:262–266, July–August 1986   6–3

It is well recognized that American football can be harmful to the knees. The cost of knee injuries can be measured in terms of time lost from academics, loss of sport experience, and sometimes, chronic disability. Prophylactic knee bracing has been suggested as a possible means of reducing the number and severity of knee injuries. The effectiveness of this preventive program was assessed.

The authors reviewed team rosters, Athletic Treatment Center daily log sheets, the National Athletic Injury/Illness Reporting System, and medical records for the University of Arizona intercollegiate teams over an 8-year period. The records of 4 academic years without preventive bracing were compared with the records of 4 academic years with preventive bracing. All linemen, offensive and defensive as well as linebackers and tight ends, were considered players at risk and were required to use the Anderson Knee Stabler. Each player at each practice session or game was counted as one "exposure to injury", and during the 4 years of brace use there were 28,191 exposures; during the 4 years without brace use there were 29,293 exposures. The data were evaluated from the perspectives of days lost from practice or games, player's position, the type and severity of injury, and the rate of injury per 100 players per season.

Players at risk showed no trend to change in injury rate. Furthermore, of the players at risk, the type and severity of injury in nonbraced and braced groups were similar. In players at risk, there was a twofold increase in knee ligament injury rate per 100 players when compared with rates for the entire team. However, the number of season-ending injuries was not changed. Practice time missed for third-degree medial ligament and medial meniscus injuries was lower in the braced group, but this is likely to have been due to improved treatment techniques initiated in 1981. Since 1981, there have been seven NCAA rule changes directed at reducing knee injuries.

Neither rule changes nor knee braces nor the combination thereof have had any apparent effect on the trend toward knee injury among college football players.

The Effects of Lateral Knee Stabilizing Braces on Running Speed and Agility

William E. Prentice and Todd Toriscelli (Univ. of North Carolina, Chapel Hill, and Marietta College, Marietta, Ohio)
Athletic Training 21:112–113, 186, 1986   6–4

Recently, much interest has developed regarding the use of lateral knee stabilizing devices for the purpose of reducing the occurrence of injury to the knee joint. These braces are most often used in football, and the limited experimental data have dealt primarily with the effectiveness of the braces in preventing knee injuries related to football. In addition to questions dealing with the effectiveness of the braces in reducing injury frequencies, there are also questions regarding the effects of the lateral knee stabilizing braces on performance. The goal of the present study was to compare the effects of three lateral knee stabilizing braces on performance.

The study population consisted of 20 male students, aged 19 to 22 years, who were tested during three separate testing sessions wearing either the Anderson Knee Stabler, the McDavid Knee Guard, or the Don Joy Knee Defender. A fourth session in which no braces were worn served as a control. The subjects were tested with regard to forward running speed, backward running speed, and agility, and during each session subjects were asked to perform a 40-yd forward sprint, a 20-yd backward sprint, and an agility drill using directional changes, carioca, etc., all at maximum speed. The times were recorded by a Lafayette Photoelectric Cell and Light

Timing Unit, and data were analyzed using a repeated-measures completely randomized block ANOVA. It was found that all three braces tested significantly reduced forward running speed relative to the control group; however, no differences existed among the three braces. In addition, speed during backward running and the agility run were unaffected by brace application. The implications of this study with regard to performance must be a consideration when examining the effectiveness of these braces in injury reduction.

▶ After my statements in the introduction to this chapter and after reading the previous three articles, this article may not seem as significant. However, what it may do is shed some light on why the present braces available are not effective. This study indicates that forward running speed is reduced, and this may be one cause that reduces their prophylactic benefits.—F. George, A.T.C., P.T.

▶ The following two articles have to do with the health care of the high school athlete. I have written many times on the need for athletic trainers on the high school level and the solution to this dilemma. The most feasible solution is the faculty-athletic trainer—a person who would teach a regular class schedule and then after school hours serve as an athletic trainer. The first of the following articles indicates that in most instances coaches are responsible for the health care of the high school athlete. The article also concludes that these coaches are not qualified to be making the decisions regarding health care, which they do.

The numbers of injuries which occur on the high school level are significant. Something must be done to reduce these injuries and to provide proper evaluation and care of the injuries. The faculty-athletic trainer will help solve the problem.—F. George, A.T.C., P.T.

Knowledge of Care and Prevention of Athletic Injuries in High Schools
P. Joanne Rowe and Donna M. Robertson (Augusta College, Augusta, Ga., and Univ. of Alabama, Tuscaloosa)
Athletic Training 21:116–119, Summer 1986   6–5

At present coaches are responsible not only for producing winning teams and teaching proper techniques, but also for keeping athletes healthy and free of injuries. The authors contend that many coaches may not have the knowledge to carry out this last function. Between 1976 and 1981 there were 42,534 reported sports injuries by males and females. This high number suggests that hundreds of decisions are being made on a daily basis with regard to the care and prevention of athletic injuries by individuals who may be unqualified to make such decisions. The goal of the present study was to determine current knowledge and the effect on the care and prevention of athletic injuries by those individuals designated as athletic trainers in the high schools of Alabama.

The authors mailed a questionnaire and survey to all high school athletic directors in the state (n = 479), who were asked to forward the material to the individual in their school who was responsible for care and treatment of athletic injuries. There were 135 responses, and 127 were used in the sample. It was noted that 88.9% of the sample was comprised of coaches, of whom 58.2% had physical education backgrounds. The respondents scored above the pass-level criteria (70%) on diet/nutrition and heat-related areas, while scoring markedly below the criteria on anatomy, care and prevention, conditioning, and equipment. The percentage of individuals meeting the criteria level of passing for the six categories of anatomy, care and prevention, conditioning, diet/nutrition, equipment, and heat-related factors was found to be 27%.

More than 73% of these 127 individuals who are responsible for the care and treatment of injured athletes are possibly making incorrect decisions on the health care of athletes 70% of the time. The authors suggest that this be a major area of concern for parents of athletes, as well as for school personnel.

A National Survey of Employment Opportunities for Athletic Trainers in the Public Schools

William E. Prentice, and Brad Mishler (Univ. of North Carolina, Chapel Hill, and Marietta College, Marietta, Ohio)
Athletic Training 21:215–219, Fall 1986   6–6

There has been considerable debate among members of the National Athletic Trainers Association (NATA) as to whether American educational and internship programs are providing optimal job marketability for graduating athletic trainers. In 1980, the Board of Directors of NATA determined that, by 1990, all NATA-approved undergraduate athletic training programs must have either a "major" or an "equivalency" in athletic training; but this decision, ironically, may have jeopardized employment opportunities for student trainers in public schools.

A study was undertaken to determine what combination of academic preparation and/or professional qualifications optimize job marketability for the athletic trainer in public schools, and what level of responsibility and salary could be expected after one obtains employment in the public schools. A 20-item questionnaire was sent to 2,000 high school principals selected at random. Seven hundred and seventy-seven questionnaires were returned. Of the 777 schools responding, only 22.7% currently employed an athletic trainer, and of these only 57.4% were certified by the NATA. Of the schools not employing an athletic trainer, only 19.4% indicated a desire to have one in the future.

Of those who planned to hire trainers, 78.3% required the individual to undertake additional teaching responsibilities, especially in science and mathematics. Only 20% would be hired as athletic trainers exclusively. Certification by the NATA was preferred, although there was no preference as to the level of degree held by the trainer. The principals preferred an individual with 1 to 3 years' experience as an athletic trainer. Starting salaries for trainers with a bachelor's degree who would also teach full time ranged from $13,000 to $16,000. Those with a master's degree could expect $16,000 to $20,000 initially. In addition to the salaries, the schools would pay stipends for athletic training responsibilities of $500 to $2,000 for the school year.

Consideration in Planning Small College Athletic Training Facilities
Eric A. Forseth (Mount Vernon Nazarene College, Mount Vernon, Ohio)
Athletic Training 21:22–25, Spring 1986   6–7

There is an increasing need to design and plan athletic training facilities, and it is evident that pre-design and planning are as important as building cost-effective, functional facilities. Close cooperation with the architect is important, as is the consideration of the individual college situation, which may dictate budgetary and building size constraints. Program needs, enrollment, and available finances are also critical factors.

Optimal use of space is necessary in correctly planning athletic training facilities. Appropriate utilization of space can increase the versatility of a training facility. Vertical stacking of storage cabinets in a corner (Fig 6–1) will spare prime space for peak-load traffic. The hydrotherapy area should be an integral part of each training facility.

Administrators of athletic training programs should become familiar

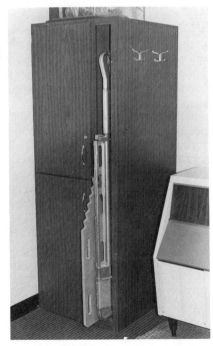

Fig 6–1.—A 7-ft. high stacked corner cabinet with an adjacent space 6 in. x 7 ft. for backboard and scoop stretcher storage. (Courtesy of Forseth, E.A.: Athletic Training 21:22–25, Spring 1986.)

with current trends and consider long-range goals. Otherwise, facilities that are currently functional may become outdated.

▶ It is especially important that the architect and trainer work closely together. The builder and architect must understand that a hydrotherapy area must have a water supply and proper floor drains. Whirlpools always overflow and they are noisy. If possible, a glass enclosure for the hydrotherapy area is a must. Doors must be large enough to allow extended stretchers to be carried through safely without having to tilt the stretcher. There must be easy access for an ambulance. The planning process must be long and slow and every detail checked and rechecked. I was especially impressed with the design of the stacked corner cabinet with space for the backboard and stretcher. See above figure.—F. George, A.T.C., P.T.

An Athletic Training Program in the Computer Age
Richard Ray and Tanya L. Shire (Hope College, Holland, Mich.)
Athletic Training 21:212–214, Fall 1986   6–8

At Hope College, five specific computer applications are used in the athletic training department. All five programs are accessible from any computer terminal. Student programmers wrote much of the customized software to meet the specific needs of the athletic training department. The authors discuss how these programs are used at this institution.

The first computer application is the Orthotron II Testing and Data Storage Program, which is used to calculate agonist-antagonist ratios, right-left strength deficit percentages, and strength/body weight ratios. It also keeps track of records on rehabilitating athletes on a daily basis.

The second computer application is a relational database system that allows the user to create data entry forms on the videoscreen. This database is used by trainers as a daily treatment log and keeps track of what equipment was used and which exercises were done by the athlete.

The third computer program in use is the Nutritional Analysis System. The program allows a person to enter the type and quantity of foods eaten into the computer and the program calculates the amount of macronutrients and micronutrients, percent of RDA, calories consumed, and the amount of projected fat weight that will be gained or lost per week.

The fourth program is the Body Composition Calculator. It provides a simple method for determining an athlete's percent fat and ideal weight based on skinfold or hydrostatic weighing measurements.

The fifth program is used for teaching and administration, including the preparation of budget projections, bid lists for supplies, inventory records, memos and letters, and other administrative documents.

The authors encourage others to consider the use of computers in their athletic training programs.

▶ Computers have definitely arrived in many training rooms across the country. The authors have described a very complete program utilizing a computer to maintain injury files, inventories, isokinetic testing data, and nutrition and body composition information. Computer Science majors in most of our universities can help develop the necessary software to run these programs. The computer can be a timesaving device once its applications are learned and can perform many calculations and other functions otherwise not possible.

Before you rush out to buy a computer, I recommend that you first decide what you want to use it for. Then select the software that will accomplish this. Only then should you select the computer that will run the software you have selected.—F. George, A.T.C., P.T.

Evaluation of Warm-Up for Improvement in Flexibility
Henry N. Williford, Jennifer B. East, Furman H. Smith, and Lou Ann Barry (Auburn Univ., Montgomery, Ala.)
Am. J. Sports Med. 14:316–319, July–August 1986   6–9

Stretching exercises are usually performed as a warm-up prior to exercise because it is believed that stretching will increase flexibility, decrease the incidence of musculotendinous injuries, improve performance, and/or prevent muscle soreness. Although there is evidence to suggest that stretching can increase flexibility, there is concern as to which stretching techniques or procedures should be used for optimal gains in flexibility. The goal of the present study was to evaluate the effect of warming the joints by jogging and then stretching on increases in joint flexibility.

The study population consisted of 51 students who were participants in a physical conditioning class. The subjects were assigned to a jog and then stretch (JS), stretch and no jog (S), or a control group. Both the JS and S groups carried out a series of stretching exercises 2 days per week for 9 weeks, and the JS group jogged for 5 minutes prior to stretching. The subjects were pretested and post-tested for shoulder, hamstring, trunk, and ankle flexibility with a Leighton flexometer. Significant increases in flexibility occurred for all of the joint angles evaluated for both the JS and S groups with the exception of trunk flexibility for the JS group. In addition, there was a significant gain in ankle flexibility in the JS group compared with the S and C groups. The S group had a marked gain in trunk flexibility compared with the JS group.

Both the JS and the S groups were effective in improving flexibility, but when the gain scores were compared, the results were variable. These results support the claim that increases in flexibility can occur as a result of a static stretching training program. However, the results do not support the claim that warming the muscle prior to stretching by jogging will lead to significant increases for all of the joint angles evaluated. The authors suggest that both methods offer possible advantages associated with improving joint flexibility.

▶ When do I stretch—before, after, or during my exercise program? How much do I stretch? What type of flexibility exercises should I do? Do PNF techniques provide the best results? Are flexibility exercises good for me or bad for me? Do they really work or am I wasting my time? Should they hurt? How much should they hurt? Does warming up help? How much is necessary?

Most of these questions have been answered within the past few years and seem much less controversial. I reread some of my comments from the 1984 YEAR BOOK OF SPORTS MEDICINE and find that we haven't made significant changes in our stretching programs since then. Some basic principles we adhere to are as follows: (1) The heart is a muscle which must be warmed up and cooled down before and after vigorous exercise. (2) All muscles should be warmed up gently before flexibility exercises are done. (3) Flexibility done in moderation when the muscles are warmed up can be beneficial. (4) Some flexibility exercises should be avoided. (5) Attempts should be made to stretch muscle bellies and not tendons. This can be done by slightly relaxing the joints that the stretched tendons pass over. (6) Never stretch a cold muscle. (7) Most of the flexibility program should be done at the end of a workout as part of the cool-down period.—F. George, A.T.C., P.T.

Skeletal Muscle Atrophy During Immobilization
H.-J. Appell (Deutsche Sporthochschule, Cologne, West Germany)
Int. J. Sports Med. 7:1–5, February 1986   6–10

Atrophy of skeletal muscle, a consequence of immobilization, is probably most accurately measured by calculating the diameter of cross-sectional fibers. Most investigators have employed this technique, and data from their immobilization experiments are reviewed.

Of main interest is work done on the ultrastructural appearance of atrophy. The myofibrils are the primary structures involved in atrophy; most changes occur within the first week. The fibrils beneath the sarcolemma are disrupted. Mitochondrial changes occur next, followed by degeneration of the sarcoplasmic reticulum. The properties and responses of muscles can be restored following immobilization, however, by means of training.

Although research has characterized some aspects of the appearance of muscle atrophy following immobilization, areas of confusion remain. The question of the type of fiber most susceptible to atrophy is not yet clearly resolved. Further ultrastructural studies in humans are required to determine if animal results will prove applicable. The cellular events during recovery from immobilization, as well as optimal recovery training protocols, remain to be determined.

Morphology of Immobilized Skeletal Muscle and the Effects of a Pre- and Postimmobilization Training Program
H.J. Appell (Deutsche Sporthochschule, Cologne, West Germany)
Int. J. Sports Med. 7:6–12, February 1986   6–11

Immobilization of limbs during treatment of sports injuries leads to muscle atrophy. A series of experiments with mice were performed to determine the effect of duration of immobilization on atrophy, and to examine the ultrastructural basis of the atrophy and the effects of muscle training on atrophy.

Hind limbs were immobilized with plaster casts for different periods of time and with and without prior and subsequent treadmill training. The muscle was examined in fiber cross-sections. During the first week of immobilization, the most pronounced reduction in fiber diameter was seen. During prolonged immobilization, only moderate atrophy occurred. Red fibers were more susceptible than white fibers to this atrophy. Some fibers underwent segmental necrosis, whereas some fibers regenerated while immobilized. Training following immobilization increased fiber diameter. However, there were severe ultrastructural alterations in these muscles. Training before immobilization reduced immobilization-induced atrophy to negligible levels.

Postimmobilization training should be undertaken with caution to prevent damage to the weakened muscle. Preimmobilization training can probably prevent the muscle from developing severe atrophy.

▶ Muscle atrophy (Abstract 6–10) is a perplexing problem for trainers and therapists. Why do some muscles atrophy more than others? Why do they atrophy so fast? The author has described what happens in total and on a microscopic level. He states that red fibers are more susceptible to atrophy than white muscle fibers. He suggests that preimmobilization training may reduce the amount of atrophy that occurs. This lends strong support whenever possible for preoperative quadriceps and hamstring strengthening programs (Abstract 6–11).—F. George, A.T.C., P.T.

Isokinetic Dynamometry: Implications for Muscle Testing and Rehabilitation
Louis R. Osternig
Exerc. Sports Sci. Rev. 14:45–80, 1986   6–12

Isokinetic exercise has become increasingly popular as a modality of rehabilitative medicine. Isokinetic rehabilitative devices, developed in the late 1960s, make it possible to study mechanical properties of muscle under conditions of constant velocity. Mass production and marketing of these devices has resulted in their widespread use in rehabilitation, conditioning, and research. The author reviews the role of isokinetic exercise in rehabilitation, discusses aspects of muscle testing with isokinetic dynamometry, and reviews the literature.

Isokinetic dynamometers are passive devices which resist applied forces and control the speed of exercise at a predetermined rate. These devices also provide a record of applied force throughout a given joint's range of motion.

Isokinetic exercise is generally thought to be safe since isokinetic dynamometers have been shown to be highly reliable in test-retest analyses done with inert weights. However, there are limitations in the interpretation and utilization of measurements from such devices since there are still some questions at this time as to whether submaximal or maximal warm-ups are essential to ensuring stable measures. Consequently, it seems prudent to recommend submaximal warm-ups prior to maximal testing in order to reduce the possibility of muscle strain, especially in novice subjects and patients undergoing rehabilitative testing.

Isokinetic dynamometers have provided clinicians and researchers with information that used to be very difficult to obtain. Continued research will further improve the accuracy of interpreting dynamic muscle function tests.

▶ Isokinetic exercise is one of many types of exercise we use in our rehabilitation programs. We have continued to make changes in our protocols and exercise regimens as we learn more and more about isokinetics, the machines, and how to use them. We have used an isokinetic dynamometer in our preseason testing examination to help us determine strength ratios and strength deficits, and strength/body weight ratios. We use the computer to calculate these figures for us. We also use these figures if an athlete is injured to determine preinjury and postinjury differences and to monitor our rehabilitation program. In injury rehabilitation testing we look at many more figures, speeds, and angles in determining the level of rehabilitation achieved.—F. George, A.T.C., P.T.

Isokinetic Shoulder Strength of High School and College-Aged Pitchers
Gordon J. Alderink and Donald J. Kuck (Grand Valley State College, Allendale, Mich., St. Joseph Mercy Hosp., Ann Arbor, Mich.)
J. Orthop. Sports Phys. Ther. 7:163–172, January 1986   6–13

Currently available isokinetic exercise devices allow the clinician not only to assess the strength of major muscle groups, but to rehabilitate those groups following musculoskeletal injuries. The advantages, indications, and efficacy of isokinetic testing have been well established, as have the reliability and validity for the measurement of torque. To date, most of the isokinetic strength data of normal individuals have focused on the lower extremity, particularly the quadriceps femoris and hamstring muscle groups. The goal of the present study was to provide descriptive data on the isokinetic shoulder strength of baseball pitchers.

The study population consisted of 24 high school and college baseball pitchers whose ages ranged from 14 to 21 years. The authors used the Cybex II and U.B.X.T. to test the strength of the shoulder abductors/adductors, flexors/extensors, horizontal abductors/adductors, and external/internal rotators at 90, 120, 210, and 300 degrees per second. There were no consistent differences between dominant and nondominant arm strength, except for the shoulder adductors and shoulder extensors. The shoulder abductors were found to be approximately 50% as strong as the adductors and extensors. There was a 1:1 ratio between the horizontal abductors/adductors, and the external rotators were approximately two thirds as strong as the internal rotators. Finally, there was a positive correlation between total body weight and shoulder strength.

This information is relatively new to the literature and should provide clinicians with some training and rehabilitation guidelines.

▶ Many of us are quite familiar with isokinetic testing of the knee joint and how to interpret the data we receive. However, there have been relatively few studies done on the shoulder joint, and much of the data we receive is difficult to interpret. The authors have given us some parameters to follow in shoulder testing and what results and rations may be considered normal. We have not been as consistent in our shoulder testing results as with our knees. Perhaps as we test more shoulders and become more proficient in the testing and interpretation of the results, this consistency will improve.—F. George, A.T.C., P.T.

Alternative to Shoulder Girdle Protection
Dave Carrier (Michigan State Univ.)
Athletic Training 21:228–229, Fall 1986   6–14

Modern football shoulder pads are very protective through designs intended to absorb and disperse great amounts of shock on impact, but provide only limited protection of the lateral aspect of the shoulder girdle. Many shoulder girdle and proximal upper arm injuries result from a lateral blow in football, and various attempts have been made to fabricate special pads to protect the vulnerable areas.

Jofa hockey shoulder pads, made of lightweight material, articulate well with the athlete's upper body (Fig 6–2). The deltoid cap is made of hard

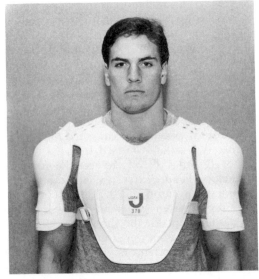

Fig 6–2.—Jofa jockey shoulder pads. (Courtesy of Carrier, D.: Athletic Training 21:228–229, Fall 1986.)

plastic that provides rigid protection to the shoulder girdle and deltoid areas. The proximal end of the cap is connected by an adjustable lace to the main part of the pad, and the distal end is held in place by an elastic strap that does not restrict performance. The pad also has adjustable chest straps. The football shoulder pads fit well over the hockey pads, although a larger pair than the athlete would normally wear may be needed.

This shoulder pad combination is a simple and effective means of obtaining further protection of the shoulder girdle and proximal arm in football players, without hindering their ability to perform.

▶ After reading this article, I ordered a pair of these hockey pads to try. Unfortunately, the season ended before I could use them. It seems like a very good idea. As the author states, we as trainers have been fabricating our own type of protective pad for these injuries, sometime successfully, sometimes not. This appears to be a simple solution to a difficult problem. If it works satisfactorily, I'm sure I will order a number of these pads.—F. George, A.T.C., P.T.

Manipulation in the Treatment of Tennis Elbow
Shirley Kushner and David C. Reid (Univ. of Alberta)
J. Orthop. Sports Phys. Ther. 7:264–272, March 1986   6–15

Tennis elbow is the gradual onset of elbow pain resulting from wrist extension with pronation or supination, aggravated by gripping. Repeated wrist extensor action appears chiefly responsible. Activities other than tennis, such as piano playing and snow shoveling, may cause tennis elbow. Resisted wrist extension and radial deviation with the elbow fully extended usually will cause pain in the proximal extensor muscle mass. If the fingers are held in flexion and wrist extension is resisted, pain may occur at the elbow.

Treatment is aimed at relieving inflammation, reducing overload forces, promoting healing, and increasing upper limb strength and flexibility. Exercise is always a mainstay of treatment. Eccentric training recently was reported to be effective when combined with passive stretching. Good results also are obtained using strengthening exercises for the wrist extensors, with the elbow initially flexed and gradually progressing to extension as pain allows.

Manipulations (table) should be used only in the context of a comprehensive treatment regimen. Mill's manipulation is the most commonly used procedure. Cyriax presently recommends manipulation with the patient sitting, the shoulder abducted and internally rotated, and the forearm fully pronated. The Kaltenborn manipulation was designed for lateral epicondylitis, and Stoddard's manipulation was developed for chronic cases of tennis elbow. Mennell used a manipulation similar to that of Mill to break adhesions.

▶ More and more trainers and therapists are using some techniques of joint

COMPARISON OF MANIPULATION TECHNIQUES

AUTHOR	MILLS[22,23]	CYRIAX 1.[4]	CYRIAX II[5,6] (MILLS)	KALTENBORN[13]	MENNELL[21]	STODDARD[32]
LESION	Frayed or detached orbicular ligament in acute cases. Adhesions in chronic cases.	Partial tear at tenoperiosteal junction of extensor carpi radialis brevis.	Inadequate healing. Scar in extensor carpi radialis brevis at tenoperiosteal junction.	Lateral epicondylitis.	Painful scar in common extensor tendon.	Adhesions binding origin or extensor digitorum communis to radial collateral ligament.
POSITION	Lying. General anaesthetic	Sitting. No anaesthetic Following 5-10 minutes of deep friction.	Sitting. Following 10-15 minutes deep friction.	Sitting or supine. No anaesthetic.	Standing. Prior injection of local anaesthetic.	Supine.
MANIPULATION	Forced extension elbow. Wrist and fingers flexed. Forearm pronated.	Elbow fully extended. Forearm supinated. Fixation at radial elbow. Varus thrust at lateral wrist.	Shoulder abducted and medially rotated. Forearm pronated, wrist flexed. Fixated at wrist. Extensor thrust at elbow.	Fixation at wrist. Varus thrust at extended elbow.	Fully flexed and pronated wrist and elbow. Elbow extension with forced over pressure.	Shoulder abducted 90°. Pronate and supinate to identify maximum tension in extensor digitorum communis. Varus thrust at elbow by forearm adduction.
INDICATION	Minimal loss of range of motion elbow extension. Tested with full wrist and finger flexion in pronation. Local epicondylar or radiohumeral joint tenderness.	Pain over the lateral epicondyle or common extensor tendon origin.	Tenoperiosteal variety. Pain on resisted wrist extension and radial deviation	Lateral epicondylitis. Restricted movement of the radial head.	Painful area at common extensor origin on palpation.	Chronic cases. No response to hydrocortisone injection Pain on gripping.
CONTRAINDICATION	Gross limitation of extension. Full range of motion.		Loss of full elbow extension. Osteoarthrosis. Loose bodies, traumatic arthritis.	Inability to fully extend.		Acute condition. Rest pain. Restriction of elbow extension.
FREQUENCY	Usually one manipulation.	Three times per week. Average of four treatments. Range:1-9 treatments.	2-3 times per week until cure. Range 4-12 sessions.			

(Courtesy of Kushner, S., and Reid, D.C.: J. Orthop. Sports Phys. Ther. 7:264-272, March 1986. © by Williams & Wilkins, 1986.)

mobilization. The authors have described these techniques for treatment of tennis elbow. I would recommend that these techniques be used only by those with extensive education and experience in joint mobilization. The techniques described are vigorous and even though I feel I have some education and experience in joint mobilization, these are techniques I don't use. I feel better using a more traditional approach to this particular injury. I have had some satisfactory results using deep friction massage for lateral epicondylitis.—F. George, A.T.C., P.T.

Instrumented Testing of Functional Knee Braces
Charles Beck, David Drez, Jr., John Young, W. Dilworth Cannon, Jr., and Mary Lou Stone (Louisiana State Univ., New Orleans, McNeese State University, Lake Charles, La., and Univ. of California at San Francisco)
Am. J. Sports Med. 14:253–256, July–August 1986   6–16

Functional knee braces are designed to provide stability for unstable knees. Despite the wide use of such devices, there are few objective data available concerning their effectiveness. The ability of seven functional knee braces to control anterior tibial displacement was studied in three patients with severe anterior cruciate ligament (ACL) laxity of the right knee.

Testing of anterior tibial displacement was done using the Medmetric KT-1000 Device and the Stryker Knee Laxity Tester. Seven functional knee braces designed to control ACL were tested, including CTi, Don Joy 4-Point, Feanny, Generation II, Lenox Hill, Lerman, and RKS. All measurements were carried out over a 10-hour period, and uninvolved knees were used as controls. The involved knees were tested in and out of each of the braces and each test was repeated three times on each subject. Of the seven braces tested, three were the "off the shelf" variety and four were custom built. It was found that one of the "off the shelf" braces (Don Joy 4-Point) consistently demonstrated greater effectiveness than the other two (Lerman and Feanny). Of the custom built braces, the Generation II and CTi consistently performed better than the others.

Of the seven functional knee braces tested, some were more effective in controlling anterior tibial displacement in the ACL-deficient knee than were others. Many questions still remain unanswered as to how these braces can contribute to the nonoperative and operative treatment regimens of ACL-deficient knees.

▶ In the discussion which followed this article, the question is presented as to the appropriateness of using these braces to enable an athlete with grade 3 anterior lateral rotatory instability to return to high-level competition. The authors' response is that it "depends on positioning and a lot of functional tests."

Once we are satisfied with the level of rehabilitation reached in the clinic, we take the athletes on the field and run them through a series of functional tests to determine the effectiveness of the brace and of their rehabilitation.

Athletes with these injuries gradually return to activity and competition. Very often their practice schedule must be altered to avoid certain exercises or to avoid undue stresses on the knee.—F. George, A.T.C., P.T.

The Lenox Hill Brace: An Evaluation of Effectiveness in Treating Knee Instability
Mark R. Colville, Christopher L. Lee, and Jerome V. Ciullo (Wayne State Univ.)
Am. J. Sports Med. 14:257–261, July–August 1986   6–17

The treatment of the patient with anterior cruciate ligament (ACL) injury is a controversial topic in sports medicine. It is particularly difficult to treat this injury when the patient is a young athletic individual who is not an elite athlete and who does not have severe symptoms of instability. Although many orthopedic surgeons do not consider these patients candidates for reconstruction, the patients often continue to participate in sports and are at increased risk for reinjury. On the basis of these considerations, these patients are frequently fitted with a knee brace in an attempt to prevent reinjury. The Lenox Hill brace was one of the first custom-made knee braces and is one of the most widely used. The goal of the present study was to determine on physical examination what objective changes the brace caused, what effect the brace had on instability, and what effect the brace had on athletic performance.

The study population consisted of 45 patients with 47 injured knees who were an average of 22 years of age at the time of injury. All 47 knees were demonstrated to have an absent or functionless ACL at arthroscopy or athrotomy. All of the patients were fitted with a Lenox Hill brace and then were examined objectively and subjectively to assess its effectiveness. The brace failed to significantly reduce maximal anterior subluxation of the tibia, but did increase resistance to displacement. In addition, rotatory instability was improved an average of one grade by the brace, while varus/valgus laxity was unchanged. Subjectively, patients experienced a decrease in episodes of giving way, and athletic performance was improved in 69% of patients. Increased symptoms of instability correlated positively with greater measured laxity and low resistance to tibial displacement.

The brace, while not effective in controlling absolute laxity, significantly reduced symptoms of instability in the nonelite athlete, possibly through increasing relative resistance to subluxation. Overall, 91% of the patients were satisfied with the brace and felt that it was beneficial for them.

▶ This article, along with the previous article, indicates that these braces may not increase knee stability as much as we would like to think they do. The article also indicates that in many cases the patients like these braces and feel they are beneficial to them. In general I am an advocate of these braces and use them in our athletic program. Every once in a while we have an athlete who cannot return to high-level competition even after a complete rehabilitation program and with this type of brace.—F. George, A.T.C., P.T.

Modification of Quadriceps Femoris Muscle Exercises During Knee Rehabilitation

T.J. Antich and Clive E. Brewster (Kerlan-Jobe Orthopaedic Clinic, Ingelwood, Calif.)

Phys. Ther. 66:1246–1251, August 1986   6–18

Rehabilitation of the quadriceps femoris is the key to full recovery after immobilization of or surgery on the knee. Muscle strengthening regimens frequently are interrupted by complaints of pain on exercise, and convalescence often is prolonged as a result. Modifications of standard quadriceps exercises often allow pain-free exercise and the more rapid progression of rehabilitation. Isotonic quadriceps exercises, done either through the full active range of motion or in terminal extension, are preferred to straight leg raising.

Patellofemoral contact points at various degrees of knee flexion (Fig 6–3) are an important consideration in pain-free rehabilitation. The most effective medication of quadriceps set exercise for reducing patellofemoral pain is active ankle dorsiflexion before quadriceps contraction. Patients with an anterior cruciate ligament (ACL) rupture or who are post-ACL reconstruction should use at least a small wedge when performing quadriceps exercises. Actively inverting the foot may benefit patients with patellar malalignment when dorsiflexion alone is ineffective. Patients with patellofemoral joint symptoms may obtain pain relief by doing isometric hip adduction exercises before knee-extension exercises. Electromuscular stimulation may reduce peripatellar pain due to weakness of the vastus medialis oblique muscle. As a last resort, the knee may be treated with ice before exercise is performed. Patients with increased anterior tibial excursion because of ACL insufficiency on isotonic quadriceps exercises should contract the hamstring muscles for 1 second before lifting the leg.

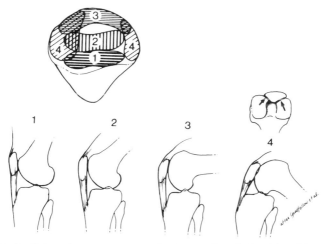

Fig 6–3.—Patellofemoral contact areas at varying degrees of knee flexion. Adapted from Goodfellow et al. (Courtesy of Antich, T.J., and Brewster, C.E.: Phys. Ther. 66:1246–1251, August 1986. Reprinted from Physical Therapy with the permission of the American Physical Therapy Association.)

Less painful quadriceps strengthening exercises will promote rehabilitation of the knee.

▶ The authors have presented us with some solutions to the problem of attempting to rebuild quadriceps strength in the presence of patellofemoral joint problems. In postsurgical or post-cast patients remember to restore patella mobility before vigorous exercise is attempted. The patient should do these stretching techniques many times during the day. As many times as a quadriceps setting exercise is done, then a patella stretch should also be done, until complete mobility of the patella is restored.—F. George, A.T.C., P.T.

Case Study: A Treatment Approach for a Resistant Knee Extension Contracture
Dan Riddle (Humana Hosp. Audubon, Louisville, Ky.)
J. Orthop. Sports Phys. Ther. 7:159–162, January 1986   6–19

Knee extension contractures are a common problem and can result in problems in regaining function. This case study describes a function-limiting knee extension contracture subsequent to an intra-articular femur fracture in an athletic man, aged 37 years. The fracture was first treated by surgical intervention and standard physical therapy without satisfactory results.

A new nonsurgical treatment program was then initiated. The patient was treated three times per week for 8.5 months. The treatment consisted of a 10-minute warm-up on a bicycle ergometer followed by 15 minutes of hot packs at the maximum tolerable temperature. The patient was then positioned on an N-K table for passive stretch at maximum temperature for 40 minutes and then with ice packs for 15 minutes. Ultrasound and deep friction massage were used during the heat stretch. A home exercise program was also initiated. The patient was discharged with 0 to 130 degrees of active knee flexion in the sitting position, which was maintained at 4-month follow-up.

This case study presents a novel treatment for a common problem. Although traditional surgical and physical therapy treatment failed in this case, the use of alternating temperature during passive stretch caused the regaining of functional knee flexion. Additional research is required to determine whether this is a superior method for the treatment of knee extension contractures.

▶ Every once in awhile we come across a knee that resists all attempts to improve range of motion. We have used the procedure the author describes, with some success. The patients usually tolerate the increased stretching using heat then cold very well. We also pay special attention to patellofemoral joint mobility in these resistant cases. I have mentioned these exercises in my comments after the previous article.—F. George, A.T.C., P.T.

Evaluation of Knee Extensor Mechanism Disorders: Clinical Presentation of 112 Patients

T.J. Antich, Celeste Criswell Randall, Roxie A. Westbrook, Matthew C. Morrissey, and Clive E. Brewster (Kerlan-Jobe Orthopaedic Clinic, Inglewood, Calif., Sports Medicine Inc., Ardmore, Pa., and Univ. of Wisconsin, La Crosse)

J. Orthop. Sports Phys. Ther. 8:248–254, November 1986   6–20

Pain may arise from many structures of the extensor mechanism of the knee, but a common site is the inferior patellar pole at the attachment of the proximal infrapatellar tendon. A physical therapist records data on patients referred with infrapatellar tendinitis, chondromalacia patella, or peripatellar pain (Fig 6–4). A total of 112 patients seen in 1983–1984 were evaluated.

About two thirds of patients had unilateral involvement. Chondromalacia was diagnosed in half the patients, infrapatellar tendinitis in 21%, and peripatellar pain in 14%. Both infrapatellar tendinitis and chondromalacia were considered present in 12% of cases. The largest group of patients were full-time amateur athletes who were active at least five times a week. Running was most prevalent, followed by basketball and tennis. Fewer than one third of patients had a history of trauma at the onset of symptoms. Both "aching" and sharp pain were frequent; pain usually was activity-related. Stair-climbing was painful for nearly 80% of patients. Significant hamstring and quadriceps tightness was documented in the involved extremity. The inferior patellar pole was most tender to palpation, followed by medial peripatellar structures. Biomechanical malalignment was not documented in most patients.

It appears necessary to carefully evaluate flexibility, quadriceps imbalance, and biomechanical alignment in patients with extensor mechanism disorders. Exercises emphasizing the vastus medialis oblique should be emphasized.

▶ The authors have stressed the importance of the strength of the vastus medialis oblique muscle and its importance in proper tracking of the patella. They have also indicated that tight hamstring muscles may cause the quadriceps to overwork, thus setting up an overuse syndrome for the extensor mechanism of the knee.

We have approached this problem from many different directions, and that is why thorough evaluations of these patients is essential. Muscle strength and flexibility as well as the biomechanical structure of the entire lower extremity are evaluated. The patients are evaluated for osthotics; knee sleeves with and without patella holes are tried; knee sleeves with sublexation straps are tried; patella tendon straps are tried. We evaluate Q angles very carefully with these patients. Abnormal Q angles can be a cause of the problem. We have used ice, ultrasound, EMS, NSAIDs, and deep friction massage. We have altered workout schedules. Some of the things we try work on some of the patients.— F. George, A.T.C., P.T.

EXTENSOR MECHANISM DISORDERS STUDY

NAME _____ DATE _____

DIAGNOSIS _____

HISTORY

1. SEX: M   F   2. AGE _____   3. RACE: B   W   O   SP

4. SPORT(S) _____   5. STATUS: PRO   FTA   PTA

6. DURATION OF SYMPTOMS _____   WEEKEND

7. INVOLVED: R L BI

8. ANTECEDENT TRAUMA: Y N

9. PAIN: SHARP   DULL   ACHING   THROBBING
          CONSTANT   INTERMITTENT

       AFTER ACTIVITY   BEFORE ACTIVITY   DURING ACTIVITY   AT REST

10. PAIN WITH: WALKING _____   RUNNING _____   U > D   U < D   U = D
               UPSTAIRS _____   DOWNSTAIRS _____

11. MEDICATIONS _____ , _____ mg. QD, BID, TID, QID

12. PAST MEDICAL HISTORY: OSGOOD-SCHLATTERS DISEASE
                            PATELLAR SUBLUXATION
                            PATELLAR DISLOCATION
                            PATELLAR TENDINITIS

PHYSICAL EXAM

                         20 UP   5 UP   15 DOWN
1. GIRTH: INVOLVED ( ) _____   _____   _____ (in cm)
              UNINVOLVED ( ) _____   _____   _____ (in cm)

2. HAMSTRING ROM: INVOLVED _____   UNINVOLVED _____

3. KNEE ROM: INVOLVED   HYPEREXTENSION _____   FLEXION _____
                 UNINVOLVED HYPEREXTENSION _____   FLEXION _____

4. QUADRICEPS TONE: INVOLVED QUADS_____   INVOLVED VMO_____

                       UNINVOLVED QUADS_____   UNINVOLVED VMO_____

5. PAIN WITH QUADRICEPS SETTING: INVOLVED _____   UNINVOLVED _____

6. PAIN WITH 90° ARC: INVOLVED_____   CONC _____   ECC _____
                         UNINVOLVED_____   CONC _____   ECC _____

7. PALPATION   INV   UNINV
    MEDIAL PATELLAR FACET   _____   _____   8. ALIGNMENT   INV   UNINV
    LATERAL PATELLAR FACET   _____   _____   G. VALGUM   _____   _____
    MEDIAL RETINACULUM   _____   _____   G. VARUM   _____   _____
    LATERAL RETINACULUM   _____   _____   SQUINTING   _____   _____
    INFERIOR POLE   _____   _____
    MEDIAL I.P. TENDON   _____   _____   9. TORQUE AT 45°
    LATERAL I.P. TENDON   _____   _____   INV   UNINV
    TIBIAL TUBERCLE   _____   _____   QUADS   _____   _____
                                                 HAMS   _____   _____

NOTES

Fig 6–4.—Initial evaluation form. (Courtesy of Antich, T.J., et al.: J. Orthop. Sports Phys. Ther. 8:248–254, November 1986. © by Williams & Wilkins, 1986.)

Knee Rehabilitation Following Anterior Cruciate Ligament Injury or Surgery

Bernard F. DePalma and Russell R. Zelko (Cornell Univ.)
Athletic Training 21:200–206, Fall 1986   6–21

Rehabilitation after primary repair of the anterior cruciate ligament (ACL) is essential to a successful return to participation in running and jumping sports. If a good rehabilitation program is not available, the function of the involved knee may be significantly impaired even though the operation itself was successful. The authors discuss the basics of a sound knee rehabilitation program following severe injury and/or surgery of the ACL that has been used for 4 years with a 100% success and return to participation rate. The program is based on research, practical application, and strength and power lifting principles. Although some athletes wear protective braces for their first year back in sports, most prefer not to wear a brace because they feel it is unnecessary after completing this program.

The program is divided into 12 phases and takes a year to complete. The goal is to obtain full flexion, full extension with no hyperextension, affected leg hamstring strength and power greater than affected leg quadriceps strength and power, and unaffected leg hamstring strength and power.

This program is based on data from an earlier report in which the load elongation characteristics of a sprain of the ACL were studied. The early part of the program is based on time and control of forces to protect the ligament and allow healing time. The program includes the use of whirlpool, swimming, and stationary cycling in the early phases and rope jumping, sprinting, and mental imagery in the later phases.

▶ The authors have presented a unique, aggressive, and successful ACL rehabilitation program. Recently many of us have become more aggressive in our ACL rehabilitation programs, i.e., initiating range of motion exercises sooner, less time in a cast, more vigorous exercises at an earlier date. The authors are ahead of us in all of these areas, and we are making some changes in our program because of their reported success.

An extremely high goal which the authors have set and achieved is hamstring strength equal to quadriceps strength. I suspect a good deal of the success of their program is because that particular goal has been achieved. The authors have also included a "squatting" exercise in their program. This is an exercise which many of us have avoided in ACL rehabilitation. After discussing this with the authors I have introduced the squat into our program, paying strict attention to the way the exercise is performed.—F. George, A.T.C., P.T.

Strengthening Exercises for Old Cruciate Ligament Tears

Yelverton Tegner, Jack Lysholm, Marketta Lysholm, and Jan Gillquist (Univ. Hosp., Linköping, Sweden)
Acta Orthop. Scand. 57:130–134, April 1986   6–22

Strength training is part of the rehabilitation program for patients with cruciate ligament injuries. This article examines a 3-month thigh and calf muscle-strength training program in 53 patients with old, but still troublesome, cruciate ligament injuries.

Significant improvement was seen in strength, performance, knee score, and activity level with these patients following the training program. Most of these patients were improved enough not to require surgery.

A strength training program can be an alternative to ligament reconstructive surgery in patients with old cruciate ligament injuries. Longer follow-up is needed to study the incidence of other problems occurring with this method of treatment.

▶ The importance of rebuilding the strength of the entire lower extremity even in old ACL injuries is stressed. The authors also state that the results of a 3-month strength training program last for at least 2 years. Proper and complete rehabilitation is an essential ingredient in achieving success with the ACL patient. Most of the problems I see are because of poor or inadequate rehabilitation.—F. George, A.T.C., P.T.

Dynamic Joint Control Training for Knee Ligament Injuries
Hidetoshi Ihara and Akikazu Nakayama (Kyushu Rosai Hosp. and Kyushu Rehabilitation College, Kitakyushu City, Japan)
Am. J. Sports Med. 14:309–315, July–August 1986   6–23

Special attention to training the muscles about the knee is necessary to treat knee ligament injuries properly, whether a conservative or surgical approach is taken. A dynamic joint control training program has been based on use of the Kin-Com Isokinetic Dynamometer. Four patients with "giving way" of one knee during sports activity were trained. All were women, aged 16 to 40 years; three played basketball, and one played volleyball. Three patients had bucket-handle medial meniscal tears and old partial anterior cruciate ligament (ACL) ruptures on the problem side. All had partial meniscectomy without surgery on the ACL. Five women, aged 20 years, without knee problems served as a control group.

Four weekly training sessions were held during 3 months, each consisting of five 5-minute segments. Subjects were told to react to sudden forward movement of the input arm of the dynamometer with contraction of the hamstring (Figs 6–5 and 6–6). Estimates of peak torque time and rising torque value of the hamstring showed significant improvement in trained subjects. Isometric muscle strength did not correlate with peak torque time. All patients had clinical improvement in giving way. Three of them now are able to play basketball and volleyball, and the remaining patient can participate in recreational sports.

Dynamic joint control training using an unstable board involves functional development of the feet to grasp the ground, maintenance of equilibrium, improved reaction to sudden added force, and rapid transference of body weight between the legs. There is concern that such training might

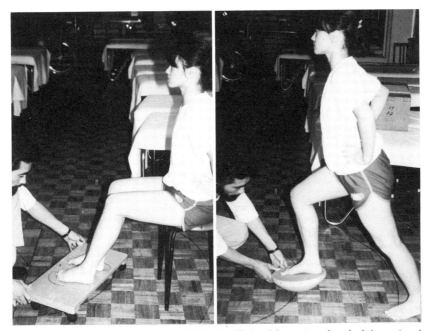

Fig 6–5.—The therapist moves the unstable board suddenly while a patient plants both feet on it and tries to resist the force.

Fig 6–6.—The patient places one leg on an unstable board and tries to maintain equilibrium against the force added by a therapist.

(Courtesy of Ihara, H., and Nakayama, A.: Am. J. Sports Med. 14:309–315, July–August 1986.)

strain a weak ligament, but the training has aided the rehabilitation of patients with torn knee ligaments.

▶ We have all been familiar with the use of balance boards in ankle rehabilitation programs. The authors have described a method of using balance boards and additional forces supplied by the therapist in knee rehabilitation programs. The purpose of these exercises is to improve dynamic control of the knee musculature. They have a small study group but have reported favorable results.—F. George, A.T.C., P.T.

A Performance Test to Monitor Rehabilitation and Evaluate Anterior Cruciate Ligament Injuries

Yelverton Tegner, Jack Lysholm, Marketta Lysholm, and Jan Gillquist (Univ. Hosp., Linköping, Sweden)
Am. J. Sports Med. 14:156–159, March–April 1986   6–24

Anterior cruciate ligament (ACL) injuries occur commonly in young athletes, and the lesion may preclude future participation in sports and may even influence activities of daily life. Therefore, the target for rehabilitation after knee injury is gradual return to the preinjury activity level.

The authors point out that a test for measuring knee function would be useful in guiding rehabilitation and a gradual return to sports. The goal of the present study was to present such a test and to provide reference values.

The reference group included 66 healthy male amateur soccer players with no knee or ankle problems (mean age, 23 ± 5 years), and the patient group included 26 men, all with an unoperated ACL tear (mean age, 27 ± 6 years). All patients had undergone clinical examination and arthroscopy at least 2 months prior to the test. The performance test simulating components of sports included a one-leg hop, running in a figure eight (straight running and turn running measured separately), running up and down a spiral staircase, and running up and down a slope. It was found that the subjects with the ACL injuries performed significantly less well than did the uninjured subjects. The test items of special interest were running in the figure eight, stair running, and slope running, all of which placed special demands on the knee.

A performance test of this design may be useful for monitoring rehabilitation and for evaluating the patient's condition. The authors note that before sports can be resumed at the original level, normal strength and normal performance should be regained.

▶ The tests which the authors describe are a major portion of our knee rehabilitation program. On the field, supervised drills include jogging, straight-ahead running, running and cutting, circles and figure eights, and carioca. When the injured athlete performs these drills satisfactorily, the difficulty of the exercises progresses. The athlete would then begin jumping over dummies or through the ropes. If a contact sport is involved, he would begin hitting dummies and sleds and progress to one-on-one drills. His performance and progression are monitored carefully at all times. He should never be allowed to scrimmage until he feels confident and performs well in the one-on-one drills.—F. George, A.T.C., P.T.

Strain Within the Anterior Cruciate Ligament During Hamstring and Quadriceps Activity

P. Renström, S.W. Arms, T.S. Stanwyck, R.J. Johnson, and M.H. Pope (Univ. of Vermont and Univ. of Göteborg, Sweden)
Am. J. Sports Med. 14:83–87, January–February 1986   6–25

Rehabilitation following anterior cruciate ligament (ACL) surgery is controversial. Rehabilitation exercises of the thigh muscles are believed to play an important role. This study measured ACL strain during simulated activity in the hamstring alone, in the quadriceps alone, and in combined activity. Seven cadaverous knees were examined.

Sutures applied to load cells were attached to the tendons. Loads were applied manually to the hamstrings and with an Instron testing machine to the quadriceps. Strain was measured with a Hall effect transducer.

Isometric hamstring activity decreased ACL strain relative to the passive strain at all positions tested. At flexion angles of 0 to 45 degrees, isometric quadriceps activity significantly increased strain within the ACL. The strain in the ACL during simultaneous activity of both hamstring and quadriceps was significantly higher than during passive normal motion from full extension to 30 degrees of flexion.

Therefore, hamstring exercises are not detrimental to ACL reconstruction and can be included early in the rehabilitation program following ACL surgery. However, the hamstrings are unable to mask the potentially harmful effects of simultaneous quadriceps contraction on repaired ACLs unless the angle of flexion exceeds 30 degrees.

▶ The authors have stressed the importance of hamstring strengthening exercises in anterior cruciate ligament rehabilitation programs. They have also warned against quadriceps strengthening exercises especially from 0 to 30 degrees of knee flexion. It is important to teach co-contraction of hamstrings and quadriceps to alleviate some of the stress placed on the ACL when the knee is extended. The following two articles describe the use of the Johnson Anti-Shear Device, which is designed to alleviate stress on the ACL when isokinetic knee extension exercises are performed.—F. George, A.T.C., P.T.

Validation of the Johnson Anti-Shear Accessory as an Accurate and Effective Clinical Isokinetic Instrument
Kent E. Timm (St. Luke's Hosp., Saginaw, Mich.)
J. Orthop. Sports Phys. Ther. 7:298–303, May 1986   6–26

The Johnson Anti-Shear Accessory (JASA) was designed to limit stress on the anterior cruciate ligament (ACL) of the knee and allow isokinetic

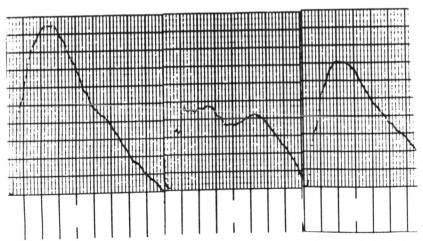

Fig 6–7.—Experiment I, torque curves. *Left,* uninvolved extremity quadriceps; *middle,* involved extremity quadriceps with Cybex knee input shaft; *right,* involved extremity quadriceps with Johnson Anti-Shear Accessory. (Courtesy of Timm, K.E.: J. Orthop. Sports Phys. Ther. 7:298–303, May 1986. © by Williams & Wilkins, 1986.)

evaluation and exercise. Two experiments were performed with the JASA and the Cybex II-CDRC isokinetic system, to validate the JASA in limiting anterior tibial shear during isokinetic activity and to be an accurate means of Cybex testing and isokinetic exercise.

A study of ten patients with nonacute physician-diagnosed ACL involvement used a Cybex II-CDRC protocol of five test knee extension/flexion repetitions at velocities of 60 to 300 degrees per second, preceded by a warm-up of three gradient submaximal and one maximal isokinetic contractions. Significant differences were found between the JASA and the standard Cybex knee input shaft for both the quadriceps and hamstrings (Fig 6–7). In ten subjects in the second study, no significant difference was found between the JASA and standard Cybex system.

The JASA effectively controls anterior tibial shear during isokinetic activity, and it is an accurate means of isokinetic evaluation and exercise.

Clinical Use of the Johnson Anti-Shear Device: How and Why to Use It
Terry Malone (Indiana Central Univ., Indianapolis)
J. Orthop. Sports Phys. Ther. 7:304–309, May 1986   6–27

The Johnson Anti-Shear Device was introduced in 1983. This device presents a method of controlling the anterior shear forces developed during isokinetic exercise on a Cybex-II or Orthotron system. The antishear device permits the therapist to alter the amount of anterior shear developed during exercise and thereby allows the therapist to individualize the rehabilitation protocol. The goal of the present article was to describe the clinical utilization of the Johnson Anti-Shear Device.

The author makes seven recommendations for the use of this device. First, initial pivot position should be midway, thereby equally dividing proximal and distal contact forces. Second, the patient should work submaximally until comfortable with the device. Third, the upper pad should be covered with temper foam; this allows a better fit between the tibia and the pad and renders the exercise more comfortable. Fourth, some patients should work only the quadriceps when using the double pad. This is especially the case when dealing with patients who are very lax and have severe secondary capsular involvement. Fifth, the torque values generated from a single pad should not be compared with those of the antishear or double pad device. Sixth, one should be very careful when using very proximal pivot placements, because great proximal placement may be very painful, especially after intra-articular surgeries. Seventh, it is important to tailor the use of the antishear device to the individual patient.

The clinical use of the Johnson Anti-Shear Device will allow the therapist to develop safer quadriceps exercise programs for their patients with injury to the anterior cruciate ligament.

▶ In Abstract 6–26 the authors detail the problem of building quadriceps strength with ACL injuries. The Johnson Anti-Shear device was designed to alleviate this problem. The following two articles (Abstracts 6–27 and 6–28) describe this device and its clinical use and validation. The authors in Abstract 6–27 have concluded that the Johnson Anti-Shear device does do what it is designed to do and that is control anterior tibial shear during isokinetic exercise. It is also concluded that it is an accurate means of isokinetic evaluation and exercise.

The author Terry Malone in Abstract 6–27 has provided us with some recommendations for the use of this device. He stresses the importance of comparing torque values only when the anti-shear device is used on both legs being tested. A most important piece of advice is to use the anti-shear device for extension exercises only, because of the "anterior shifting force on the proximal pad through hamstring contraction".—F. George, A.T.C., P.T.

A Comparison of Two Progressive Weight Training Techniques on Knee Extensor Strength
Bert H. Jacobson (Oklahoma State Univ.)
Athletic Training 21:315–318, Winter 1986   6–28

Strength is a highly valued commodity in sports, but isotonic strength development techniques have not received the same scientific scrutiny as cardiovascular development techniques. A new mode of isotonic resistance training has recently been developed which uses an isotonic exercise in which a single set of repetitions is performed to the point of absolute failure in the concentric phase and near failure in the eccentric phase. The author evaluated the effects on the strength of a preselected joint movement of two different isotonic progressive weight training techniques.

The study was done with 45 college-aged men who were randomly divided into three groups of 15 subjects each. All subjects trained three times a week on alternate days for 10 weeks on a Nautilus Leg Extension machine. One group performed a commonly used weight training program consisting of a minimum of three sets of six repetitions at progressively altered load increments of 80% 1 maximum repetition (1MR). This regimen has been shown to increase strength significantly. The second group performed a single set of 8 to 12 repetitions at progressively altered load increments of 60% to 65% 1MR to complete failure in both the concentric and eccentric phase of the exercise. The third group served as a control.

Both groups had a significant gain in strength in comparison to the control group. However, there was no significant difference in strength gain between the two experimental groups.

If a program of single sets of MR is as effective in producing strength gains as a program that uses multiple sets, a great deal of time could be saved by using the single-set program.

▶ MR or "manual resistance" technique means that a partner applies additional force by pushing on a weight or bar during the eccentric phase of the exercise. The theory is that a muscle can generate more force in an eccentric contraction than in a concentric contraction. Therefore, if the force is increased during the eccentric phase of the exercise, greater strength gains can be made. There needs to be a great deal more research in this area, however this article gives us a basis to work with in our conditioning programs. Please understand the author is stating the same results can be achieved in less time not with less work. This manual resistance technique is a very intense workout. Usually with an increase in intensity there is an accompanying increase in frequency of injuries sustained. I would recommend its use for those with experience in weight training and not for the beginner.—F. George, A.T.C., P.T.

Proprioceptive Neuromuscular Facilitation Versus Weight Training for Enhancement of Muscular Strength and Athletic Performance
Arnold G. Nelson, Roger S. Chambers, Carl M. McGown, and Keith W. Penrose (Brigham Young Univ.)
J. Orthop. Sports Phys. Ther. 7:250–253, March 1986   6–29

Virtually all athletic training routines include progressive resistive exercise, usually in the form of weight training. This inclusion is due in part to several carefully controlled research studies which have indicated that weight training improves performance. However, proprioceptive neuromuscular facilitation (PNF) is another form of progressive resistive exercise which is commonly used by physical therapists. These PNF exercises are designed to promote or hasten the neuromuscular response of the proprioceptors, and PNF patterns have a spiral, diagonal direction and are in line with the topographic arrangement of the muscles. Hence, PNF exercises are very similar to actions and movements found in various sports. The effects of a traditional weight training program and PNF were compared.

The study population consisted of 30 healthy female college students who were randomly assigned to one of three groups: weight training, PNF, and control. The weight training and PNF women trained 3 days per week for 8 weeks. All of the subjects were tested for changes in knee and elbow extensor strength, throwing distance, and vertical jump. The weight training group increased strength by 19.3% for knee extension and 20.4% for elbow extension, while the PNF group increased strength by 22.1% for knee extension and by 29.1% for elbow extension. Weight training led to an increase in throwing distance of 12.8% and of vertical jump of 9.9%, while PNF led to an increase in throwing distance of 25% and of vertical jump of 16%.

It is concluded that PNF may be superior to weight training in athletic performance enhancement and, therefore, a better modality for athletic conditioning and injury rehabilitation.

The Use of Proprioceptive Neuromuscular Facilitation Techniques in the Rehabilitation of Sport-Related Injury
William E. Prentice and Elaine F. Kooima (Univ. of North Carolina, Chapel Hill)
Athletic Training 21:26–31, Spring 1986   6–30

Proprioceptive neuromuscular facilitation (PNF) is an approach to therapeutic exercise based on the principles of functional human anatomy and neurophysiology. PNF employs proprioceptive, cutaneous, and auditory input to cause functional improvement in motor output, and it can be a vital element in the rehabilitation process of many sports-related injuries. PNF techniques have been recommended as a means of increasing strength, as well as flexibility and range of motion. The goal of the present study was to provide a guide for the sports therapist using the principles and techniques of PNF as a component of a rehabilitation program.

There are certain principles of PNF which must be superimposed on any of the specific techniques. It is thought that application of the following principles may assist in promoting a desired response in the patient being treated. First, the patient must be taught PNF patterns learning the sequential movements from starting position to terminal position. Second, it is important to look at the moving limb, because this visual stimulus offers the patient feedback for directional and positional control. Third, verbal cues are used to coordinate voluntary effort with reflex responses. Fourth, manual contact with appropriate pressure is essential for influencing direction of motion and facilitating a maximal response, since reflex responses are greatly affected by pressure receptors. Fifth, proper mechanics and body positioning by the therapist are essential in applying pressure and resistance.

Sixth, the amount of resistance given should facilitate maximal response, which will permit smooth, coordinated motion; the appropriate resistance depends upon the capabilities of the patient. Seventh, rotational movement is a critical component of all PNF patterns because maximal contraction is not possible without it. Eighth, normal timing is the sequence of muscle contraction which takes place in any normal motor activity resulting in coordinated movement. Ninth, timing for emphasis is used primarily with isotonic contractions. Tenth, specific joints may be faciliated by using traction or approximation. Eleventh, giving a quick stretch to the muscle prior to muscle contraction facilitates a muscular response of greater force through the mechanisms of the stretch reflex.

Specific techniques of PNF include both strengthening and stretching techniques. The exercise patterns are three component movements which include flexion/extension, abduction/adduction, and internal/external rotation. It is concluded that the principles and techniques of PNF when used appropriately with specific patterns can be an extremely effective tool for rehabilitation of sports-related injury. PNF may be used as a method of strengthening weak muscles or muscle groups as well as for improving range of motion. The authors recommend that the specific techniques selected for use should depend on individual patient need and may be modified accordingly.

▶ The authors of Abstract 6–29 state that PNF might be superior to WT for training programs and rehabilitation because "PNF patterns improve motor skill through positive motor transfer." We have used PNF techniques in both our flexibility program and our injury rehabilitation program with a good deal of success. We have had difficulty instituting PNF into our conditioning programs because in many cases we do not have enough strength to provide adequate resistance to a strong athlete. PNF techniques can be time consuming, and this becomes an important factor if these techniques are to be used with a 100-man football squad. Please refer to Abstract 6–28.

The authors of Abstract 6–30 describe in detail the principles and techniques of PNF patterns. They recommend its use in the rehabilitation of athletic injuries. The athletes, as other patients do, appreciate the individual attention given them when doing PNF exercises. Because of this they put a great deal of energy and effort into these exercises, and this may partly contribute to the success of PNF.—F. George, A.T.C., P.T.

Fatigue Response in Human Quadriceps Femoris Muscle During High Frequency Electrical Stimulation

Michael G. Parker, Matthew Berhold, Robert Brown, Steven Hunter, Matthew R. Smith, and Robert O. Runhling (Univ. of Utah)
J. Orthop. Sports Phys. Ther. 7:145–153, January 1986   6–31

Electrical muscle stimulation is used in physical therapy. Nevertheless, the physiologic mechanism explaining the resulting increase in muscular strength is unclear. Rather than intensity of training, muscle fatigue may be the important contributing factor. This study assessed the effects of two patterns of high frequency electrical stimulation on the dynamic peak torque decline of the human quadriceps muscle group in 12 healthy subjects.

The patterns of decline of torque with and without electrical stimulation are shown in Figure 6–8. The mean peak quadriceps torque declines are shown in Figure 6–9. There was a significant difference between the dif-

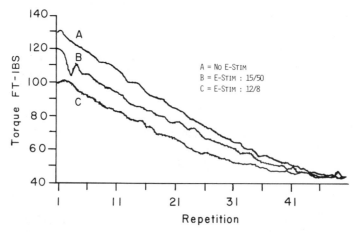

Fig 6–8.—Decline in peak quadriceps torque following electrical stimulation. Curve A: $Y = 138 \cdot (10^{-0.0105 \cdot R})$; curve B: $Y = 117.5 \cdot (10^{-0.0095 \cdot R})$; curve C (fast): $Y = 104.7 \cdot (10^{-0.0095 \cdot R})$; curve C (slow): $Y = 72.8 \cdot (10^{-0.004824 \cdot R})$. (Courtesy of Parker, M.G., et al.: J. Orthop. Sports Phys. Ther. 7:145–153, January 1986. © by Williams & Wilkins, 1986.)

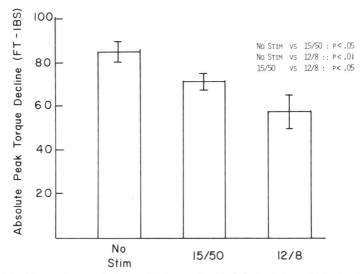

Fig 6–9.—Mean peak torque declines ± (SE) for no prior electrical stimulation and following the 15/50 and 12/8 patterns of stimulation. (Courtesy of Parker, M.G., et al.: J. Orthop. Sports Phys. Ther. 7:145–153, January 1986. © by Williams & Wilkins, 1986.)

ferent regimens. Greater amounts of electrical stimulation produced a greater amount of fatigue. High frequency current appears to selectively fatigue fast twitch (FT) muscle fibers.

Because of their larger nerve fiber diameter, the FT motor units are more rapidly recruited during an electrical stimulus. This could explain the greater muscle fatigue at lower training intensities. Therefore, selective stimulation of FT muscle fibers may be important in explaining the mechanism of strength increase following application of high frequency electrical current. Further research is required to determine which stimulation pattern provides the greatest strength increases.

▶ In the 1986 YEAR BOOK OF SPORTS MEDICINE, I selected six articles on the subject of electrical stimulation. My comments referred to studies which indicate that strength gains may be achieved and other studies indicating no improvement in strength. A letter I referred to claims we are in fact using TENS units in these studies and in most clinics and not true galvanic ES units. There are many variables which must be considered when evaluating these studies. The authors of this study (Abstract 6–31) suggest that it is the stimulation of fast twitch muscle fibers which accounts for the increase in strength noted in their study.—F. George, A.T.C., P.T.

Comparative Study Using Four Modalities in Shinsplint Treatments

Wayne Smith, F. Winn, and R. Parette (USCG Training Ctr., Cape May, N. Jersey, and Natl. Inst. for Occupational Safety and Health, Cincinnati)
J. Orthop. Sports Phys. Ther. 8:77–80, August 1986   6–32

"Shinsplints" is a term used to describe many overuse injuries of the lower leg, and the literature includes many variations in the treatment of this condition. Traditional treatment involves use of ice and heat in conjunction with biomechanical correction and supportive exercises. Furthermore, some investigators have suggested that shinsplints are due to muscle inflammation induced by overuse, and as such would respond to the application of an anti-inflammatory medication to the involved muscles. There are several means available for administration of medication to muscles, including mechanical application (phonophoresis) and electrical application (iontophoresis). The effects of ice massage, ultrasound, iontophoresis, and phonophoresis in the treatment of shinsplints were compared.

The study population consisted of 50 patients (age range, 18 to 25 years) with shinsplint syndrome who were randomly assigned into five groups of 10. The criterion for identification of shinsplints was palpable pain along the medial aspects of the tibia. Group 1 received iontophoretic treatments of dexamethasone sodium phosphate (4 mg/ml) and 1 cc of 4% lidocaine hydrochloride; group 2 received 10 minutes of ice massage; group 3 received continuous ultrasound and phonoelectrophoretic treatments using a mixture of 33 mg of Decadron and 16 cc of 2% lidocaine gel; group 4 received continuous ultrasound alone; group 5 was the control group. It was found that none of these treatment modalities was superior to another; however, all were clearly superior to a control treatment program.

The appropriate treatment modalities for shinsplints should be a function of the restoration of the individual's range of motion, the number of treatments that can be provided, and the availability of the treatment mode.

▶ What is the best method of treating shinsplints? A lecture on this subject will certainly attract large numbers of coaches, trainers, and runners at any sports medicine symposium. I'm sorry that I don't have a simple answer for the question. The problem and its causes must be evaluated carefully. Shinsplint pain doesn't occur in everyone for the same reason. There may be one or more contributing factors, and each one must be corrected.

Running surfaces and shoes must certainly be considered. Changes in either may be a cause or cure of shinsplint pain. Always watch for the athlete who has been running on grass when he changes sports or events and begins to run on a hard surface. Evaluate for the need of orthotics or a new and better supportive shoe. Go on the field or track and evaluate the runner's technique. We have found many of our athletes with this problem do not have a high enough knee lift in their running stride. This will cause the anterior lower leg muscle to work harder to lift the toe to clear the ground when running. Weak anterior lower leg muscles and tight posterior leg muscles may also contribute to the problem.—F. George, A.T.C., P.T.

Subject Index

A

Abuse
  cocaine, acute cardiac events in, 146
  drug, female athletes as targets for, 352
Acetazolamide
  exercise performance and muscle mass
    at high altitude and, 161
Acromioclavicular
  dislocation, study of treatments, 260
  joint, ligamentous system study, 258
Adolescence
  amenorrhea during, in athlete, 356
  diabetes type I during, and physical
    fitness, 96
  football playing during, mouth
    protectors and oral trauma, 211
  protein excretion during, urinary, 344
  sports injuries during, 346
  swimming during, effect of
    menstruation cycle phase on, 357
Adrenal
  activity monitoring during male
    marathon run, 121
  medulla deficiency, hemodynamic and
    hormonal responses to exercise in,
    95
Adrenaline
  cardiovascular response alteration to
    endurance trained subjects to, 51
  -induced platelet aggregation and alpha-
    2-adrenoreceptor density, 48
β-Adrenergic blockade
  in leukocytosis, exercise-induced, 46
$β_2$-Adrenergic mechanism
  in skeletal muscle (in rat), 44
β-Adrenoceptor blockade
  muscle contractile performance during,
    47
α-2-Adrenoreceptor density
  platelets and, 48
Aerobic
  capacity after infectious mononucleosis,
    177
  dance injuries, epidemiology of, 208
  exercise in paraplegia, 169
  training, exercise tolerance and
    echocardiography in
    postmenopausal women, 30
Age
  -related blood pressure response to
    dynamic work with small muscle
    masses, 35
Aged
  hot weather, exercise and the kidneys,
    175

measurement of customary physical
    activity before and after retirement,
    173
Air
  Force recruits, sudden cardiac death in,
    16
  ionization, cardiorespiratory variables
    and attention span, 61
Alcohol
  lipoprotein cholesterol and
    apolipoprotein A-1 after, 79
  running and, 152
Aldosterone
  during swimming and running, 53
Allograft (*see* Graft)
Altitude
  extreme (*see* Extreme altitude)
  high (*see* High altitude)
  sickle cell trait and exercise, 168
Amenorrhea
  in athlete
    during adolescence, 356
    bone mineral density after resumption
      of menses, 359
  in runners, women
    diet and bone status in, 361
    highly trained, nutritional intakes and
      status, 362
Amphetamines
  athletic performance and, 148
Anabolic (*see* Steroids, anabolic)
Anaerobic
  capacity, lactic, test development in,
    102
Anaphylactic syndromes
  exercise causing, 105
Androgyny
  psychological, of female college athletes,
    380
Anemia
  of athlete, 67
  long-term, and central circulation
    during exercise, 65
  swimming, endurance, hemolysis and
    iron depletion, 68
Ankle
  injuries
    clinical observations, 330
    diagnostic dilemmas in, 317
  instability, repair with periosteal
    ligament transfer, 329
  magnetic resonance imaging of, high-
    resolution, 326
  sprains (*see* Sprains, ankle)
Anxiety
  catecholamines at rest and exercise
    during, 50

Apicitis
  patellar, predisposition in athletes, 285
Apolipoprotein A-1
  after alcohol and exercise, 79
Arthralgia
  patellofemoral, thermography of, in
    athletes, 279
Arthroscopy
  complications of, 306
  for cruciate ligament reconstruction,
    315, 316
  curettage in osteochondrosis dissecans
    of knee, 308
  of hip, 271
  knee, under local anesthesia
    as outpatient procedure, 307
    study of, 307
  for meniscus repair, 309
    assessment of healing parameters, 314
    evaluation with repeat arthroscopy,
      310
    intra-articular, with posterior
      incision, 314
  for osteochondral lesions of talus, 322,
    323
  in patellar retinacular release, 280
  of shoulder, appraisal, 240
  of talar dome fracture, 321
Arthrotomography
  glenohumeral, in shoulder instability,
    244
Asthma
  exercise causing, 55
    gastrointestinal regulatory peptides in,
      59
    prevention, 57
Athlete(s)
  amenorrhea of (*see* Amenorrhea, in
    athlete)
  anemia of, 67
  competitive, and sudden death causes
    in, 15
  endurance, left atrial enlargement in, 23
  esophageal function in, and moderate
    exercise, 170
  hamate fracture of hook, 225
  hypothyroid, TSH and prolactin
    responses to TRH in, 97
  injured, psychology of, 338
  metatarsophalangeal joint injuries in,
    318
  patellar apicitis predisposition in, 285
  patellar chondropathy predisposition in,
    285
  patellofemoral arthralgia, thermography
    of, 279
  with plantar fasciitis, surgery results,
    319

  quadriplegia in, transient, and
    congenital cervical stenosis, 220
  rotator cuff tears, surgery of, 256
  stress and, 178
  ulnar collateral ligament reconstruction,
    230
  women
    college, psychological androgyny of,
      380
    with menstrual irregularity,
      musculoskeletal injury increase in,
      358
    as targets for drug abuse, 352
  young
    Putti-Platt procedure for shoulder
      dislocation in, 250
    ventricular tachycardia in, 19
Athletic
  drinks, gastric emptying of, 118
  injury, in high schools, knowledge of
    care and prevention, 386
  performance
    amphetamines and, 148
    caffeine and, 148
    proprioceptive neuromuscular
      facilitation vs. weight training in,
      410
  program, university, and drug testing,
    32
  trainers in public schools, opportunities
    for, 387
  training
    facilities, for small college, planning
      of, 388
    program in computer age, 389
Atrium
  left, enlarged in former endurance
    athletes, 23
Atrophy
  skeletal muscle, during immobilization,
    391
Attention
  span and air ionization, 61
Autograft (*see* Graft)
Axillary nerve
  shoulder procedures and, 239

B

Baseball
  pitchers, isokinetic shoulder strength of,
    393
Basketball
  players, female and male, comparison of
    cruciate ligament laxity between,
    353

Beta-blockade
enzymatic adaptation to physical
training during (in rat), 44
exercise capacity in trained men during,
41
in hypertension (*see* Hypertension, beta-
blockade in)
pistol shooting performance and, 40
Beta-endorphin-like immunoreactivity and
pleasantness after running, 179
Biceps
tendon, ultrasound of, 254
Bicycle
accidents
injuries of adult cyclists, 212
maxillofacial fractures in, 212
helmet use by children, 347
Biomechanical
consequences of sport shoe design,
183
study to contrast karate with boxing,
183
Biomechanics
of knee menisci, 196
of long jump, 188
of running, 184
Blockade
beta- (*see* Beta-blockade)
beta-adrenergic, and exercise-induced
leukocytosis, 46
beta-adrenoceptor, muscle contractile
performance during, 47
Blood
cells (*see* Red blood cell)
flow, quadriceps, exercise and
hypoxemia, 30
loss, gastrointestinal, during marathon
run, 124
pressure
in hypertension during beta-blockade,
39
physical activity and, in young
women, 34
response abnormality during exercise,
37
response to dynamic work with small
muscle masses, 35
Body
mass and thermal responses in water,
112
Bone
block iliotibial band transfer in cruciate
ligament repair, 295
density and long-distance running, 132
mineral content and physical activity in
women, 69
mineral density
physical fitness and, 70

after resumption of menses in
amenorrheic athletes, 359
pegs, cortical, in osteochondral fracture
of knee, 292
soft tissue fixation to, 334
status in amenorrheic runners, 361
temporal response to unloading, 72
Boxers
retinal injuries and detachment in, 217
Boxing
contrasted with karate by
biomechanical study, 183
medical and public health aspects of,
331
Boytchev procedure
for shoulder instability, 248
Braces
joint counterforce, for tennis player,
229
for knee
in football, 384
functional, instrumented testing of,
397
Lenox Hill, effectiveness of, 398
to prevent football player injuries,
209, 383
prophylactic, in college football, 384
stabilizing, running speed and agility
with, 385
Lenox Hill, effectiveness for knee
instability, 398
Brachial plexus
stretch injuries, 235
Bracing
knee, to prevent sports injuries, 208
Brain
damage, due to climbs to extreme
altitude, 163
Breakdancer
pulmonary embolism of, 143
Breath
holding in divers, reappraisal of, 138
Breathing
loaded, sense of effort during, and
caffeine, 150
Bronchospasm
exercise causing, 58
Bursitis
prepatellar, in wrestlers, 277

C

Caffeine
athletic performance and, 148
effect
on loaded breathing, 150
on respiratory muscle endurance, 150

exercise performance after, in habitual
  caffeine users, 148
treadmill running and, incremental, 149
Calcaneofibular ligament
  rerouting peroneal tendons under, 327
Capsulorrhaphy
  DuToit staple, for shoulder dislocation,
  249
Carbohydrate
  beverages, ingesting during exercise in
    the heat, 86
  strenuous exercise when fed, muscle
    glycogen during, 89
Carbonic anhydrase
  liberation, during exercise, 74
Cardiac (*see* Heart)
Cardiopulmonary
  stress testing, 24
Cardiorespiratory
  variables and air ionization, 61
Cardiovascular
  disease, physical activity, life styles and
    longevity, 13
  effects of repeated sauna bathing, 109
  events and cocaine, 146
  response alteration to adrenaline in
    endurance trained subjects, 51
  risk factors, and vigorous physical
    activity, 26
  surgery, exercise training after, 20
Catecholamines
  during anxiety, 50
  in hypertension during beta-blockade,
  39
  during swimming and running, 53
Cell(s)
  blood (*see* Red blood cell)
  fat, epinephrine and physical training,
  84
  muscle, leakage of myoglobin after
    exercise, 75
  sickle cell trait, exercise and altitude,
  168
Cervical
  stenosis, congenital, as transient
    quadriplegia in athletes, 220
Children
  bicycle helmet use by, 347
  exercise and, overview of, 341
  infant swimming classes, 342
  scuba diving, 348
  sports injuries of, 346
  swimming training, echocardiography
    in, 341
Cholesterol
  increase after endurance training in
    female runners, 80
  lipoprotein
    after alcohol and exercise, 79

physical activity and, 79
  in weight-trained and endurance-
    trained women, 376
Chondromalacia
  patellae, radiography of, 276
Chondropathy
  patellar, predisposition in athletes, 285
Chronic compartment syndrome, 262
Circulation
  central, during exercise, anemia and
    retransfusion, 180
Clavicle
  fracture (*see* Fracture, clavicle)
Clavicular
  harness, modified, for shoulder
    dislocation, 246
Climbers (*see* Extreme altitude)
Cocaine
  abuse, acute cardiac events in, 146
  cardiovascular events and, 146
Collagen
  fibrils, organization in tendon, 153
Compartment decompression
  repeat, with partial fasciectomy, 265
Compartment syndrome
  chronic, 262
    anterior, of leg, 263
    tibialis posterior, exertional, 264
Competition
  iron status of female field hockey
    players and, 364
Computer
  age, athletic training program in, 389
Computerized knee model
  in Müller femorotibial ligament
    reconstruction, 298
Concussion
  in football, college, 217
Conditioning
  exercise decreasing premenstrual
    symptoms, 358
  sports, and physiological differences
    between genders, 334
Contractions
  muscular, endurance capacity of
    untrained people in, 372
Contracture
  knee, resistant extension, 400
Coronary
  heart disease, high risk, exercise ECG
    in, 26
Cruciate ligament
  anterior (*see below*)
  laxity, comparison between male and
    female basketball players, 353
  old tears, strengthening exercises for,
  403
  posterior, injuries in athlete, results of
    nonoperative treatment, 305

testing, objective, 194
Cruciate ligament, anterior
    autograft of patellar tendon origin, 299
    injuries
        to counsel or to operate? 293
        monitoring rehabilitation in, 405
    injury or surgery, knee rehabilitation
        after, 403
    instability, Insall procedure results in,
        295
    reconstruction
        with arthroscopy, 315, 316
        with "ligamentization," 300
        with semitendinosus tendon and
            iliotibial tract, 296
        tendon graft in, allogeneic, 301
    repair with bone block iliotibial band
        transfer, 295
    replacement
        (in dog), 304
        with patellar tendon allograft, 303
    strain during hamstring and quadriceps
        activity, 406
    tear, acute nonoperated isolated, 294
    transplant, study of, 302

D

Dance
    aerobic, epidemiology of injuries, 208
Death
    sudden (*see* Sudden death)
Decompression
    accidents after deep-sea diving, causing
        inner ear trauma, 135
    acute, nephrotic syndrome after, 137
Decompression
    sickness, ulnar palsy complicating, 136
Dehydration
    exercise, fluid balance in, 116
Diabetes mellitus
    hemodynamic and hormonal responses
        to exercise in, 95
    type 2, and long-term exercise, 92
Diet
    in amenorrheic runners, 361
Dislocation
    acromioclavicular, treatment study, 260
    patella, natural history, 281
    peroneal tendons, recurrent, 327
    shoulder
        anterior subcoracoid, external
            rotation method, 246
        clavicular harness for, modified, 246
        locked posterior, 251
        recurrent, DuToit staple
            capsulorrhaphy for, 249

    recurrent, Putti-Platt procedure in
        young athlete, 250
    of tibiofibular joint, 266
        recurrent, 268
        recurrent, stabilization by ligament
            reconstruction, 267
Divers
    breath holding in, reappraisal of, 314
    Japanese male breath-hold, wet-suit
        diving of, 113
    scuba, pediatric, 348
Diving
    deep-sea, inner ear trauma due to
        decompression accidents after, 135
    scuba, medical standards for, 137
    wet-suit, in Japanese male breath-hold
        divers, 113
Drinks
    athletic, gastric emptying of, 118
    glucose-electrolyte, various, and fluid
        balance, 116
Drug(s)
    abuse, female athletes as targets for,
        352
    testing in university athletic program,
        151
    therapy, and ventricular tachycardia in
        young athlete, 19
DuToit staple capsulorrhaphy
    for shoulder dislocation, 249
Dynamometry
    isokinetic, 392
Dystrophy
    reflex sympathetic, 336
        of knee, 337

E

Ear
    inner, trauma due to decompression
        accidents after deep-sea diving, 135
Echocardiography
    aerobic training and exercise tolerance,
        in postmenopausal women, 30
    of atrial enlargement, left, in endurance
        athlete, 23
    in swimming training in children, 341
Edema
    pulmonary, at high altitude, 165
Elbow
    joint, ulnar collateral ligament tears,
        231
    tennis, manipulation in, 395
Elderly (*see* Aged)
Electrical stimulation
    fatigue in quadriceps femoris muscle
        during, 412

Electrocardiography
  exercise
    false positive, exercise ^{201}Tl
      scintigraphy in, 28
    in high risk for coronary heart
      disease, 26
    in ischemic heart disease, 27
Electrolyte
  -glucose drinks, various, and fluid
    balance in exercise, 116
Electro-mechanical response times
  force development rate in males and
    females and, 370
Electromyography
  analysis, tennis stroke and grip size,
    189
  of joint counterforce braces on tennis
    player, 229
  of shoulder muscles
    activity and fatigue during repetitive
      work, 200
    during swimming, 199
Embolism
  pulmonary, of breakdancer, 143
Endocrine
  effects of repeated sauna bathing, 111
β-Endorphin
  -like immunoreactivity and pleasantness
    after running, 179
Endurance
  athletes, left atrial enlargement in, 23
  capacity of untrained people in
    muscular contractions, 372
  events, and muscle damage, 353
  swimming, hemolysis, anemia and iron
    depletion, 68
  trained subjects
    adrenaline in, cardiovascular response
      alteration in, 51
    alpha-2-adrenoreceptor density and,
      48
  -trained women, HDL-C in, 376
  training in runners, cholesterol increase
    after, 80
Enzyme
  adaptation to physical training under
    beta-blockade (in rat), 44
  efflux and skeletal muscle damage, 62
Epilepsy
  exercise in, 168
Epinephrine
  fat cells and physical training, 84
Ergogenic
  aids, vitamins and minerals as, 156
Erythrocyte (see Red blood cell)
Esophagus
  function in athletes, and moderate
    exercise, 170

Ethanol
  reducing myoglobin release during
    isokinetic exercise, 77
Ethical
  dilemma for U.S. physicians, anabolic
    steroids as, 144
Exercise
  acute, and hemostasis, 64
  aerobic, in paraplegia, 169
  in aged, hot weather and kidneys, 175
  anaphylactic syndromes due to, 105
  asthma due to (see Asthma, exercise
    causing)
  blood pressure response during,
    abnormal, 37
  bronchospasm due to, 58
  capacity in trained men, and beta-
    blockade, 41
  carbonic anhydrase, muscle, liberation
    during exercise, 74
  catecholamines during anxiety and, 50
  children and, overview, 341
  cholesterol and apolipoprotein A-1
    after, 79
  circulation and, central, anemia and
    retransfusion, 65
  conditioning, decreasing premenstrual
    symptoms, 358
  dehydration, fluid balance in, 116
  ECG (see Electrocardiography, exercise)
  in epilepsy, 168
  fitness-type, and iron status in women,
    363
  in glucose tolerance, 93
  glycogen and, muscle, 88, 89
  growth hormone secretion after, 355
  in the heat, ingesting carbohydrate
    beverages during, 86
  hormone and hemodynamic responses
    to, 95
  in hypertension during beta-blockade, 38
    blood pressure and catecholamines
      after, 39
  immunity to disease and, 171
  in insulin resistance, 93
  isokinetic muscle, ethanol reducing
    myoglobin release during, 77
  knee joint laxity due to, 272, 273
  leukocytosis due to, and adrenergic
    blockade, 46
  long-duration, oral glucose during, 91
  long-term
    in diabetes type 2, 92
    muscle cell leakage of myoglobin
      after, 75
  McArdle's disease and, 63
  menstrual disturbances due to,
    managing, 355

Exercise
  moderate, and esophageal function in
    athletes, 170
  myocardial infarction and (in rat), 17
  pain in lower leg, 262
  performance
    after caffeine in habitual caffeine
      users, 148
    at high altitude and acetazolamide,
      161
  prolactin secretion after, 355
  prolonged, triglyceride clearance after,
    81
  prostaglandin synthesis during, renal,
    157
  protein excretion during adolescence
    and, 344
  quadriceps blood flow and hypoxemia,
    30
  quadriceps femoris muscle, during knee
    rehabilitation, 399
  rehydration, fluid balance in, 116
  scintigraphy, [201]T1, in false positive
    exercise ECG, 28
  sickle cell trait and altitude, 168
  after sleep loss, stress hormonal
    response in, 98
  strengthening, for old cruciate ligament
    tears, 403
  strenuous, when fed carbohydrate,
    muscle glycogen during, 89
  stress and the athlete, 178
  stretch-shortening cycle, 373
  submaximal, intense, and hyperoxia,
    103
  tolerance, aerobic training and
    echocardiography in
    postmenopausal women, 30
  training
    after cardiovascular surgery, 20
    hypertension and, 33
    lipids and lipoproteins after, 83
    in special patient populations,
      172
  vasodilation during, thermoregulatory,
    and menstrual cycle, 99
  ventricular tachycardia after, 18
  verapamil and, 43
  vigorous, and sudden death, 14
  in vitamin E deficiency and vitamin C
    supplements, 101
  women going easy on, 352
Exertional
  tibial posterior compartment syndrome,
    264
Extensors
  of knee, isokinetic torque levels in
    soccer players, 197

Extreme altitude
  climbers, ventilation control in, 166
  climbs to, causing brain damage, 163
Extremities
  lower
    compartment syndrome of, chronic
      anterior, 263
    exercise pain in, 262
  upper
    force, speed and power output in,
      during horizontal pulls, 205
    strength in young women, 374

F

Fasciectomy
  partial, in repeat compartment
    decompression, 265
  plantar, in athletes, surgery results, 319
  in chronic anterior compartment
    syndrome of leg, 263
Fat
  cells, epinephrine and physical training,
    84
Fatigability
  sex differences in, 367
Fatigue
  McArdle's disease and, 63
  in quadriceps femoris muscle during
    electrical stimulation, 412
  in shoulder muscles during repetitive
    work, 200
Femorotibial
  ligament reconstruction, Müller, 298
Femur
  neck
    bone mineral density and physical
      fitness, 70
    fracture, distraction type stress, 271
  osteochondral defects, fresh
    osteochondral allografts in, 289
Field hockey
  players, female, iron status of, effects of
    physical training and competition
    on, 364
  team, Canadian Women's Olympic,
    physiological monitoring of, 378
Fitness
  physical (*see* Physical fitness)
  -type exercise, and iron status in
    women, 363
Flexibility
  improvement, warm-up for, 390
Flexors
  knee, isokinetic torque levels in soccer
    players, 197

Fluid
  balance in exercise dehydration and
    rehydration, 116
Foot
  injuries, diagnostic dilemmas in, 317
  midfoot osteochondritis dissecans, 320
Football
  college
    concussion in, 217
    players, braces to prevent knee injury
      in, 383, 384
    players, lumbar spondylolysis and
      spondylolisthesis in, 223
  knee braces in, 384
  player
    adolescent, mouth protectors and oral
      trauma, 211
    knee braces to prevent injury, 209
Force
  development rate, and electro-
    mechanical response times, 370
  of upper extremity during horizontal
    pulls, 205
Fracture
  clavicle
    outcome, 261
    ununited, surgery of, 261
  femoral neck, distraction type stress,
    271
  hamate, of hook, in athletes, 225
  knee, osteochondral, cortical bone pegs
    in, 292
  maxillofacial, in bicycle accidents, 212
  olecranon, stress, in javelin throwers,
    232
  of radius
    distal end, 226
    head, closed, results of excision, 234
    head, comminuted, reduction and
      fixation, 233
    results of delayed excision, 235
  talar dome, arthroscopy of, 321
Friction
  iliotibial band friction syndrome, 270
Frostbite
  ketanserin for, 176

G

Gastric (*see* Stomach)
Gastrointestinal
  blood loss during marathon run, 124
  hemorrhage in competitive runners, 125
  peptides in asthma due to exercise, 59
Gender (*see* Sex)
Glenohumeral
  arthrotomography in shoulder
    instability, 244

Glenoid
  labrum damage, anterior, in swimmers,
    242
Glucose
  -electrolyte drinks, various, and fluid
    balance in exercise, 116
  oral, during long-duration exercise, 91
  tolerance, and exercise, 93
Glycogen, muscle
  exercise and, 89
  during strenuous exercise when fed
    carbohydrate, 89
Golf
  swing, rotator cuff function during, 202
Gonadotropin
  -releasing hormone in male marathon
    runners, 122
Graft
  autograft, cruciate ligament, of patellar
    tendon origin, 299
  fresh osteochondral allografts in
    osteochondral defect of femur,
    289
  tendon, allogeneic, in cruciate ligament
    reconstruction, 301
Growth
  hormone secretion after exercise, 355
Gymnastic
  activities, spinal injury during, 222

H

Hamate
  fracture, of hook, in athletes, 225
Hamstring
  activity, strain within anterior cruciate
    ligament during, 406
Harness
  modified clavicular, for shoulder
    dislocation, 246
HDL-C
  in weight-trained and endurance-trained
    women, 376
Health
  hazards of windsurfing on polluted
    water, 141
  public, aspects of boxing, 331
Heart
  (*see also* Cardiovascular)
  disease
    coronary, high risk, exercise ECG in,
      26
    ischemic, exercise ECG in, 27
  events in cocaine abuse, 146
  rate, overshoot, incidence, 32
  size, not decreasing after exercise
    cessation, 21

sudden cardiac death in Air Force
   recruits, 16
Heat
   exercise in the, ingesting carbohydrate
      beverages during, 86
   stroke at Mekkah pilgrimage, 106, 107
Helmet
   bicycle, use by children, 347
Hemolysis
   swimming, anemia and iron depletion,
      68
Hemorrhage
   gastrointestinal, in competitive runners,
      125
Hemorrheology
   sauna effects on, 108
Hemostasis
   exercise and, 64
High altitude
   exercise performance at, and
      acetazolamide, 161
   medicine, 158
   muscle mass at, and acetazolamide,
      161
   pulmonary edema, 165
   transient ischemic attacks at, 162
High schools
   athletic injuries in, knowledge of care
      and prevention, 386
Hip
   arthroscopy of, 271
Hockey (*see* Field hockey)
Hormone(s)
   gonadotropin-releasing, in male
      marathon runners, 122
   growth, secretion after exercise, 355
   responses to exercise, 95
   stress, response to exercise after sleep
      loss, 98
Hot weather
   exercise, and kidneys in aged, 175
Hyperoxia
   exercise and, intense submaximal, 103
Hypertension
   beta-blockade in
      blood pressure and catecholamines
         after exercise during, 39
      exercise during, 38
   exercise training and, 33
   in runners, 130
Hypothalamic
   gonadotropin-releasing hormone in
      male marathon runners, 122
Hypothyroid
   athlete, TSH and prolactin responses to
      TRH in, 97
Hypoxemia
   exercise and quadriceps blood flow,
      30

I

Iliopatellar band
   anatomy, 289
Iliotibial band
   friction syndrome, 270
   transfer, bone block, in cruciate
      ligament repair, 295
Iliotibial tract
   anatomy, 289
   in cruciate ligament reconstruction, 296
Imaging (*see* Magnetic resonance imaging)
Immunity
   to disease and exercise, 171
Indomethacin
   renal prostaglandin synthesis during
      exercise and, 157
Infant
   swimming classes, 342
Infarction
   myocardial, and exercise (in rat), 17
Infectious mononucleosis
   aerobic capacity after, 177
Insall procedure
   in anterior cruciate ligament instability,
      result, 295
Insulin
   resistance, and exercise, 93
Intestine (*see* Gastrointestinal)
Intraarticular contact areas
   after meniscectomy and repair in
      meniscal tears, 287
Ionization
   air, cardiorespiratory variables and
      attention span, 61
Iron
   depletion, endurance swimming,
      hemolysis and anemia, 68
   status
      of female field hockey players, 364
      poor, of women runners training for
         marathon, 365
      in women, and fitness-type exercise,
         363
Ischemic
   heart disease, exercise ECG in, 27
   transient ischemic attacks at high
      altitude, 162
Iselin's disease, 347
Isokinetic
   dynamometry, 392
   instrument, Johnson anti-shear
      accessory as, 407
   muscle exercise, ethanol reducing
      myoglobin release during, 77
   shoulder strength of pitchers, 393
   torque levels for knee in soccer players,
      197

training, muscular power in young
women after, 375
Isometric
muscular contractions, endurance
capacity of untrained people in,
372
Isotope
uptake and skeletal muscle damage, 62

J

Javelin throwers
olecranon stress fracture, 232
Johnson anti-shear accessory
as isokinetic instrument, 407
use of, how and why, 408
Joint
acromioclavicular, ligamentous system
study, 258
control training in knee ligament
injuries, 404
counterforce braces for tennis player,
229
disease, degenerative, and running, 131
elbow, ulnar collateral ligament tears,
231
knee
instability, 291
laxity due to exercise, 272, 273
metatarsophalangeal, injuries in
athletes, 318
shoulder, load and muscular activity
during lifting, 199
tibiofibular (*see* Dislocation, tibiofibular
joint)
Jump
long, biomechanics of, 188

K

Karate
contrasted with boxing by
biomechanical study, 183
Ketanserin
for frostbite, 176
Kidney
in aged, hot weather and exercise, 175
function and marathon running, 120
prostaglandin synthesis during exercise,
157
Knee
arthroscopy (*see* Arthroscopy, knee)
braces (*see* Braces, of knee)
bracing to prevent sports injuries, 208
contracture, resistant extension, 400
cruciate ligament, anterior, instability,
Insall procedure result in, 295

extensor mechanism disorders,
evaluation, 401
extensor strength, and weight training
techniques, 409
extensors and flexors, isokinetic torque
levels for, in soccer players, 197
fracture, osteochondral, cortical bone
pegs in, 292
injuries in wrestling, 210
instability, Lenox Hill brace for, 398
joint
instability, 291
laxity due to exercise, 272, 273
ligament injuries, joint control training
in, 404
magnetic resonance imaging of (*see*
Magnetic resonance imaging, knee)
meniscus, microstructure and
biomechanics, 196
meniscus tears, CT evaluation, 285
model, computerized, in Müller
femorotibial ligament
reconstruction, 298
osteochondrosis dissecans, arthroscopic
curettage in, 308
reflex sympathetic dystrophy of, 337
rehabilitation
after cruciate ligament injury or
surgery, 403
quadriceps femoris muscle exercises
during, 399
stress, after meniscectomy and repair in
meniscal tears, 287

L

Lactate
blood, lack of influence of menstrual
cycle on, 360
Lactic
anaerobic capacity, test development in,
102
Lead
levels in long-distance road-runners, 129
Leg (*see* Extremities)
Legionella pneumophila
from Canadian hot springs, 177
Lenox Hill brace
effectiveness for knee instability, 398
Leukocytosis
exercise causing, and adrenergic
blockade, 46
Life
styles, physical activity, cardiovascular
disease and longevity, 13
Lifters
power, ingesting anabolic steroids,
lipoprotein alteration in, 155

Lifting
  shoulder joint load and muscular
    activity during, 199
Ligament
  calcaneofibular, rerouting peroneal
    tendons under, 327
  cruciate (*see* Cruciate ligament)
  femorotibial, reconstruction, Müller,
    298
  knee, injuries, joint control training in,
    404
  ligamentous system of acromioclavicular
    joint, 258
  periosteal, transfer for lateral ankle
    instability, 329
  reconstruction in tibiofibular joint
    dislocation, 267
  ulnar collateral (*see* Ulnar collateral
    ligament)
Limb (*see* Extremities)
Lipids
  after exercise training, 83
Lipoprotein
  alteration in power lifters ingesting
    anabolic steroids, 155
  cholesterol (*see* Cholesterol, lipoprotein)
  exercise training and, 83
Locomotion
  mechanical efficiency in, 373
Longevity
  physical activity, life styles and
    cardiovascular disease, 13
Lumbar
  spondylolysis and spondylolisthesis in
    college football players, 223

M

McArdle's disease
  pathophysiology, 63
Magnetic resonance imaging
  high-resolution, of ankle, 326
  knee injury
    high-resolution MRI, 275
    traumatic, 274
  knee, normal, anatomy, 277
  knee, 1.5-T surface-coil, 274
  of rotator cuff tears, 252
  of shoulder, normal, 244
Marine
  -acquired infections, 139
Maxillofacial
  fracture in bicycle accidents, 212
Meals
  swimming accidents and, 134
Medial tibial syndrome, 262
Mekkah pilgrimage
  heat stroke at, 106, 107

Meniscectomy
  effects in meniscal tears, 287
Meniscus
  of knee, microstructure and
    biomechanics, 196
  repair (*see* Arthroscopy, for meniscus
    repair)
Meniscus tears
  diagnosis with new manipulative test,
    286
  effect of meniscectomy and repair, 287
  of knee, CT evaluation, 285
Menses
  resumption in amenorrheic athletes,
    bone mineral density after, 359
Menstrual cycle
  thermoregulatory vasodilation during
    exercise and, 99
Menstruation
  abnormality
    women athletes with, musculoskeletal
      injury increase in, 358
    in women runners, prolactin and GH
      secretion in, 355
  cycle lack of influence on blood lactate,
    360
  disturbances due to exercise,
    management, 355
  phase, effect on swimmers during
    adolescence, 357
  premenstrual symptoms, conditioning
    exercise decreasing, 358
Metatarsophalangeal joint
  injuries in athletes, 318
Microcalorimetry
  for thermogenesis in skeletal muscle
    measurement, 47
Midfoot
  osteochondritis dissecans of, 320
Mineral(s)
  bone mineral content and physical
    activity in women, 69
  density (*see* Bone, mineral density)
  as ergogenic aids, 156
Mitochondrial
  oxidation, vitamin E deficiency and
    vitamin C supplements, 101
Model
  knee, computerized, in Müller
    femorotibial ligament
    reconstruction, 298
Monitoring
  adrenal and testicular, during male
    marathon run, 121
  physiological, of Canadian Women's
    Olympic Field Hockey Team,
    378
  rehabilitation in anterior cruciate
    ligament injury, 405

Mononucleosis
infectious, aerobic capacity after, 177
Morphometry
of collagen fibril organization in tendon, 153
Mountain
sickness on Mount Everest, and phenytoin, 160
Mountaineering
accidents, necropsy study, 216
Mouth
protectors and oral trauma in adolescent football players, 211
Müller
femorotibial ligament reconstruction, 298
Muscle
carbonic anhydrase liberation during exercise, 74
cell leakage of myoglobin after exercise, 75
contractile performance during beta-adrenoceptor blockade, 47
contractions, endurance capacity of untrained people in, 372
damage and endurance events, 353
glycogen (*see* Glycogen, muscle)
isokinetic exercise, ethanol reducing myoglobin release during, 77
mass at high altitude, and acetazolamide, 161
power in young women after isokinetic training, 375
quadriceps femoris
exercises during knee rehabilitation, 399
fatigue during electrical stimulation, 412
respiratory, endurance and caffeine, 150
shoulder (*see* Shoulder, muscle)
skeletal
atrophy during immobilization, 391
beta₂-adrenergic mechanism in (in rat), 44
damage, study of, 62
immobilized, morphology of, 391
muscle fiber type changes after injuries and immobilization of, 332
profiles of swimmers, 206
thermogenesis in, measurement of, 47
small muscle masses, dynamic work with, blood pressure response to, 35
strength, and proprioceptive neuromuscular facilitation vs. weight training, 410
in tennis stroke, EMG analysis of, 189

testing, isokinetic dynamometry for, 392
torso, activity in relaxed standing, 193
Musculoskeletal
injuries, increase in women athletes with menstrual abnormality, 358
Myocarditis
sudden death and sports, 16
Myocardium
infarction, and exercise (in rat), 17
Myoglobin
muscle cell leakage of, after exercise, 75
release, ethanol reducing, during isokinetic exercise, 77

N

Necropsy
in mountaineering accidents, 216
Nephrotic syndrome
minimal change, after decompression, 137
Nerve
axillary, and shoulder procedures, 239
Neurapraxia
of spinal cord with transient quadriplegia, 219
Neuromuscular facilitation, proprioceptive
muscular strength and athletic performance, 410
in sport-related injury rehabilitation, 410
Nutrition
intake in highly trained amenorrheic runners, 362

O

Ocean
marine-acquired infections, 139
Old age (*see* Aged)
Olecranon
stress fracture in javelin throwers, 232
Olympic Committee, U.S.
experience with bronchospasm due to exercise, 173
Oral
trauma, and mouth protectors for adolescent football players, 211
Orienteers
elite, injuries in, 132, 133
Osteoarthritis
long-distance running and, 132
Osteochondral
defects of femur, osteochondral allografts in, 289

fracture of knee, cortical bone pegs in, 292
lesions of talus, arthroscopy for, 322, 324
Osteochondritis dissecans
of midfoot, 320
Osteochondrosis dissecans
of knee, arthroscopic curettage in, 308
Osteoporosis
physical activity and, 69
Oxidation
mitochondrial, vitamin E deficiency and vitamin C supplements, 101
Ozone
exposure, work performance and $\dot{V}O_{2max}$, 60

P

Pain
of ankle sprain, 328
exercise, in lower leg, 262
patellofemoral, study of, 278
after stepping and skeletal muscle damage, 62
Palsy
ulnar, complicating decompression sickness, 136
Paraplegia
aerobic exercise in, 169
Patella
apicitis, predisposition in athletes, 285
chondropathy, predisposition in athletes, 285
dislocation, natural history, 281
instability and chondromalacia, radiography of, 276
prepatellar bursitis in wrestlers, 277
retinacular release, arthroscopic, 280
Patellar tendon (*see* Tendon, patellar)
Patellofemoral
arthralgia, thermography of in athletes, 279
pain, study of, 278
reconstruction, 282
subluxation, retinacular release in, 282
Performance (*see* Athletic, performance)
Periosteal
ligament transfer for ankle instability, 329
Peroneal tendons
dislocation, recurrent, 327
Phenytoin
mountain sickness on Mount Everest and, 160

Physical activity
blood pressure and, in young women, 153
bone mineral content and, in women, 69
cholesterol and, lipoprotein, 79
customary, measurements in aged before and after retirement, 173
life styles, cardiovascular disease and longevity, 13
osteoporosis and, 69
vigorous, and cardiovascular risk factors, 26
Physical fitness
bone mineral density in femoral neck and lumbar spine and, 70
in diabetes type I, in adolescents, 96
Physical training
enzymatic adaptation to, during beta-blockade (in rat), 44
epinephrine and fat cells, 84
iron status of female field hockey players and, 364
Physician(s)
sports, going public on anabolic steroids, 145
U.S., anabolic steroids as ethical dilemma for, 144
Pistol
shooting performance and beta-blockade in, 40
Pitchers
isokinetic shoulder strength of, 393
Plantar fasciitis
in athletes, surgery results, 319
Platelet
activation after marathon run, 126
alpha-2-adrenoreceptor density and, 48
Postmenopausal women
aerobic training, exercise tolerance and echocardiography in, 30
Power
muscular, in young women after isokinetic training, 375
output of upper extremity during horizontal pulls, 205
Premenstrual symptoms
conditioning exercise decreasing, 358
Prepatellar
bursitis in wrestlers, 277
Prolactin
after exercise, 355
response to TRH in hypothyroid athlete, 97
Proprioceptive (*see* Neuromuscular facilitation, proprioceptive)
Prostaglandin
renal, synthesis during exercise, 157

Prosthesis
  synthetic, in cruciate ligament
    replacement (in dog), 304
Protein
  excretion, urinary, during adolescence,
    344
Psychological
  androgyny of female college athletes,
    380
Psychology
  of injured athlete, 338
Pubic
  stress symphysitis in female distance
    runner, 354
Public health
  aspects of boxing, 331
Public schools
  athletic trainers in, opportunities for,
    387
Pulmonary
  cardiopulmonary stress testing, 24
  edema at high altitude, 46
  embolism of breakdancer, 143
Pulls
  horizontal, force, speed and power
    output of upper extremities during,
    205
Putti-Platt procedure
  for shoulder dislocation in young
    athlete, 250

Q

Quadriceps
  activity, strain within anterior cruciate
    ligament during, 406
  blood flow, exercise and hypoxemia, 30
  femoris (*see* Muscle, quadriceps
    femoris)
Quadriplegia
  transient
    congenital cervical stenosis and, in
      athletes, 220
    in neurapraxia of spinal cord, 219

R

Radiography
  of patella in instability and
    chondromalacia, 276
Radius (*see* Fracture, radius)
Reconstruction
  cruciate ligament (*see under* Cruciate
    ligament)
  femorotibial ligament, Müller, 298
  ligament, in tibiofibular joint
    dislocation, 267

patellofemoral, 282
  of rotator cuff, 257
  ulnar collateral ligament in athletes, 230
Recreation
  spinal cord injury due to, 218
Red blood cell
  survival rates, marathon running failing
    to influence, in women, 367
  volume, mean, in long distance runners,
    127
Reflex
  sympathetic dystrophy, 336
    of knee, 337
Rehabilitation
  dynamometry for, isokinetic, 392
  knee (*see* Knee, rehabilitation)
  monitoring, in anterior cruciate
    ligament injury, 405
  sport-related injury, proprioceptive
    neuromuscular facilitation in, 410
Rehydration
  exercise, fluid balance in, 116
  in wrestling performance, and rapid
    weight loss, 115
Renin
  during swimming and running, 53
Resonators
  for MRI in rotator cuff tears, 252
Respiratory
  muscle endurance and caffeine, 150
Retina
  injury and detachment in boxers, 217
Retinacular release
  patellar, arthroscopic, 280
  in patellofemoral subluxation, 282
Retransfusion
  central circulation during exercise and,
    65
Revascularization
  in cruciate ligament transplant, 302
Rotator cuff
  function during golf swing, 202
  results and reconstruction with, 257
  tear
    chronic, 255
    magnetic resonance imaging of, 252
    surgery in athletes, 256
    surgery, muscle-shoulder strength and
      motion range after, 257
  ultrasound of, 254
    pitfalls, 253
Rowing
  mechanical efficiency, 190
  terrestrial, 142
Runners
  amenorrhea, diet and bone status in,
    361
  competitive, gastrointestinal bleeding in,
    125

distance, female, pubic stress
symphysitis in, 354
endurance training, cholesterol increase
after, 80
hypertension in, 130
long-distance
lead levels in, 129
mean red cell volume in, 127
marathon
collapsed, enigma of, 119
male, hypothalamic gonadotropin-
releasing hormone in, 122
sacroiliac dysfunction in, 224
treadmill, novice, kinematic
accommodation of, 186
women
with abnormal menstruation,
prolactin and GH secretion in, 355
amenorrheic, highly trained,
nutritional intake and status of,
362
training for marathon, poor iron
status of, 365
Running
alcohol and, 152
biomechanics of, 184
joint disease in, degenerative, 131
long-distance, bone density and
osteoarthritis, 132
marathon
failure to influence RBC survival
rates, 367
gastrointestinal blood loss during,
124
kidney function and, 120
in male, adrenal and testicular
monitoring during, 121
platelet activation after, 126
thrombin activity increase after, 126
women runners training for, poor
iron status of, 365
pleasantness after, and beta-endorphin-
like immunoreactivity, 179
renin, aldosterone and catecholamines
during, 53
speed and agility with lateral knee
stabilizing braces, 385
treadmill, incremental, and caffeine,
149

S

Sacroiliac
dysfunction in runners, 224
Salivary
sampling to monitor male marathon
run, 121

Sauna
bathing, repeated
cardiovascular and metabolic effects,
109
endocrine effects of, 111
effects on hemorrheology, 108
Scintigraphy
exercise ^{201}T1, in false positive exercise
ECG, 148
Scuba diver
pediatric, 348
Sex
differences
in fatigability, 367
physiological, and sports
conditioning, 334
in strength, 367, 369
-related blood pressure response to
dynamic work with small muscle
masses, 35
Shinsplint
treatments, four modalities, 413
Shoe
sport, design, biomechanical
consequences of, 183
Shoulder
arthroscopy, appraisal, 240
complex, examination of, 236
dislocation (*see* Dislocation, shoulder)
girdle protection, alternative to, 394
instability
Boytchev procedure for, 248
glenohumeral arthrotomography in,
244
joint load and muscular activity during
lifting, 199
magnetic resonance imaging of, normal
shoulder, 244
muscle(s)
activity and fatigue in, during
repetitive work, 200
strength after rotator cuff tear
surgery, 257
during swimming, EMG of, 199
procedures and axillary nerve, 239
strength, isokinetic, of pitchers, 393
Sickle cell
trait, exercise and altitude, 168
Sit-to-stand
movement pattern, kinematic study,
192
Skeletal
muscle (*see* Muscle, skeletal)
musculoskeletal injuries, increase in
women athletes with menstrual
irregularity, 358
Ski
jumpers, Nordic, injury patterns in,
215

Sleep
  loss, exercise after, stress hormonal
    response to, 98
Soccer
  Australian female soccer players,
    physiological characteristics of, 379
  players, isokinetic torque levels for knee
    extensors and flexors in, 197
Soft tissue
  fixation to bone, 334
  injuries, acute, literature review, 335
Speed
  of upper extremity during horizontal
    pulls, 205
Spine
  cord injury
    activity in, 207
    cervical, neurapraxia with
      quadriplegia, 219
    due to sports and recreation, 218
    during windsurfing, 141
  injuries during gymnastic activities, 222
  lumbar, bone mineral density and
    physical fitness, 70
Splint
  shinsplint treatment, four modalities,
    413
Spondylolisthesis
  in college football players, 223
Spondylolysis
  lumbar, in college football players, 223
Sports
  conditioning, and physiological
    differences between genders, 334
  injuries
    during childhood and adolescence,
      346
    knee bracing to prevent, 208
  physician, goes public on anabolic
    steroids, 145
  precision, beta-blockade in, 39
  -related injury, rehabilitation,
    proprioceptive neuromuscular
    facilitation in, 410
  spinal cord injury due to, 218
  sudden death and myocarditis, 16
  women in, price of participation, 351
Sprain
  ankle
    classification by anatomical
      structures, 148
    lateral, early mobilizing, 328
Sprinting
  wheelchair, seat position in, 191
Squash
  sudden death and, 14
Standing
  relaxed, torso muscle activity during,
    193

Stenosis
  cervical, congenital, as transient
    quadriplegia in athletes, 220
Stereologic
  analysis of collagen fibril organization
    in tendon, 153
Steroids
  anabolic
    Australian sports physician goes
      public, 145
    collagen fibril organization in tendon
      and, 153
    as ethical dilemma for U.S.
      physicians, 144
    power lifters ingesting, and
      lipoprotein alteration, 155
Stomach
  (See also Gastrointestinal)
  emptying of athletic drinks, 118
Strain
  of anterior cruciate ligament during
    hamstring and quadriceps activity,
    406
Strength
  knee extensor, and weight training
    techniques, 409
  muscle, proprioceptive neuromuscular
    facilitation vs. weight training in,
    410
  sex difference in, 367
  shoulder, isokinetic, of pitchers, 393
  shoulder-muscle, after rotator cuff tear
    surgery, 257
  tensile, and water content in patellar
    tendon replacement of cruciate
    ligament (in dog), 304
  training program in women, 375
  of upper extremity in young women,
    374
Strengthening
  exercises in old cruciate ligament tears,
    403
Stress
  athlete and, 178
  fracture of femoral neck, distraction
    type, 271
  hormonal response to exercise after
    sleep loss, 98
  in knee after meniscectomy and repair
    of meniscal tears, 287
  olecranon fracture in javelin throwers,
    232
  symphysitis, pubic, in female distance
    runner, 354
  test, cardiopulmonary, 24
Stretch
  brachial plexus stretch injuries, 235
  -shortening cycle exercises, locomotion
    mechanical efficiency and, 373

Stroke
heat, at Mekkah pilgrimage, 106, 107
Sudden death
cardiac, in Air Force recruits, 16
causes in competitive athletes, 15
exercise and, vigorous, 14
myocarditis and sports, 16
Sulindac
renal prostaglandin synthesis during
exercise and, 157
Sunbeds
UV-A, for cosmetic tanning, 180
Swimmers
adolescent, effect of menstrual cycle
phase on, 357
glenoid labrum damage, anterior, 242
skeletal muscle profiles of, 206
Swimming
accidents, influence of water
temperature and meals on, 134
classes for infants, 342
endurance, hemolysis, anemia and iron
depletion, 68
renin, aldosterone and catecholamines
during, 53
shoulder muscles during, EMG of, 199
training, echocardiography in, in
children, 341
Sympathetic dystrophy
reflex, 336
of knee, 337
Symphysitis
pubic stress, in female distance runner,
354

T

Tachycardia
ventricular
exercise causing, 18
in young athlete, 19
Talar
dome fracture, arthroscopy of, 321
Talus
compression syndrome, 324
osteochondral lesions, arthroscopy for,
322, 323
Tanning
cosmetic, UV-A sunbeds for, 180
Tendon
biceps, ultrasound of, 254
collagen fibril organization in, 153
gracilis, in cruciate ligament
reconstruction with arthroscopy,
316
graft, allogeneic, in cruciate ligament
reconstruction, 301

patellar
in cruciate ligament reconstruction
with "ligamentization," 300
in cruciate ligament replacement, 303
in origin of cruciate ligament
autograft, 299
in replacement of cruciate ligament
(in dog), 304
peroneal, recurrent dislocation, 327
semitendinosus, in cruciate ligament
reconstruction, 296
with arthroscopy, 316
Tennis
elbow, manipulation in, 395
player, joint counterforce braces for,
229
stroke, EMG analysis and grip size, 189
Testes
activity monitoring during male
marathon run, 121
Thallium-201
scintigraphy, exercise, in false positive
exercise ECG, 28
Thermal
responses in water, body mass and
morphology, 112
Thermogenesis
in skeletal muscle, measurement of, 47
in patellofemoral arthralgia in athletes,
279
Three wheeler
as unstable, dangerous machine, 214
Thrombin
activity increase after marathon run,
126
Tibia
medial tibial syndrome, 262
Tibiofibular joint (*see* Dislocation,
tibiofibular joint)
Tomography, computed
of meniscus tears of knee, 285
Torque
levels, isokinetic, for knee in soccer
players, 197
Trainers
athletic, in public schools, opportunities
for, 387
Training
aerobic, exercise tolerance and
echocardiography in
postmenopausal women, 377
athletic facilities, for small college,
planning of, 388
athletic, program in computer age, 389
endurance
HDL-C in women after, 376
in runners, cholesterol increase after,
80
exercise (*see* Exercise, training)

high-frequency, moderate-intensity, in
sedentary women, 377
isokinetic, muscular power in young
women after, 375
joint control, in knee ligament injuries,
404
for marathon, women runners, poor
iron status of, 365
physical (*see* Physical training)
pre- and postimmobilization, program,
391
strength, program for women, 375
swimming, echocardiography of, in
children, 341
weight (*see* Weight, training)
Transfer
periosteal ligament, for ankle lateral
instability, 329
Transplantation
cruciate ligament, study of, 302
Treadmill
running, incremental, and caffeine,
149
TRH
TSH and prolactin responses to, in
hypothyroid athlete, 97
Tricycle
adult, as unstable, dangerous machine,
214
Triglyceride
clearance after prolonged exercise,
81
TSH
response to TRH in hypothyroid
athlete, 97

U

Ulnar
collateral ligament
reconstruction in athletes, 230
tears of elbow joint, 231
palsy complicating decompression
sickness, 136
Ultrasound
of biceps tendon, 254
of rotator cuff, 254
pitfalls, 253
Ultraviolet
-A sunbeds for cosmetic tanning,
180
Unloading
bone temporal response to, 72
Urinary
protein excretion during adolescence,
344

V

Vasodilation
thermoregulatory, during exercise, and
menstrual cycle, 99
Vehicle
accidents, all-terrain, 213
Ventilation
in extreme altitude climbers, 166
Ventricle
tachycardia (*see* Tachycardia,
ventricular)
Verapamil
exercise and, 43
Vessels (*see* Cardiovascular)
Vitamin(s)
C supplements, exercise and
mitochondrial oxidation, 101
E deficiency, exercise and mitochondrial
oxidation, 101
as ergogenic aids, 156
V_{O_2Max}
not decreasing after exercise cessation,
21
after ozone exposure, 60

W

Walking
stride length alteration and racewalking
economy, 187
Warm-up
for flexibility improvement, 390
Water
content and tensile strength in patellar
tendon replacement of anterior
cruciate (in dog), 304
temperature and swimming accidents,
134
thermal responses in, body mass and
morphology, 112
Weight
loss, rapid, and rehydration in wrestling
performance, 115
-trained women, HDL-C in, 376
training
in muscular strength and athletic
performance, 410
techniques and knee extensor
strength, 409
Wheelchair
sprinting, seat position in, 191
Windsurfing
on polluted water, health hazards of,
141
spinal cord injury during, 141

Women
athletes with menstrual irregularity, musculoskeletal injury increase in, 358
Australian soccer players, physiological characteristics of, 379
Canadian Olympic Field Hockey Team, physiological monitoring of, 378
college athletes, psychological androgyny of, 380
going easy on exercise, 352
iron status, and fitness-type exercise, 363
middle-aged, high-frequency, moderate-intensity training in, 377
runners (*see* Runners, women)
in sports, price of participation, 351
strength training program for, 375

young
muscular power in, after isokinetic training, 375
upper extremity strength in, 374
Work
dynamic, with small muscle masses, blood pressure response to, 35
intensity, study of, 203
performance after ozone exposure, 60
pure positive and pure negative, mechanical efficiency of, 203
repetitive, shoulder muscle during, activity and fatigue in, 200
Wrestlers
bursitis in, prepatellar, 277
Wrestling
knee injuries in, 210
performance test, rapid weight loss and rehydration in, 115

Author Index

A

Aalto, T., 285
Abbott, R.J., 141
Adams, L.L., 207
Adams, R.P., 103
Adams, W.C., 60
Adelaar, R.S., 184
Adelsberg, S., 189
Akeson, W.H., 299, 300
Alberty-Ryöppy, A., 292
Albohm, M.J., 353
Albright, J.P., 210, 244, 277
Alburger, P.D., 316
Alderink, G.J., 393
Al-Harthi, S.S., 106
Allen, M.J., 262
Alojada, N., 358
Al-Orainey, I.O., 106
Altschule, M.D., 119
Amiel, D., 299, 300
Amsterdam, E.A., 377
An, K.-N., 258, 304
Anderson, A.F., 286
Andrews, J.R., 321
Andriacchi, T., 298
Angel, D., 277
Anisette, G., 281
Antich, T.J., 399, 401
Antonelli, D., 199
Antonelli, D.J., 202
Appell, H.-J., 391
Appenzeller, O., 107
Apple, F.S., 365
Arborelius, U.P., 199
Arends, B.G., 43
Arms, S.W., 406
Armstrong, R.B., 333
Arnoczky, S.P., 303, 304
Aro, H., 271
Aronson, V., 156
Arvidsson, H., 271
Arvidsson, I., 271
Asami, T., 190
Ashlock, M.A., 303
Aura, O., 203, 373

B

Baker, C.L., 321
Baker, E.R., 358
Baker, L.L., 326
Ballantyne, D., 14
Banner, H.J., 143
Baratz, M.E., 287
Barkan, A., 122
Barnes, M.R., 262
Barnett, A., 95
Barrack, R.L., 272
Barry, L.A., 390
Bassett, F.H., III, 302

Bassett, L.W., 274
Bassey, E.J., 173
Bayer, M., 257
Beaupré, A., 196
Beauville, M., 84
Beck, C., 397
Becker, D., 207
Beilin, L.J., 39
Beitins, I.Z., 122
Bekaert, S., 61
Bell, D.G., 370
Bell, R.H., 281
Bell, S., 265
Belliato, R., 135
Benade, A.J.S., 155
Benazet, J.P., 329
Bender, P.R., 98
Benson, W.E., 217
Bentley, G., 276
Bergdolt, E., 48
Bergfeld, J.A., 305
Berhold, M., 412
Berkowitz, M.S., 225
Bern, M.M., 64
Berry, M., 148
Besser, M.I.B., 307
Betz, R.R., 316
Biden, E., 334
Biga, N., 120
Bikle, D.D., 72
Bilfield, B.S., 285
Birrer, R.B., 158
Bjerg-Nielsen, A., 260
Bjorkengren, A., 326
Blackett, W.B., 160
Blecher, A., 173
Blier, P., 50
Bloch, D.A., 132
Blom, P.C.S., 88
Blum, S.M., 363
Bocek, Z., 124
Bohannon, R.W., 375
Bohl, W.R., 225
Boileau, R.A., 363
Bolle, R., 59
Boniface, R.J., 194
Boran, K.J., 16
Borgat, C., 16
Borms, J., 341
Bouhour, J.B., 16
Bowen, G.S., 208
Bowling, R.W., 236
Boyden, T.W., 30
Bradwell, A.R., 161
Brahams, M.A., 225
Brand, M., 125
Brenes, G., 207
Brewster, C.E., 399, 401
Brisson, G., 50
Broberg, M.A., 235
Brodsky, A.E., 324
Brooks, G.A., 101
Brooks-Gunn, J., 357
Brown, R., 412

Brown, R.D., 375
Brunberg, J.A., 274
Bryan, W.J., 239
Buckley, W.E., 217
Burd, B., 342
Burhol, P.G., 59
Burk, D.L., Jr., 274
Burke, K.L., 380
Burke, M., 21
Butler, F.K., 136
Butler, J.E., 318

C

Caiozzo, V.J., 206
Caldwell, J.R., 131
Campagna, N.F., 252
Campbell, L.G., 97
Cannon, W.D., Jr., 397
Cantwell, J.D., 146
Capito, C., 250
Cardou, A., 196
Carr, D.B., 107
Carrera, G.F., 252
Carrier, D., 394
Carter, V.S., 256
Casale, T.B., 105
Casanova, M., 135
Cashman, P.A., 103
Caspari, R.B., 315
Casscells, S.W., 309
Catsos, P.D., 361
Cazorla, G., 53
Celsing, F., 65
Chad, K.E., 379
Chaitman, B.R., 27
Chambers, R.S., 410
Chan, K.W., 137
Chan, M.K., 137
Chandler, J.B., 244
Chang, F.E., 355
Chang, W.J., 139
Chao, E.Y.S., 258
Chayoth, R., 34
Chen, H.-i., 98
Chesner, I., 161
Chestnut, C.H., III, 359
Chillag, K., 273
Choukroun, R., 196
Christensen, H., 200
Christensen, N.J., 30
Christensen, P., 260
Ciullo, J.V., 398
Clancy, M., 316
Clancy, R., 280
Clanton, T.O., 318
Clarke, D.H., 367
Clarke, R.P., 255
Clement, T., 160
Cofield, R.H., 258
Coggan, A.R., 89
Cohen, J.C., 155

434

Coleclough, A.A., 183
Collins, K.A., 250
Colpitts, M., 160
Colquhoun, D., 379
Colville, M.R., 398
Cook, N.J., 121
Cook, T.C., 79
Coote, J.H., 161
Costanzo-Nordin, M.R., 146
Costill, D.L., 88
Coward, D.B., 310
Cowart, V.S., 168
Cowell, L.L., 169
Coyle, E.F., 89
Craig, E.V., 258
Crampes, F., 84
Crielaard, J.M., 102
Cross, M., 250
Crow, R.S., 26
Cruise, R.J., 376
Cullinane, E.M., 21, 81
Cumming, D.C., 97
Cutler, J.A., 26

D

Daczkewycz, R., 249
Dahlström, S., 271
Daniel, D.M., 334
Danzl, D.F., 246
Davidson, D.M., 206
Davis, G.L., 64
Dearwater, S.R., 207
Defer, G., 170
deKlerk, N., 39
Delman, A., 372
Del Pizzo, W., 306
de Lumen, B., 101
Dembert, M.L., 348
De Meyer, F., 61
Denoncourt, P.M., 308
DePalma, B.F., 403
Depester, N., 61
Deuster, P.A., 362
Devereaux, M.D., 279
Dewailly, E., 141
Diamond, P., 50
Diehl, D.M., 364
Diehr, P.H., 209, 383
Diffey, B.L., 180
Diamakopoulos, P., 308
Dodds, W.G., 355
Dodek, A., 130
Dodelson, R., 157
Dohlmann, B., 116
Domagala, E., 81
Dorchy, H., 96
Dorey, F., 274
Dover, E.V., 80
Dowd, G.S.E., 276
Doyle, D., 216
Drawbert, J.P., 384
Drez, D., Jr., 397
Drinkwater, B., 359

Drygas, W.K., 126
Duda, M., 144, 352
Dunbar, W.H., 310
Duncan, B., 347
Durstine, J.L., 80
Dutka, B.J., 177
Dykes, P.W., 161

E

East, J.B., 390
Eberl, S., 70
Edelman, R., 96
Edmonds, V.E., 218
Edwards, N.L., 131
Edwards, R.H.T., 62
Eggert, A., 318
Ehsani, A.A., 93
Eichner, E.R., 67, 68, 168
Eifler, W.J., 26
Eisenman, P.A., 175
Eisman, J.A., 70
Ekblom, B., 51, 65
Ekholm, J., 199
Ekstrand, J., 197
El-Khoury, G.Y., 244
Ellman, H., 257
Elrod, B., 256
Epstein, S.E., 15
Erhard, R., 236
Eriksson, E., 271, 307, 332
Ernst, E., 108
Escobar, P.L., 336
Eskola, A., 261
Espiner, E., 95
Estes, M., III, 146
Evans, P., 177
Evans, W.J., 361
Ewing, J.W., 310
Ewy, G.A., 41

F

Faber, W.M., 155
Facečić-Sabadi, V., 341
Fagher, B., 47
Farine, I., 322
Fay, J.J., 285
Fentem, P.H., 173
Feray, C., 329
Ferkel, R.D., 306
Fernie, G.R., 183
Finerman, G.A.M., 274
Fisher, E.C., 361
Fisher, R.L., 125
Fisher, S.M., 148
Flannigan, C., 14
Foley, M.E., 112
Foray, J., 176
Foreyt, J.P., 79
Forseth, E.A., 388
Forster, P.J.E., 161

Forsythe, W.A., 148
Fortmann, S.P., 26
Foster, C., 20
Foster, D.T., 210, 277
Foutch, R., 160
Fox, J.M., 336
Foxcroft, W.J., 60
France, P., 384
Franchimont, P., 102
Francis, A.M., 249
Franz, I.-W., 46
Frederick, E.C., 183
French, H.G., 233
Freund, B.J., 30, 41
Friberg, O., 285
Friedman, M.J., 336
Fries, J.F., 132
Frisk-Holmberg, M., 38
Froncisz, W., 252
Fronsoe, M.S., 80
Fu, F.H., 194, 287
Fujimaki, E., 246
Fukuda, K., 258
Fukunaga, T., 190
Fuller, C., 367
Furberg, C.D., 26

G

Gagna, G., 329
Galbraith, S.L., 216
Gallimore, G.W., Jr., 275
Gardner, G.M., 257
Gargiulo, J.M., 357
Garneau, R., 196
Garnica, R.A., 375
Garon, M.W., 211
Garrett, J.C., 289
Garrick, J.G., 208
Garrigues, M., 84
Genieser, N.B., 143
Genuario, S.E., 219
Gerard, E.S., 206
Gérardin, H., 196
Gerbino, P.G., 280
Gerrard, D.F., 170
Giachino, A.A., 268
Gibson, M., 298
Gillespie, W.J., 64
Gillien, D.M., 208
Gillquist, J., 197, 403, 405
Girardin, B.W., 376
Gisolfi, C.V., 86
Gleis, G.L., 246
Glisson, R.R., 302
Globus, R.K., 72
Glodava, A., 235
Godfrey, J.J., 202
Gohil, K., 101
Gold, R.H., 274
Goldberg, I., 234
Goletz, T.H., 282
Goodyear, L.J., 80
Gore, D.R., 257

Gotto, A.M., Jr., 79
Grainger, J.A., 97
Grana, W.A., 273, 278
Graves, J., 367
Grayman, G., 213
Gregg, J.R., 320, 347
Grieve, D.W., 205
Grobler, S.R., 129
Groppel, J.L., 229
Grosjean, M., 102
Guezennec, C.Y., 53
Guidotti, S.M., 157
Guidouin, R., 196
Gumaa, K., 107

H

Ha'Eri, G.B., 248
Hagberg, J.M., 33, 93
Hagege, A., 176
Häggmark, T., 307, 332
Hajek, P.C., 326
Hakki, A.-H., 28
Haller, R.G., 63
Hällgren, R., 77
Hander, G., 257
Hanson, P., 172
Harmon, M., 372
Harms, S.E., 275
Harnett, C.A., 157
Harr, S., 213
Harrelson, G.L., 118
Harrington, R., 30
Harris, B., 121
Harrison, J.M., 375
Hartung, G.H., 79
Hartzman, S., 274
Harwood, F.L., 300
Haskell, W.L., 26, 83
Hasler, K., 48
Haupt, H.A., 151
Hawkins, R.J., 251, 281, 294
Hay, J.G., 188
Hayashi, K., 183
Haynes, C.D., 214
Hazleman, B.L., 279
Healy, B., 17
Hedin, G., 75
Helmig, P., 281
Hemmert, M.K., 89
Henning, C.E., 314
Henry, J.H., 282
Herbert, P.N., 81
Hermanson, B.K., 209, 383
Hetrick, G.A., 41
Hewson, G.F., Jr., 384
Heyduck, B., 126
Heyward, V.H., 369
Higgins, J.R., 16
Hirai, A., 99
Hirashita, M., 99
Hirata, K., 99
Hirose, H., 246, 301
Hirovonen, J., 111

Hirt, S., 192
Hixson, E.G., 215
Hjemdahl, P., 51
Hochman, J.S., 17
Hodgdon, J.A., 272
Hodgson, J.L., 334
Hoffmann, B., 35
Höglund, C., 23
Holloszy, J.O., 93
Holly, R.G., 377
Honda, Y., 166
Hong, S.K., 113
Horoshovski, H., 322
Houser, M.T., 344
Housset, E., 176
Houts, P.S., 358
Hrilainen, A., 292
Hsieh, C.-C., 13
Huber, D.J., 244
Hudson, A.R., 183
Hughston, J.C., 289
Hulkko, A., 232
Hunter, S., 412
Hurley, J., 249
Huttunen, P., 111
Hvass, I., 328
Hvidsten, D., 59
Hyde, J.S., 252
Hyde, R.T., 13
Hyrkäs, T., 212

I

Iaquinto, J., 316
Ihara, H., 404
Ikram, H., 95
Ilkhanipour, K., 194
Inoue, M., 301
Irving, G.A., 120
Irving, J.M., 173
Irving, R.A., 120
Ishikawa, M., 246
Iskandrian, A.S., 28
Isner, J.M., 146
Ivy, J.L., 89

J

Jacobs, I., 370
Jacobs, P., 367
Jacobs, R., 212
Jacobson, B.H., 409
Jahn, M.F., 344
Jahre, C., 219
Jamjoom, A., 107
Jandrain, B., 91
Jansson, E., 332
Jenssen, T.G., 59
Jesmanowicz, A., 252
Ji, L.L., 44
Jilka, S.M., 41
Jobe, F.W., 199, 202, 230, 256

Johannes-Ellis, S.M., 369
Johannessen, S., 377
Johansson, C., 132
Johnson, C.L., 310
Johnson, L.F., 124
Johnson, R.J., 406
Johnstone, G.F., 274
Jolly, B.L., 314
Jones, D.A., 62
Jones, H.H., 132
Joyner, M.J., 41
Judlin, D., 295
Jupiter, J.B., 226
Jürgensen, U., 328

K

Kadakia, S.C., 124
Kalenak, A., 358
Kaliner, M., 105
Kallio, V., 92
Kamon, E., 334
Kanal, E., 274
Kane-Marsch, S., 28
Kantor, M.A., 81
Kaplan, N., 277
Karpakka, J., 109
Karpowicz, W., 115
Karuza, A., 160
Katagiri, T., 246
Kathol, M.H., 244
Katsas, G., 146
Katz, R.M., 57
Kavanaugh, J.H., 285
Keahey, T.M., 105
Keene, J.S., 317
Keith, J.F., III, 348
Kellett, J., 335
Kelsen, S.G., 150
Kerlan, R.K., 256
Kertzer, R., 364
Keul, J., 48
Khalil, M.A., 324
Khogali, M., 107
Kiburz, D., 212
Kiens, B., 30
Kim, M.H., 355
Kimura, H., 166
Kimura, T., 301
Kleiner, J.B., 299, 300
Klinzing, J.E., 115
Kneeland, J.B., 252
Knirk, J.L., 226
Knudsen, B., 116
Kobayashi, A., 344
Kobayashi, N., 246
Kobryn, U., 35
Kochan, R.G., 44
Komatsu, T., 113
Komi, P.V., 203, 373
Konda, N., 113
Kooima, E.F., 410
Körner, L.M., 263
Kramer, E.L., 143

Kregel, K.C., 86
Kronmal, R.A., 209, 383
Krüger, A., 179
Kruse, P., 40
Kuck, D.J., 393
Kujala, U.M., 285
Kumar, V.P., 293
Kunitomo, F., 166
Kuriyama, T., 166
Kuroda, S., 231
Kushner, S., 395
Kusnierkiewicz, J., 93
Kvist, M., 285
Kyle, S.B., 362

L

Laajam, M.A., 106
Lachmann, S.M., 279
Lacroix, M., 91
Ladd, A.L., 220
Ladefoged, J., 40
Laisney, M., 134
Lamb, R., 192
Lamont, L.S., 360
Lampe, J.W., 365
Lampman, R.M., 122
Lane, N.E., 132
Lange, R.H., 317
Lanir, A., 277
Lankenner, P.A., Jr., 280
Laporte, R.E., 79, 207
Lardy, H.A., 44
Larsen, E., 260
Larson, D., 125
Larson, E., 334
Lawley, M.J., 306
Leach, R.E., 319
Ledent, P., 102
Ledoux, M., 50
Lee, C.L., 398
Lefebvre, P.J., 91
Léger, H., 295
Lehman, R.C., 320, 347
Lehmann, M., 48
Lehtonen, A., 92
Leiper, J.B., 372
Lennon, D.L.F., 44
Leppäluoto, J., 109, 111
Leppilampi, M., 74
Levin, S., 150
Levine, E., 158
Levine, R., 158
Lewis, D.A., 334
Lewis, S.F., 63
Lhoste, F., 53
Lidell, C., 77
Liedholm, H., 47
Linde, F., 133, 328
Lindqvist, C., 212
Linson, M.A., 266
Lipscomb, A.B., 286
Lipski, M., 158
Litt, I.F., 356

Livesey, J., 95
Lloyd, T., 358
Lohman, T.G., 69, 364
Lombardo, J.A., 148
Lombardo, S.J., 230, 256
Longley, S., 131
Lory, D., 135
Lui, H., 377
Lundin, L., 77
Lutz-Schneider, V., 376
Luyckx, A.S., 91
Lysholm, J., 403, 405
Lysholm, M., 403, 405

M

McCabe, M.E., III, 124
McCarroll, J.R., 223
MacConnie, S.E., 122
McFarland, E.G., 304
McGown, C.M., 410
McMahon, L.F., Jr., 125
McMaster, W.C., 242
McMurray, R.G., 148
McNaughton, L., 152
McNaughton, L.R., 149
Madsen, F., 328
Magyarosy, I., 108
Malarkey, W.B., 355
Malcorps, H., 61
Malone, T., 408
Manco, L.G., 285
Mandelbaum, B.R., 274
Maquire, J.I., 217
Mar, M.H., 148
Marchetto, P., 316
Marchiori, G.E., 191
Maresky, L.S., 129
Margetts, B., 39
Maron, B.J., 15
Marshall, W.H., Jr., 132
Marshall, W.J., 141
Martens, M.A., 327
Martin, B.J., 98
Martin, P.E., 187
Martinez, E., 41
Martinsson, A., 51
Maslowski, A., 95
Mason, J., 212
Massey, B.H., 69
Masuyama, S., 166
Matsuo, A., 190
Matthaei, H., 179
Mattila, K., 92
Maughan, R.J., 372
Medved, R., 341
Medved, V., 341
Melson, G.L., 253, 254
Mendes, D.G., 277
Mendini, R.A., 384
Mendoza, F.X., 251
Mengato, P., 91
Meredith, C.N., 361
Merkle, A., 211

Merritt, T.R., 294
Metz, K.F., 79
Meyer, F.M., 141
Meyers, J.F., 315
Meyerstein, N., 34
Micheli, L.J., 280, 346
Michna, H., 153
Middleton, W.D., 252, 253, 254
Mikosz, R., 298
Miller, C., 145
Miller, G., 146
Miller, J.M., 223
Milles, J.J., 161
Minei, J.P., 304
Misamore, G.W., 294
Mishler, B., 387
Möller, M., 197
Monahan, T., 352
Monti, M., 47
Morey-Holton, E., 72
Morgan, C.D., 309
Morgan, D.H., 376
Morgan, D.W., 187, 376
Moritz, U., 47
Morrey, B.F., 235, 304
Morrison, D.A., 30
Morrison, R.G., 331
Morrissey, M.C., 401
Moser, P.B., 362
Mosora, F., 91
Mouton, W.L., 138
Moyer, R.A., 316
Moynes, D.R., 199, 202
Mueller, E., 244
Mulier, J.C., 222
Murphy, P., 178
Murphy, W.A., 253, 254
Murray, M.P., 257
Murray, W.B., 138
Mustafa, M.K.Y., 107
Myllynen, P., 261, 292
Mysnyk, M.C., 210, 277

N

Nagasaka, T., 99
Nagata, A., 246
Nagle, F.J., 44
Nakayama, A., 404
Nash, H.L., 171
Nauman, J., 131
Neaton, J.D., 26
Neer, C.S., II, 251
Nelson, A.G., 410
Nelson, M.E., 361
Németh, G., 199
Neumann, C.H., 326
Newham, D.J., 62
Ngoi, S.S., 293
Nicholls, G., 95
Nielsen, B., 116
Nielsen, S., 291
Nielsen, U., 40

Niemann, J., 179
Nikolaou, P.K., 302
Nikula, P., 232
Nilson, K., 359
Nirschl, R.P., 229
Nisell, R., 199
Noakes, T.D., 91, 120, 155, 367
Northcote, R.J., 14
Norwood, L.A., 289
Noyez, J.F., 327
Nuber, G.W., 199
Nunomura, T., 99
Nuzik, S., 192
Nyström, J., 65

O

Obeid, M.T., 106
Öberg, B., 197
Ogilvie-Harris, D.J., 240
Okita, S., 166
Olha, A.E., 55
Olson, D.W., 270
Ono, K., 301
Orava, S., 232
Ortengren, B., 307
Österman, K., 285
Osternig, L.R., 392
Ott, S., 359
Owen, M.D., 86

P

Packer, L., 101
Paffenbarger, R.S., Jr., 13
Painter, P., 172
Pallikarakis, N., 91
Pamenter, R.W., 30
Pandolf, K.B., 112
Panush, R.S., 131
Parette, R., 413
Parisian, J.S., 323
Park, Y.S., 113
Parker, M.G., 412
Parker, R.D., 225
Parks, D.L., 246
Parolie, J.M., 305
Parr, G.R., 279
Patel, D., 308
Patel, M.K., 141
Pätiälä, H., 261
Patrick, J.M., 173
Patsch, W., 79
Paulev, P.-E., 40
Paulos, L.E., 310, 384
Pavlov, H., 219
Penrose, K.W., 410
Peronnet, F., 50
Perry, J., 199
Petri, H., 43
Pettersson, H., 131
Peura, D.A., 124

Peylan, J., 234
Phillips, M., 16
Pianta, R.M., 251
Pien, F.D., 139
Pihlstedt, P., 65
Pinto, C.V., 136
Pirnay, F., 91, 102
Pocock, N.A., 70
Podrid, P.J., 19
Poirier, C., 141
Poortmans, J.R., 96
Pope, M.H., 406
Potera, C., 351
Preece, D., 152
Prentice, W.E., 385, 387, 410
Prietto, C.A., 206
Prineas, R.J., 26
Priollet, P., 176
Prior, J.C., 358
Pritsch, M., 322

Q

Qi, W.M., 376

R

Rabb, D.M., 69
Raczka, R., 267
Rand, J.J., 215
Randall, C.C., 401
Ransch, E., 35
Rao, J.P., 249
Rauschning, W., 274
Rautaharju, P.M., 26
Raven, P.B., 169
Ray, R., 389
Read, G.F., 121
Ready, A.E., 378
Rebman, L.W., 330
Reckling, F., 212
Reed, T., 16
Reeves, R.S., 79
Reicher, M.A., 274
Reid, D.C., 395
Reid, W.A., 216
Reider, B., 298
Reinus, W.R., 253, 254
Renon, P., 135
Renström, P., 406
Requardt, H., 244
Resnick, D., 326
Riad-Fahmy, D., 121
Ribbeck, B.M., 302
Richardson, N.V., 161
Richmond, H.G., 216
Riddle, D., 400
Ritter, M.A., 223, 353
Riviere, D., 84
Roberts, W.C., 15
Robertson, D.B., 334
Robertson, D.M., 386

Robertson, R.J., 207
Robie, B.H., 219
Robinowitz, M., 16
Rockar, P.A., Jr., 236
Röcker, L., 46, 126
Roessler, B., 127
Roffman, M., 277
Rogers, P., 39
Rokkanen, P., 261
Rold, B.A., 354
Rold, J.F., 354
Romer, J.F., 369
Rönnemaa, T., 92
Rorabeck, C.H., 264
Rose, F.D., 146
Rosenberg, P.S., 255
Rosenberg, T.D., 137, 384
Rossouw, R.J., 129
Roux, R.D., 300
Rovere, G.D., 151, 208
Rowe, C.R., 296
Rowe, P.J., 386
Rowell, B.R., 30
Roxin, L.-E., 75, 77
Roy-Camille, R., 329
Rubin, B.D., 206
Runhling, R.O., 412
Ryan, J.B., 321
Ryan, L.M., 252
Ryan, M.J., 125

S

Saar, E., 34
Saartok, T., 307
Sabathier, C., 53
Sady, S.P., 21, 81
Saerens, P., 96
Sagawa, S., 113
Saillant, G., 329
Sakamaki, K., 231
Sale, D., 372
Sallis, J.F., 26
Salter, D.K., 319
Saltin, B., 30
Sambrook, P.N., 70
Sanders, R.A., 233
Sanger, J.J., 143
Sanmarco, M.E., 37
Santavirta, S., 212
Sarma, R.J., 37
Sartoris, D.J., 326
Satku, K., 293
Sauter, R., 244
Sawka, M.N., 112
Schauder, K., 239
Schelberg-Karnes, E., 273
Schieb, D.A., 186
Schmidlechner, C., 108
Schmidt, C., 131
Schmole, M., 179
Schneeberger, J., 138
Schoomaker, E.B., 362

Schork, M.A., 122
Schultz, J., 93
Schulz, J.I., 55
Schwartz, M.L., 183
Scott, G.A., 314
Scott, S.M., 310
Scranton, P.E., 220
Seaber, A.V., 302
Seals, D.R., 33
Seavey, M.S., 319
Sebik, A., 307
Selby, G.B., 68
Sennett, B., 219
Sepic, S.B., 257
Shangold, M.M., 355
Shephard, R.J., 32
Sherman, A.R., 363
Sherman, O.H., 306
Shields, C.L., Jr., 256
Shino, K., 301
Shiraki, K., 113
Shire, T.L., 389
Silver, D.D., 222
Silver, J.R., 222
Singh, A., 362
Sjøgaard, G., 116
Skinner, H.B., 272
Skipper, B., 107
Slaughter, M.H., 69
Slavin, J.L., 365
Slemenda, C.W., 79
Smith, E.L., 69
Smith, F.H., 390
Smith, M.R., 412
Smith, S.C., 364
Smith, W., 413
Snyder, S.J., 306
Sophocles, A.M., Jr., 165
Sørensen, J.P., 40
Sorsa, S., 212
Soudry, M., 277
Squires, W.G., 169
Srinivasan, I., 143
Stahl, S., 307
Stamler, J., 26
Stanwyck, T.S., 406
Stark, H., 230
Staübli, M., 127
Steadward, R.D., 191
Steenkamp, I., 367
Steiner, M.E., 273
Stewart, R.I., 138
Stillman, R.J., 69
Stini, W.A., 30
Stone, M.L., 272, 397
Stone, R.G., 314
Stork, J., 131
Strauss, M.B., 137
Ström, G., 38
Stroud, S.D., 214
Strziga, P., 108
Stuller, J., 142
Stumpf, P.G., 358
Sturner, W.Q., 146
Styf, J.R., 263
Subramanian, R., 146

Sugita, T., 166
Sullivan, M., 355
Supinski, G.A., 150
Svedenhag, J., 51
Svensson, O., 199
Sweeney, K., 146
Swensen, H.E., 274

T

Takahata, T., 99
Takala, T.E.S., 74
Tator, C.H., 218
Tatsumi, K., 166
Tegner, Y., 403, 405
Teitz, C.C., 209, 383
Terblanche, S.E., 101
Terry, G.C., 289
Thomas, D.P.P., 279
Thomas, J., 325
Thomason, P.A., 266
Thomine, J.M., 295
Thompson, C.E., 214
Thompson, P.D., 21, 81, 146
Tibone, J.E., 256
Tietjien, R., 337
Timm, K.E., 407
Tiu, S., 143
Tojima, H., 166
Tolfree, S.E.J., 62
Toner, M.M., 112
Torg, E., 347
Torg, J.S., 219
Toriscelli, T., 385
Totty, W.G., 253, 254
Trager, G.W., 213
Traven, N.D., 79
Triantafyllou, S.J., 358
Troxel, R.K., 338
Tullos, H.S., 239
Tuominen, M., 109, 111
Turksoy, R.N., 361

U

Ugelvig, J., 116

V

Väänänen, A., 109, 111
Väänänen, H.K., 74
Vadenboncoeur, L., 21
Vainionpää, S., 261
van Baak, M.A., 43
van der Linden, J., 205
van der Merwe, M., 378
Vandongen, R., 39
Van Houten, D.R., 80
VanSant, A., 192
VanWinkle, G.N., 314
Van Zyl-Smit, R., 120

Vayssairat, M., 176
Venge, P., 75, 77
Vertongen, F., 96
Vicario, S.J., 246
Vigersky, R.A., 362
Vigna, Y., 358
Virmani, R., 16
Vogelaere, P., 177
Volle, M., 50
Vøllestad, N.K., 88
Voy, R.O., 58
Vranizan, K.M., 26
Vuori, J., 74, 109, 111

W

Wait, J., 24
Walburn, J., 344
Walker, R.F., 121
Wall, P.T., 86
Wall, S.R., 97
Walsh, C.M., 191
Wang, J.B., 384
Ward, A., 172
Warren, M.P., 357
Warren, R.F., 303, 304
Washburn, R.A., 79
Watanabe, S., 166
Weber, H., 244
Webster, E., 131
Weesner, C.L., 353
Weinert, C.R., Jr., 267
Weiss, B.D., 347
Weiss, M.R., 338
Welch, M.J., 177
Werner, B., 65
West, J.B., 163
Westbrook, R.A., 401
Wheeler, L., 177
Wheeler, M.E., 64
Whieldon, T.J., 224
Whipple, T.L., 315
Whiteside, J.A., 358
Whiteside, P., 208
Wildmann, J., 179
Wiley, A.M., 240
Williamson, B., 282
Williford, H.N., 390
Wilmore, J.H., 30, 41
Wing, A.L., 13
Winiewicz, T.W., 224
Winn, F., 413
Wisneski, R.J., 219
Woelfel, A., 18
Wohns, R.N.W., 160, 162
Wolf, G.L., 274
Wood, M.B., 304
Wood, P.D., 26, 132
Woodhull-McNeal, A.P., 193
Worobetz, L.J., 170
Wright, J.R., Jr., 215
Wright, J.T., 211
Wroble, R.R., 210, 277
Wyatt, M.P., 272

Y

Yamaji, K., 32
Yamamoto, K., 190
Yaqub, B.A., 106
Yates, C., 278
Yates, C.S., 151
Yates, J.R., 246

Yeates, M.G., 70
Yin, P.D., 137
Yocum, L., 256
Yonker, R., 131
Yosipovitch, Z., 234
Young, J., 397
Young, J.C., 103
Yuguchi, Y., 166

Z

Zambraski, E.J., 157
Zarins, B., 296
Zelko, R.R., 403

TO ORDER: DETACH AND MAIL

Please enter my subscription to the journal(s) and/or Year Book(s) checked below:
(To order by phone, call **toll-free 800-621-5410**. In IL, call **collect 312-726-9746**.)

	Practitioner (approx.)	Resident	Institution
Current Problems in Surgery® (1 yr.)	____$55.00	____$29.95	____$72.00
Current Problems in Pediatrics® (1 yr.)	____$39.95	____$29.95	____$65.00
Current Problems in Cancer® (1 yr.)	____$49.95	____$29.95	____$65.00
Current Problems in Cardiology® (1 yr.)	____$49.95	____$29.95	____$65.00
Current Problems in Obstetrics, Gynecology, and Fertility® (1 yr.)	____$49.95	____$29.95	____$65.00
Current Problems in Diag. Radiology® (1 yr.)	____$49.95	____$29.95	____$72.00
Disease-A-Month® (1 yr.)	____$39.95	____$29.95	____$65.00
	Binder____$14.95 (each year)		
1987 Year Book of Anesthesia® (AN-87)	____$44.95	____$29.95	
1987 Year Book of Cancer® (CA-87)	____$44.95	____$29.95	
1987 Year Book of Cardiology® (CV-87)	____$44.95	____$29.95	
1987 Year Book of Critical Care Medicine® (16-87)	____$44.95	____$29.95	
1987 Year Book of Dentistry® (D-87)	____$45.95	____$29.95	
1987 Year Book of Dermatology® (10-87)	____$45.95	____$29.95	
1987 Year Book of Diagnostic Radiology® (9-87)	____$44.95	____$29.95	
1987 Year Book of Digestive Diseases (13-87)	____$42.95	____$29.95	
1987 Year Book of Drug Therapy® (6-87)	____$44.95	____$29.95	
1987 Year Book of Emergency Medicine® (15-87)	____$44.95	____$29.95	
1987 Year Book of Endocrinology® (EM-87)	____$45.95	____$29.95	
1987 Year Book of Family Practice® (FY-87)	____$42.95	____$29.95	
1987 Year Book of Hand Surgery® (17-87)	____$42.95	____$29.95	
1987 Year Book of Hematology (24-87)	____$39.95	____$29.95	
1987 Year Book of Infectious Diseases (19-87)	____$39.95	____$29.95	
1987 Year Book of Medicine® (1-87)	____$44.95	____$29.95	
1987 Year Book of Neonatal-Perinatal Medicine (23-87)	____$39.95	____$29.95	
1987 Year Book of Neurology and Neurosurgery® (8-87)	____$44.95	____$29.95	
1987 Year Book of Nuclear Medicine® (NM-87)	____$44.95	____$29.95	
1987 Year Book of Obstetrics and Gynecology® (5-87)	____$42.95	____$29.95	
1987 Year Book of Ophthalmology® (EY-87)	____$44.95	____$29.95	
1987 Year Book of Orthopedics® (OR-87)	____$44.95	____$29.95	
1987 Year Book of Otolaryngology-Head and Neck Surgery (3-87)	____$44.95	____$29.95	
1987 Year Book of Pathology and Clinical Pathology® (PI-87)	____$44.95	____$29.95	
1987 Year Book of Pediatrics® (4-87)	____$42.95	____$29.95	
1987 Year Book of Plastic and Reconstructive Surgery® (12-87)	____$46.95	____$29.95	
1987 Year Book of Podiatric Medicine and Surgery (18-87)	____$39.95	____$29.95	
1987 Year Book of Psychiatry and Applied Mental Health® (11-87)	____$42.95	____$29.95	
1987 Year Book of Pulmonary Disease (21-87)	____$39.95	____$29.95	
1987 Year Book of Rehabilitation (22-87)	____$39.95	____$29.95	
1987 Year Book of Sports Medicine® (SM-87)	____$42.95	____$29.95	
1987 Year Book of Surgery® (2-87)	____$47.95	____$29.95	
1987 Year Book of Urology® (7-87)	____$44.95	____$29.95	
1987 Year Book of Vascular Surgery (20-87)	____$39.95	____$29.95	

Prices quoted are in U.S. dollars. Canadian orders will be billed in Canadian funds at the approximate current exchange rate.
A small additional charge will be made for postage and handling. Illinois and Tennessee residents will be billed appropriate sales tax. **All prices quoted subject to change.**

ACCT. NO._____

NAME_____

ADDRESS_____

CITY_____ STATE_____ ZIP_____

ZAI

Printed in U.S.A.

YEAR BOOK MEDICAL PUBLISHERS
35 EAST WACKER DRIVE   CHICAGO, ILLINOIS 60601